Disease

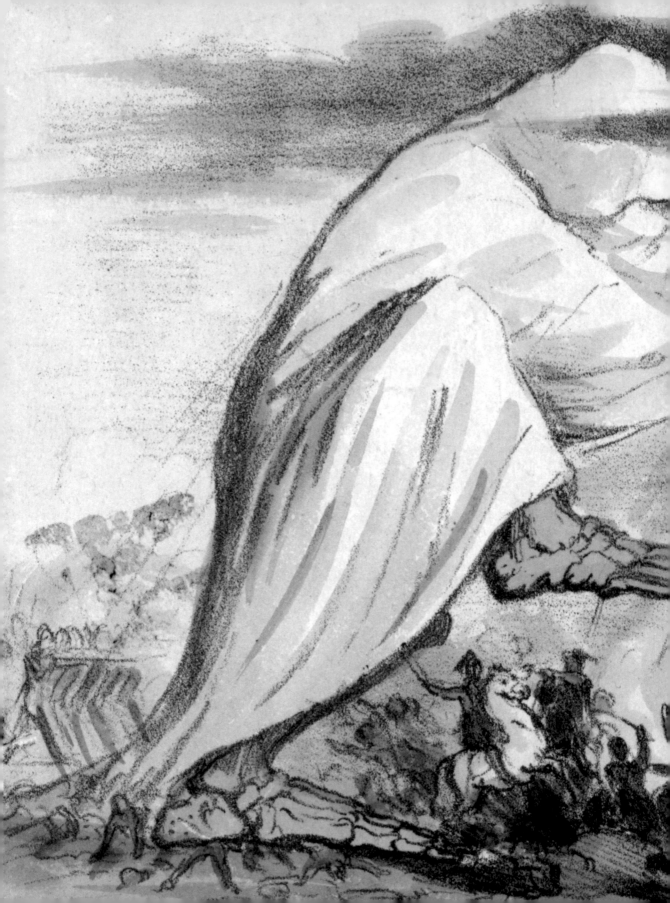

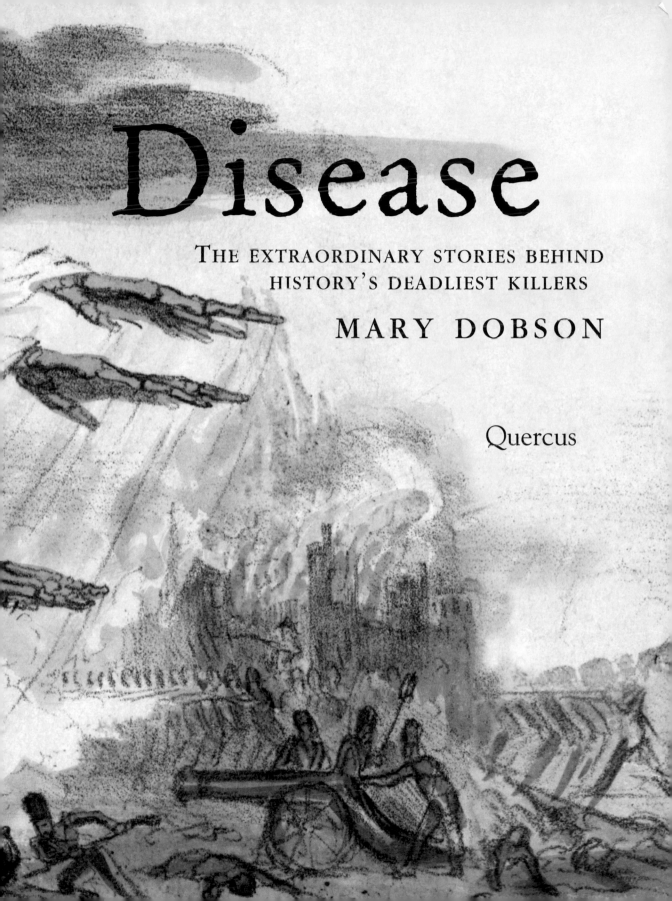

Disease

THE EXTRAORDINARY STORIES BEHIND
HISTORY'S DEADLIEST KILLERS

MARY DOBSON

Quercus

CONTENTS

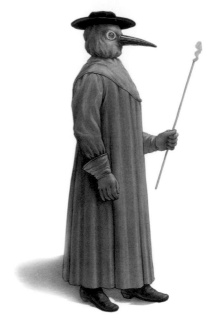

A 17th-century physician wearing a traditional plague-preventive costume.

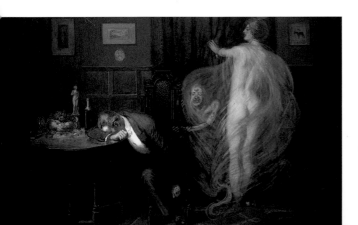

Syphilis, painted in 1910 by the artist Richard Cooper.

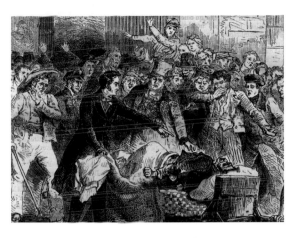

A depiction of the 1832 cholera epidemic in Paris.

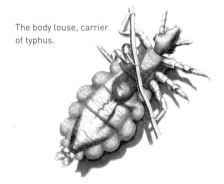

The body louse, carrier of typhus.

PREFACE

'I hope that Lord Grey and you are well; no easy thing seeing that there are about fifteen hundred diseases to which man is subject.'

SYDNEY SMITH TO LADY GREY, FEBRUARY 1836

The diseases that are encompassed within this book have affected human history in a multitude of ways over the past few millennia. Choosing 30 diseases out of the '1500' or so suggested by the English clergyman Sydney Smith (1771–1845) has been both stimulating and challenging. The final decision was based on the idea of including a varied selection of some of the world's most important diseases and covering a range of those that have had, and continue to have, a major impact in many parts of the world. While this book is essentially written from a historical perspective, I have chosen a number of diseases that now seriously affect some of the poorest countries (where, in the 21st century, life expectancy can be less than 50 years compared to over 80 years in the wealthiest nations), and have included a selection of the more unusual and mysterious diseases which have afflicted humans over the ages.

Some of those selected, such as malaria and schistosomiasis, are 'ancient' diseases – possibly first emerging as significant human diseases approximately 7000 years ago when people and domestic animals began to live in close proximity. Infections, like smallpox and measles, which are easily transmitted from person to person, may have accompanied the rise of early urban settlements from around 3000 BC. The opening up of overland and ocean trade routes, especially with the circumnavigations of the globe from the late 15th century onwards, accelerated the spread of many diseases from place to place and continent to continent. Others, notably AIDS, are 'new' to human society, emerging and spreading rapidly only in the past 50 or so years. A few have seemingly come and gone. SARS – the first serious and easily transmissible new disease to emerge in the 21st century – spread around the globe over a short period of time in 2003, disappeared and has, so far, not re-appeared.

Some of the diseases in this book, such as kuru in Papua New Guinea, have had a serious but largely local impact. Several, especially those like malaria and African trypanosomiasis (sleeping sickness) which are transmitted by insect vectors, continue to have a devastating effect on tropical and sub-tropical regions. Others, such as the Black Death of the mid-14th century, smallpox and measles from the early 16th century, the cholera pandemics in the 19th century, the Spanish influenza pandemic of 1918–19 and the current AIDS pandemic, have been catastrophes on a global scale with far-reaching consequences for societies and individuals the world over. The recent outbreak of bird flu (H5N1 influenza) presents a global threat that we hope will never happen. And one major disease covered in this book has been effectively eradicated by human intervention. In 1979, the World Health Organization announced that smallpox, one of the worst scourges of humanity, had been eradicated from the globe by a vaccine developed nearly 200 years before. We can only hope that there will further success stories and that the global burden of disease will be reduced significantly in the coming years.

The 30 diseases eventually chosen have been grouped into four categories and arranged, at least very approximately, within the groups chronologically according to their first recorded serious impact on the world. The first three groups comprise infectious diseases: bacterial diseases (from plague to encephalitis lethargica), parasitic diseases (from malaria to onchocerciasis) and viral diseases (from smallpox to SARS). The fourth group of diseases (from scurvy to heart disease) do not conform to the models of bacterial, parasitic and viral maladies and are loosely labelled 'lifestyle diseases', since factors such as diet, smoking, physical exercise and occupation play a key (though not the only) role in their causation. Indeed, for each of the diseases selected – whether primarily infectious or non-infectious – there is always a complex set of inter-related biological, genetic, environmental and social factors meaning that some people succumb, while others survive or remain untouched by the circulating pathogen or potentially fatal disorder.

In each of the chapters the aim has been to give a broad overview and chronology of the history of each disease, its impact on human societies, and estimates of numbers affected both past and present. I have also tried to include some of the key scientific and medical discoveries associated with each disease and to highlight the often remarkable human endeavours and sometimes extraordinary achievements in identifying, preventing or treating each disease. The accompanying quotes and illustrations aim to convey something of the suffering, pain, misery and bewilderment experienced by people in times of sickness over the centuries, as well as the commitment and determination of men and women in their search for solutions. In some chapters I have touched on a few of the many mysteries that have perplexed scholars, scientists, physicians and patients in their quest to understand the origins, nature and cause of disease and its effect on human societies and individuals across the globe.

The history of medicine is a rich and expanding field of wide interest. Each new scholarly or scientific study brings with it further facts, findings and figures. The application of novel techniques, such as the use of DNA probes, should make it easier in the future to identify some of the puzzling pathogens of the past and, perhaps, solve a number of historical debates. With the sequencing of the human and microbial genomes and advances in such fields as molecular medicine, we are also now in a stronger position in the 21st century than ever before to understand more clearly human predisposition and susceptibility to disease, to discover the mysterious ways of microbes, animal and insect vectors and to bring to future generations the promise of new diagnostics, vaccines and therapies. Reducing poverty and hunger, and improving sanitation, hygiene and education also still remain some of the most fundamental factors of importance for ensuring the future health and happiness of people in many parts of the world.

My sincerest thanks go to all those who have made this book possible – my acknowledgements and suggestions for further readings are given on pages 253–4.

Mary Dobson
St John's College
Cambridge

October 2007

PLAGUE

The very mention of plague induces shudders of horror in adults and school-children alike. Plague has been responsible for some of the worst catastrophes in the story of humankind, and more than once has changed the course of history. Bubonic plague is caused by a bacterium, *Yersinia pestis*, mainly transmitted to humans by wfleas from infected rodents, notably the black rat, *Rattus rattus*. Although most historians assume that this was the prime mode of transmission of most plague epidemics, some have recently questioned whether the so-called plagues of the past really were 'true' bubonic or pneumonic plague. The story of plague is at once the most gruesome and the most fascinating of medical mysteries.

'When leaving his surgery on the morning of April 16, Dr Bernard Rieux felt something soft under his foot. It was a dead rat lying in the middle of the landing.'

This unsettling moment comes near the beginning of *La Peste* (The Plague), a novel by the French philosopher Albert Camus (1913-60), first published in 1947. *'On the spur of the moment he kicked it to one side and, without giving it a further thought, continued on his way downstairs. Only when he was stepping out into the street did it occur to him that a dead rat had no business to be on his landing, and he turned back to ask the concierge of the building to see to its removal.'*

Thus a dead rat, a doctor and a concierge become bound up in one of the most compelling fictional accounts of plague, set in the late 1940s in the Algerian port city of Oran. An allegory of the Nazi occupation of France, and a metaphor of the meaning of life and suffering, the story also contains all the classic plague scenarios. A few days after Dr Rieux comes across his first dead rat, the city is overwhelmed by the creatures. From basements, cellars and sewers the rats *'emerged in long wavering files into the light of day, swayed helplessly, then did a sort of pirouette and fell dead at the feet of horrified onlookers'*. Some

timeline

540–mid-8th century First cycle of plague, possibly originating in Asia, spreads to North Africa then to the Mediterranean and the Middle East.

541–4 Plague of Justinian.

1330s–18th century Second cycle of plague, with many severe outbreaks in Europe.

1347–53 The Black Death – one of the most deadly pandemics in human history.

1665–6 The Great Plague of London.

1720–2 Plague in Marseilles – the last major outbreak in western Europe.

From 1855 Third cycle of plague, starting in Asia, with 12.6 million

deaths in India between 1898 and 1948. In the 1900s plague reaches the Pacific coast of North America, Australia and Great Britain (with a few deaths in Glasgow, Cardiff and Liverpool).

1894 Severe epidemic in Canton (Guangzhou) and Hong Kong. Alexandre Yersin (1863–1943) identifies the plague bacillus.

1895 Yersin and others in Paris develop an

anti-plague serum from the blood of horses to boost human immune systems.

1896 The Russian-born bacteriologist Waldemar Haffkine (1860–1930) sets up a small

lab in Bombay and develops a successful vaccine.

1898 The French bacteriologist Paul-Louis Simond (1858–1947), working in Bombay and Karachi, deduces

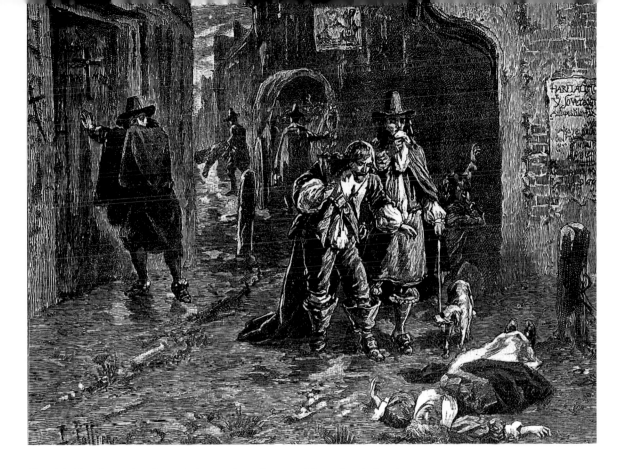

die with blood spurting from their mouths, others are bloated and already beginning to rot. Everywhere people feel underfoot the squelchy roundness of dead – or still squealing but dying – rats. On 30 April the concierge, M. Michel, dies of bubonic plague. His last words are:

'Them rats! Them damned rats!'

As plague sweeps through the city, the doctor describes the panic, the horrors, the pain of death and broken hearts, the attempts to clean up and cordon off the city, separating loved ones and fuelling despair, frustration, compassion and anguish. When the plague recedes and the gates of the city open once more, there is

Two men discover a plague victim in the street during the Great Plague of London in 1665, whilst behind them another corpse is carried out to a cart for disposal.

that rat fleas are the critical intermediary link between rats and humans.

1900–4 San Francisco suffers the first known plague epidemic in North America.

1904–7 The Plague Research Commission confirms the role of the rat and the flea in the transmission of plague.

1907–9 Plague in San Francisco, following the 1906 earthquake.

100,000 rats are captured.

1910–11 Epidemic of pneumonic plague in Manchuria in northeast Asia after hunters handle and eat the meat of infected tarabagans (Russian

marmots), in a quest to cash in on the booming trade in their fur. The epidemic spreads along newly constructed railway lines, killing 60,000 people.

1924–5 Outbreak of plague in Los Angeles.

1950s The antibiotics streptomycin and gentamycin are used to treat plague.

1994 Outbreak – possibly of

plague – in India rings alarm bells around the world.

2001 Scientists unravel the complete genetic structure of the bacillus responsible for plague.

21st century Approximately 2000 new cases and 180 deaths per year, with 98.7 per cent of cases and deaths in Africa.

'We see death coming into our midst like black smoke, a plague that cuts off the young, a rootless phantom that has no mercy for fair countenance. Woe is me of the shilling [bubo] in the armpit; it is seething, terrible, where ever it may come, a head that gives pain and causes a loud cry, a burden carried under the arms, a painful angry knob, a white lump.'

JEUAN GETHIN (d.1349), WELSH POET

rejoicing and relief. But Dr Rieux knows that *'the plague bacillus never dies or disappears for good ... and that perhaps the day would come when ... it would rouse up its rats again and send them forth to die in a happy city'.*

DEAD RATS AND MODERN IMAGINATIONS

Rats and rat fleas invariably feature together in our imaginations as the harbingers of the terrible plagues of the past. At the start of a typical epidemic, large numbers of rodents are suddenly afflicted. As in Camus' story, when the rats begin to die off, the infected rat fleas (*Xenopsylla cheopis*), frantic with hunger, search for new sources of blood, and thus turn to humans. Engorged with plague bacilli, the flea acts like a hypodermic needle, injecting the bacilli into the lymphatic system of humans.

The early signs of the disease are the hard swollen buboes (from the Greek *boubon*, 'swollen groin') in the groin, armpit or neck, close to the site of the flea bite. Plague can also become pneumonic when the bacilli enter the lungs, and when this happens the disease can be transmitted directly from person to person. Septicaemic plague is the most lethal form of all, occurring when the bacilli go straight into the bloodstream, and resulting in the haemorrhaging body being covered with ominous black 'tokens'. Untreated, bubonic plague kills up to 60 per cent of its victims, pneumonic plague some 90 per cent, and septicaemic plague virtually 100 per cent. The human flea, *Pulex irritans*, may also play a role in the subsequent inter-human dissemination of the plague – this remains a plausible but contentious theory.

WRITERS AND EYEWITNESSES

Rat 'falls' or 'die-offs' are the key feature that precipitates an outbreak of plague in humans. In India and China, folk wisdom warns that when the rats start dying, it is time to flee. But in early European descriptions of plague, there is an eerie silence about dead rats. In *A Journal of the Plague Year* (1722) Daniel Defoe (1660-1731) gives a riveting semi-fictional account of the Great Plague that visited London in 1665-6. Although he recounts a similar sequence of events as Camus does in *La Peste*, Defoe nevertheless says nothing about dying rats. The diarist Samuel Pepys (1633-1703), who actually lived through the Great Plague, also fails to mention dead rats.

During the Black Death of the mid-14th century, eyewitnesses such as Giovanni Boccaccio (1313-75) mention the myriad human corpses that littered the streets and filled the mass graves, but again there is no mention of swarms of dying rats. Further back in time, the account made in 542 by

The transmitter of plague from infected rats to humans is the flea. Fleas are tiny, flattened insects which pass the disease on when they bite their victims to obtain a meal of blood.

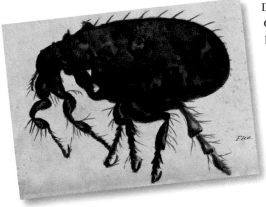

Procopius of Caesarea (c.500–c.565) of the Plague of Justinian - thought to be the first major epidemic of bubonic plague in European history - gives no clues as to whether this 'plague' was sparked off by rats and their fleas.

Camus was writing some 30 years after scientists had conclusively shown that the plague bacillus is transmitted by infected rodents and their fleas. Procopius, Boccaccio, Defoe and others were describing plague hundreds of years before that connection had been made. Their accounts of the signs and symptoms, the devastation, the human terrors and the social, economic and psychological consequences of plague are not dissimilar. But was this the same disease? Most historians would say 'yes' - but some have taken a different view (see What was the Black Death?, right)

THE FIRST GREAT PLAGUE

The word 'plague' derives from the Greek word *plege*, and the Latin word *plaga*, meaning 'blow' or 'stroke'. Like the words 'pest', 'pestilence' and 'pox', it was often used to cover a multitude of devastating epidemic diseases. The various biblical 'plagues' and some of the ancient 'plagues', such as the Plague of Athens (430–427 BC), the Plague of Orosius (AD 125), the Plague of Antoninus (164–89) and the Plague of Cyprian (250–66), were lethal epidemics but, while their identity remains uncertain, they were probably not bubonic plague.

WHAT WAS THE BLACK DEATH?

Most historians still adhere to the conventional view that the Black Death and later plague epidemics were a combination of bubonic, pneumonic and septicaemic plague, and that the black rat and its fleas (even if absent from most documentary sources) were somehow involved. Overturning conventional wisdom is not easy, especially when it relates to a story so ingrained in our minds.

But there are a number of scholars who have argued that the first and second cycles of 'plague' were not bubonic plague at all. Anthrax (a bacterial disease) or some highly contagious haemorrhagic fever, rather like the Ebola virus, are possible alternatives.

Spurred on by such debates, scientists are now excavating old plague pits in the hope of identifying the pathogenic agent responsible, and thus solving some of the mysteries. Others are looking for the remains of black rats, in the hope that they might tell us more.

The first great plague to bear the characteristic swollen buboes was the Plague of Justinian in 541–4. Spreading from Egypt to Europe, the Plague of Justinian may well have played a role in the eventual collapse of the Roman empire.

In the fourth century, the Roman empire had split in half with two capitals: Rome in the west and Constantinople in the east. By the sixth century, the western Roman empire, invaded by Goths and Vandals, had already fallen apart; in the east the emperor Justinian (r.527–65), was determined to re-conquer and unite the western and eastern realms. But his ambitions were thwarted by the plague that bears his name. The Plague of Justinian killed, at its peak, as many as 10,000 people a day in Constantinople (now Istanbul) and spread like wildfire through coastal ports and inland towns. It is estimated that perhaps one-quarter of the population of Mediterranean Europe died over the following few years.

The Byzantine chronicler Procopius of Caesarea vividly described the horrors of this epidemic, '*by which the whole human race came near to be annihilated*'.

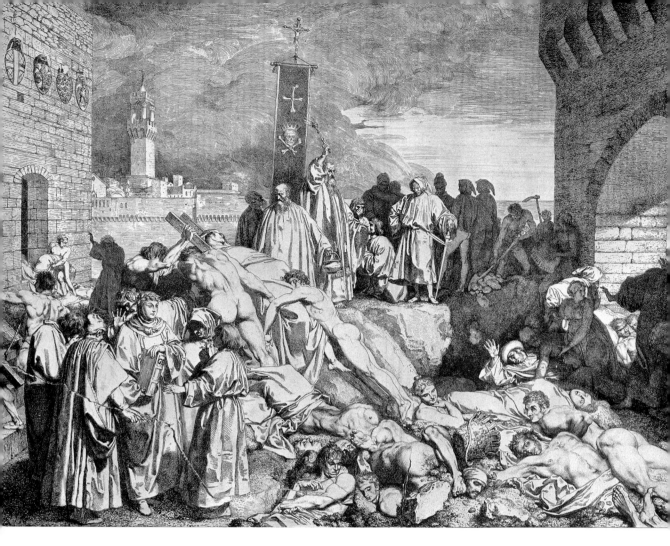

The plague devastating
Florence in 1348, an event graphically described by the Italian author Giovanni Boccaccio in *The Decameron* (1350–3), from which this illustration is taken. One observer during the Black Death likened the plague pits in which the layers of corpses were separated with sprinklings of dirt to 'cheese between layers of lasagne'.

Victims, he reported, writhed in fever, suffering agonies from grossly swollen buboes. Some became delirious and hallucinated, others died vomiting and choking on blood – possibly suggesting that both the bubonic and pneumonic forms of the disease were involved. There were too many corpses to bury. Roofs were removed from the fortified towers of Constantinople so that the dead bodies could be piled high. Some of the corpses were tossed onto rafts and allowed to drift out to sea. Panic, disorder and madness reigned. Thus began the first cycle of bubonic plague.

THE ORIGINS OF THE BLACK DEATH

The eruption of the second cycle of plague – the catastrophic Black Death, which spread from Asia to the Middle East, North Africa and Europe in the mid-14th century – is firmly imprinted on many people's imaginations. Descriptions of buboes the size of an egg or even an apple, plus blotches, boils, bruises, black pustules and the coughing up of blood, vomit and sputum suggest that the Black Death may have been a combination of bubonic, septicaemic and pneumonic plague. While there are still many unsolved riddles about the Black Death, most historians agree that in Europe alone, in the space of a few years, from 1347–53, at least 25 million people died, possibly more than one-third of the population of Europe. It was the greatest demographic crisis of the Medieval period, and in terms of the proportion killed, the single most calamitous epidemiological event in all of history.

How, where and why the Black Death started is less certain. It is possible that it erupted somewhere in the steppes of Central Asia in the 1330s and then spread westwards along the caravan routes. The most gripping (but not necessarily the most plausible) account of its introduction to Europe begins on the Crimean coast of the Black Sea at the trading post of Kaffa (now known as Theodosia), where a group of Genoese merchants were trapped by besieging Tartars.

When the attackers were struck by the plague, they were forced to retreat, leaving behind hundreds of unburied corpses. According to Gabriele de' Mussis (d.1356), as a parting shot the Tartar leader Khan Jani Beg (d.1357), *'stunned and stupefied'* by the arrival of the plague, *'ordered corpses to be placed in catapults and lobbed into the city in the hope that the intolerable stench would kill everyone inside … '*

The 'intolerable stench' did not, apparently, kill all the Genoese. Some escaped, unwittingly carrying the plague with them back to the shores of the Mediterranean. When they arrived at Messina in Sicily in the autumn of 1347 they tumbled off the ships with *'sickness clinging to their bones'*. The Black Death had reached Europe.

THE SORROW AND THE PITY
The term 'Black Death' was only coined much later, the word 'black' referring possibly to the sheer horror of the pestilence and to the blackened bodies of its victims. Contemporaries called the epidemic the 'Great Mortality' or the 'Big Sickness'. The poignant accounts they left behind ring with the terrible sorrows it brought in its wake. The Italian poet Petrarch (1304–74)

'**How many valiant men,** how many fair ladies, breakfasted with their kinsfolk and that same night supped with their ancestors in the other world.'

GIOVANNI BOCCACCIO (1313–75)

The epidemic of plague, known as the Black Death, spread rapidly through Europe in the mid-14th century. Probably carried overland from Central Asia initially via caravan trading routes, it was disseminated to major coastal ports across western Europe on merchant ships.

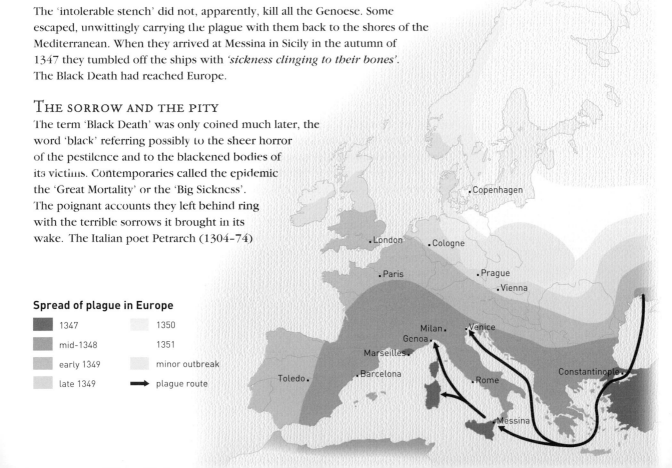

Spread of plague in Europe

- 1347
- mid-1348
- early 1349
- late 1349
- 1350
- 1351
- minor outbreak
- ➡ plague route

Copenhagen

London · Cologne

Paris · Prague · Vienna

Milan · Venice
Genoa ·
Marseilles ·
Barcelona
Toledo · Rome · Constantinople
Messina

expressed the perplexity and loneliness that must have haunted those who survived:

> *'Where are our dear friends now? Where are the beloved faces? Where are the affectionate words, the relaxed and enjoyable conversations? What lightning bolt devoured them? What earthquake toppled them? What tempest drowned them? What abyss swallowed them? There was a crowd of us, now we are almost alone.'*

A tax collector and shoemaker in Siena, Italy, called Agnolo di Tura believed, like many others, that *'This is the end of the world'*. His whole family died, *'And I, Agnolo di Tura, called the Fat, buried my five children with my own hands'*.

Everywhere – from the China Sea to the Mediterranean, across vast swathes of continental Europe and the British Isles, to the northern reaches of Scandinavia and Russia – countless bodies were buried by surviving family and friends, tossed onto rattling carts, buried in pest pits, or left to rot in the midday sun, to be devoured by wolves, pigs and dogs. In Venice the dead were dropped into gondolas and rowed out to sea with cries of *'Corpi morti, corpi morti'*.

ROTTING CORPSES AND SILENT BELLS

The smell of death was all-pervading – in the foetid breath and buboes of the afflicted, in the filthy alleys of crowded towns and villages, in the ghost ships crewed by dying sailors, in the mass graves stacked high with putrefying corpses. Giovanni Boccaccio (1313-75), describing Florence in *The Decameron* (1350-3), wrote:

> *'Many dropped dead in the open streets, both by day and by night, whilst a great many others, though dying in their own houses, drew their neighbours' attention to the fact more by the smell of their rotting corpses than by any other means. And what with these, and the others who were dying all over the city, bodies were here, there and everywhere.'*

With the sadness and stenches came a dreadful silence. In some places even the funeral bells and weeping ceased – for *'all expected to die'*. Petrarch, who had lost his beloved Laura to the plague in Avignon in 1348, noted the vast and dreadful silence hovering over the world. *'Is it possible'*, he wondered, *'that posterity can believe these things? For we, who have seen them, can hardly believe them'*.

As the 'Great Mortality' slowly retreated, there was an outpouring of macabre art and literature across Europe. The Dance of Death, the Grim Reaper, fearsome visions of

---

WHY ME? WHY HERE? WHY NOW?

Written accounts of plague epidemics dating from the Medieval and early modern periods remind us of the many ways in which people at the time wrestled to make sense of the origin, cause and spread of plague.

At one level were the divine and celestial explanations – God's reaction to the sins of humanity, or some ominous configuration of stars and planets.

There were also the 'down-to-earth' explanations: earthquakes, unusual weather and, above all, the rot and decay of rubbish accumulating in streets and dung heaps, emitting foul miasmas that poisoned the air.

And then there were the people themselves: whether sinful, smelly or sickly, humans were somehow thought to be bound up with the pestilential corruption of the world, and also capable of spreading sickness by contagious vapours from breath, buboes or clothes.

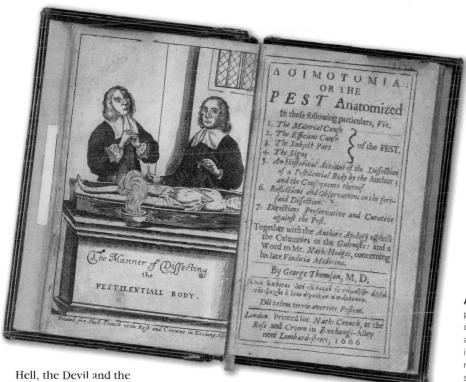

A historical account by the physician George Thomson, detailing the dissection of a plague victim. Incense is burning in the bowl as a means of camouflaging the stench of the body.

Hell, the Devil and the
Four Horsemen of the Apocalypse, and the symbol
of the skull and crossbones – all are chilling reminders of the scars that the Black
Death seared into the minds of men and women in the later Middle Ages.

PLAGUE CONTINUES TO TAKE ITS TOLL

After the ravages of the Black Death, plague did not disappear. It continued to
reap its grim harvests, and between the 14th and 18th centuries, some 50 million
Europeans are believed to have died as the plague periodically swept from
east to west.

The Great Plague of London in 1665–6 – so vividly described by
Samuel Pepys and Daniel Defoe – killed 70,000–100,000 people, or
one-fifth to one-quarter of the population of London, causing panic
and terror. 'Searchers' – often illiterate old women – sought out and
identified the sick, who were incarcerated in their homes, their doors
marked with a red cross and the words '*Lord have mercy upon us*'.
Carts collected the dead at night, and the corpses filled up mass graves
to the brim. The churches were crammed with the grieving, the
penitent and the sickly. Many who could afford to do so fled, including
not only the court, but also priests and physicians.

Whipped for Not Smoking
*During the Great Plague of London
of 1665–6 a schoolboy at Eton
College is recorded as being 'never
whipped so much in his life as he
was one morning for not smoking'
– tobacco being regarded as a
way of preventing infection.*

'*But Lord*', wrote Pepys on 16 October 1665, '*how empty the streets are, and
melancholy, so many poor sick people in the streets, full of sores, and so many
sad stories overheard as I walk, everyone talking of this dead, and that man
sick, and so many in this place, and so many in that*'.

'Now, there is a dismal solitude … shops are shut … people rare, very few walk about … and there is a deep silence in almost every place. If any voice can be heard, it is the groans of the dying, and the funeral knell of them that are ready to be carried to their graves.'

THOMAS VINCENT, DESCRIBING THE GREAT PLAGUE
OF LONDON, 1665–6

Pepys himself survived, and even at times enjoyed the occasional merrymaking. His wife, whom he sent to Woolwich, was much *'afeared'* about her pet dog, as the authorities rounded up and killed all stray dogs and cats. She also washed her hair in vinegar while Pepys, who was *'put into an ill conception of myself and my smell'*, was *'forced to buy some roll tobacco to smell and chaw - which took away the apprehension'*.

The plague spread to many other English towns and villages. When the community of Eyam in the Peak District of Derbyshire was hit, the rector, William Mompesson (1639–1709), cordoned off the village in an attempt to prevent the plague spreading to the surrounding countryside. The villagers left coins in vinegar-filled holes in gateposts along the bounds of the village to pay for food left for them by neighbours. By the autumn of 1666, over 250 of Mompesson's flock had died, possibly one-third of the population of Eyam. As one chronicler described it, *'shut up in their narrow valley, the villagers perished helplessly like a stricken flock of sheep'*. The rector's own wife was one of the victims. Mompesson survived and, reflecting on the tragedy, wrote: *'The condition of this place hath been so dreadful that I persuade myself it exceedeth all history and example. I may truly say our Town has become a Golgotha, a place of skulls … My ears never heard such doleful lamentations. My nose never smelt such noisome smells and my eyes never beheld such ghastly spectacles.'*

THE RAT RACE

The last devastating outbreak of plague in western Europe was in Marseilles, France, in 1720–2, when around 50,000 people died. On this occasion dead rats were noted: apparently 10,000 of them were gathered up by fishermen and dumped out at sea. But still no connection was established at the time between rats and bubonic plague. Thereafter, plague 'disappeared' from western Europe – or at least never reappeared, except for a few brief flurries.

Historians have long debated all sorts of theories about the disappearance of plague from western Europe. For England, the Great Fire of London in

A 17th-century physician wearing a traditional plague-preventive costume. The long, beak-like nose piece was filled with aromatic substances to combat the stench associated with plague. Although the connection between fleas and plague transmission was unknown at the time, the long robes, gloves and mask would have helped to give the wearer protection from flea bites.

'FLEE EARLY, FLEE FAR, RETURN LATE'

The advice usually given to those wishing to avoid infection during an outbreak of plague was to flee. This was often a dilemma for physicians and priests, as it meant leaving the poor and sick to face illness and death alone.

During the Black Death and later plagues, many people undertook penance and prayed for forgiveness in the hope of avoiding infection. Some took penitence to extremes, flogging themselves or one another with knotted strips of leather or iron spikes. Yet more horrific was the mass torture and murder of thousands of Jews and others in Europe accused of poisoning wells and spreading the disease. These pogroms cast a dark shadow over the era of the Black Death.

In later plague epidemics, authorities ordered cleaning up of dung heaps, and quarantining the infected. Individuals sought to save themselves by smoking tobacco, sitting under a foul-smelling latrine or sniffing roses. Viper fat, spiders' webs, toad poison, woodlice and crabs' eyes were a few of the antidotes offered for sale. When the plague threatened London, someone suggested filling a ship with peeled onions and letting it float down the Thames, in the hope that its absorbent powers would protect the city.

Those who could, such as the wealthy, fled from plague-infected areas, as this woodcut of London from 1630 shows.

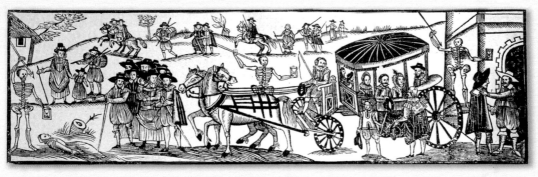

September 1666, the cleansing of urban environments, the development of resistance to plague amongst the black rats, the ousting of the black rat (*Rattus rattus*) by the brown or sewer rat (*R. norvegicus*), and changes in climate are just a few of the ideas that have been mooted, but which have generally been questioned. Quite a number of historians have highlighted the effectiveness of quarantine measures (see Quarantine, page 18), but why the cycle of plague was eventually broken still remains something of a puzzle. Although plague receded from western Europe, it continued to flare up in eastern Europe, Asia and Africa, and eventually reached North America and Australia. The third great plague pandemic originated in China in the mid-19th century, and by the 1890s was causing massive mortality in many parts of Southeast Asia. With plague raging in Hong Kong in 1894, two leading scientists were sent to find its cause.

Alexandre Yersin (1863–1943), a Swiss-born French bacteriologist, and Shibasaburo Kitasato (1852–1931), a Japanese bacteriologist who had worked with Robert Koch (1843–1910) in Berlin, were in a race to come up with an answer. Kitasato had the backing of the British authorities in Hong Kong and access to a large number of autopsies in Kennedy Town Hospital. Yersin made do with a straw hut and a few basic medical tools, and had to bribe gravediggers to allow him to cut out some buboes from the dead awaiting burial. Both scientists thought they had found the plague bacillus in the summer of 1894. It was, however, Yersin's bacillus – a gram-negative bacterium – that was identified as the correct one. He named it *Pasteurella pestis* in honour of his French patron, Louis Pasteur (1822–95). In 1954 it was renamed *Yersinia pestis*.

Yersin also developed an anti-serum that became the first 'cure' for plague. But neither Yersin nor Kitasato solved the critical piece of the puzzle – how was plague spread? Although Yersin had noticed the large number of dead rats lying on the road in infected areas of Hong Kong and had speculated that plague might be rat-borne, it was Masanori Ogata (1853–1919) working in Formosa (now Taiwan) and Paul-Louis Simond (1858–1947), a French scientist in Bombay, who in 1898 worked out that plague was transmitted from rats to humans by the bite of a flea. The idea was initially ridiculed, and it took nearly a decade before it was finally accepted by the scientific community.

POCKETS OF PESTILENCE

During this third great plague pandemic, the disease reached North America – and also Australia – for the first time. In 1900 the SS *Nippen Maru* arrived at San Francisco from China and, although it was quarantined, plague somehow reached the Chinese community. A Chinese immigrant, Chick Gin, was the first victim. He was found dead in a filthy, overcrowded 'flophouse' called the Globe Hotel with foaming, bloody spittle over his face, ashen grey skin and huge swellings around his groin and armpits. His death was quickly followed by draconian measures to quarantine, vaccinate and 'cleanse' Chinatown.

When plague struck San Francisco again after the terrible earthquake in 1906, there was, this time, an understanding of the role of the rat and its flea in the transmission of plague. The authorities set out to 'wage a war on the rats': posters encouraged people to trap and poison them, but they also warned against picking up dead rats or squashing fleas with fingers or teeth. There were 121 cases of plague and 113 deaths in the first outbreak (almost all Chinese immigrants), and 160 cases and 78 deaths in the second outbreak (this time mostly white Americans).

Los Angeles was hit in 1924–5, and as recently as the 1970s and 80s there have been curious and isolated cases of plague in parts of the USA – some of which have been traced not to rats but to prairie dogs. A

QUARANTINE The use of quarantine to prevent contagious epidemics from entering ports arose in the wake of the Black Death. In 1377 the Venetian colony of Ragusa (now Dubrovnik in Croatia) detained travellers from infected places on a nearby island for 30 days – *trentini giorni*. When this proved ineffective, the period was raised to 40 days – *quaranti giorni* – from which we derive the word 'quarantine'. The Italian states in the 14th and 15th centuries imposed stringent quarantine regulations during times of plague, and other countries soon followed suit.

The most impressive example was the Habsburg *cordon sanitaire*, which from the early 18th century ran from north of the Danube to the Balkans. It was manned by 100,000 peasants with checkpoints and quarantine stations to prevent the movement of contagious people coming into Europe from the adjacent Ottoman empire.

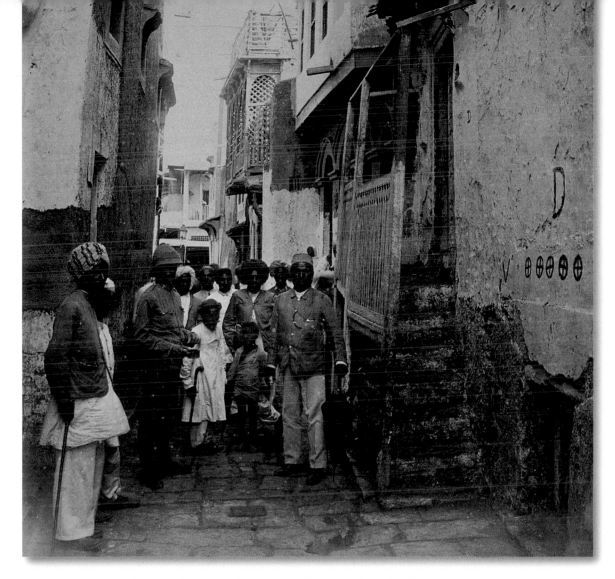

number of other small mammals are now known to harbour the plague bacillus in the wild, including ground squirrels, marmots, chipmunks and rabbits. Except for western Europe, pockets of pestilence remain in all parts of the world. As Camus' Dr Rieux reminds us, *'the plague bacillus never dies or disappears for good'*.

PLAGUE PERSISTS

Today, there are antibiotics to control plague and a vaccine that confers some protection, but plague remains endemic in many countries in Africa, eastern Europe, the Americas and Asia, with about 2000 cases a year (including some ten to 20 in the USA). When in 1994 pneumonic plague broke out in Surat, a city in the Indian state of Gujarat, there were scenes reminiscent of the Black Death: panic, people fleeing, scientists in plague-protective garb, and, above all, confusion. And while this outbreak was dealt with quickly using mass preventive vaccination and antibiotics, it reminded the world that plague is still a disease that can terrify and perplex us.

A scene outside a plague- infected house in Karachi (then in British-ruled India, now in Pakistan), photographed in 1897. Millions have died from plague in Asia over the centuries, with an estimated 12.6 million deaths from the disease between 1898 and 1948 in India alone.

LEPROSY – or Hansen's disease – is a chronic bacterial infection caused by the bacillus

Mycobacterium leprae. In serious cases it can eventually (after a long incubation period) lead to nerve, skin and bone damage. Contrary to popular belief, leprosy is the least contagious of all major communicable diseases, and there are still many puzzles about its mode of transmission. Leprosy hospitals (known as leprosaria) in the Middle Ages provided both physical and spiritual care for those suffering from this disfiguring disease. In the 19th and 20th centuries leprosy colonies were set up to isolate the infected in many parts of the world. There are now more appropriate ways to treat the disease, including effective antibiotics, and there has been an encouraging reduction in the global prevalence of leprosy over the past two decades. Cases of the disease do, however, still occur in Africa, Latin America and Asia, and continued efforts, with early detection and treatment, are needed to eliminate leprosy and overcome its stigma.

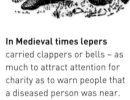

Gerhard Henrik Armauer Hansen (1841–1912), the Norwegian physician who in 1873 discovered the causative agent of leprosy, later recalled his early experience working in the National Leprosarium No. 1 in Bergen in 1868:

> *'I suffered terribly. I had never seen so much misery concentrated in one place. Gradually, though, as I commenced handling the patients, my aversion disappeared and was replaced by a great desire to learn the illness in detail … the result was that after a few months I eagerly looked forward to dealing with my ravaged patients.'*

In Medieval times lepers carried clappers or bells – as much to attract attention for charity as to warn people that a diseased person was near.

With a generous grant from the Norwegian government, Hansen conducted a comprehensive epidemiological study of leprosy in Norway. He travelled along the fjords visiting affected families, until he was finally convinced that leprosy was a communicable disease. After further clinical and experimental studies, Hansen and others were able to show that leprosy was a bacterial infection.

timeline

c.1550 BC One of the earliest accounts of possible leprosy appears in an Egyptian papyrus.

600 BC Evidence of leprosy in historical documents from India.

c.475 BC onwards A number of Chinese writings describe leprosy.

AD 758 Empress Komyo sets up the first leprosy hospital in Japan, at Nara.

c.1085 The first known leprosy hospital in England, is established at Harbledown near Canterbury.

1100–1350 Over 300 'leper' hospitals are established in England, although most are small and short-lived.

c.1350–1500 Leprosy declines across Europe.

1847 The Norwegian doctors Daniel Danielssen (1815–94) and Carl Boeck (1805–75) publish Om Spedalskhed ('On Leprosy'). They differentiate between the two main forms of leprosy and draw

a distinction between leprosy and a range of other diseases with similar symptoms, such as syphilis, scurvy, psoriasis and scabies.

1867 The Royal College of Physicians in London reports, on the basis of an empire-wide survey, that leprosy is not contagious and is best tackled by improvements in health, diet and living conditions.

The clinical manifestations of leprosy (which can take many years to appear) vary in a continuous spectrum between two polar forms. One form (known as lepromatous or multibacillary leprosy) is characterized by nodular tubercles that ultimately, if left untreated, destroy the facial features and cause permanent damage to the skin, nerves, limbs and eyes. The other form (known as tuberculoid or paucibacillary leprosy), which progresses more slowly, is a milder form, and more typically leads to patchy areas on the skin with loss of sensation.

In the late 1940s, leprosy became officially known as Hansen's disease, both in honour of the Norwegian pioneer and in order to reduce the stigma so often associated with the pejorative terms 'leprosy' and 'leper' – though the name leprosy still remains in common use in historical and medical accounts (and for historical veracity is used here).

LEPROSY IN THE MIDDLE AGES

Prior to Hansen's discovery, the history of leprosy is shrouded in myths, misconceptions and mystery. It is generally thought that leprosy is an old disease, possibly dating back to the ancient civilizations of China, India and Egypt. In Europe the disease seems to have become a serious problem in the Middle Ages. Although it is unlikely that all 'leprosy' cases were, in fact, suffering from Hansen's disease (rather than any of the other disfiguring skin diseases prevalent at the time), recent bio-archaeological evidence from skeletons in Britain dating back to at least the fourth century AD shows that some reveal the unmistakable skeletal evidence of the ravages of the disease.

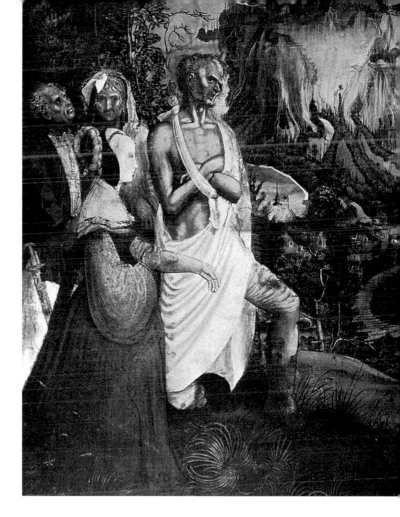

This illustration by Nikolaus Manuel Deutsch (c.1484–1530) depicts both the early stages (left) and later stages (right) of leprosy. Later stages can include permanent damage to the skin and nerves and disfigurement of the face.

1873 Norwegian physician Gerhard Henrik Armauer Hansen (1841–1912) identifies the bacillus causing leprosy under the microscope – one of the first bacteria to be identified as causing disease in humans.

1873 The Belgian priest and missionary Father Damien (1840–89) goes to Hawaii to help in a leprosy colony.

1885 In Norway an Act on Seclusion of Lepers is passed, stating that all patients have to be isolated in a separate room at home or admitted to a leprosy hospital.

1892 In South Africa a directive is passed that 'all persons with leprosy be segregated on Robben Island'.

1894 Establishment of the leprosy hospital at Carville, Louisiana, USA.

1897 The First International Congress on Leprosy, held in Berlin, Germany, recommends isolation as the appropriate policy towards leprosy.

1921 The US Public Health Service takes over operational control of the National Leprosarium at Carville.

1924 Founding of the British Empire Leprosy Relief Association (BELRA) to 'rid the empire of leprosy'. This later becomes the British Leprosy Relief Association (LEPRA).

(continued …)

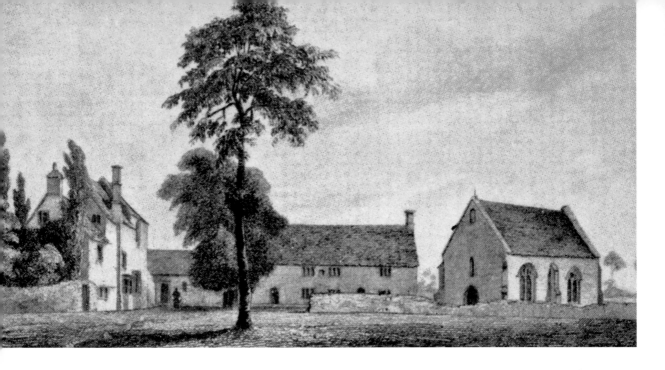

The Old Leper Hospital, St Bartholomew, Oxford, England.

Between 1100 and the Dissolution of the Monasteries in the 1530s at least 320 'leper' hospitals were founded in England by lay and religious benefactors, and usually run either by the church or towns and cities. Many leprosaria were also established in continental Europe, but it is impossible to guess at the number.

There were, undoubtedly, wide variations in the way that leprosy sufferers were identified (or misidentified) and treated in different parts of the Medieval world. A commonly held perception of Medieval England involves 'lepers', outcast from society, carrying a clapper or bell to warn people of their presence and being forcibly isolated in 'leper' hospitals for fear of spreading contagion. Recently, however, it has been suggested that this view was introduced into 19th-century accounts of English Medieval history by those who were arguing at the time for the compulsory isolation of 'lepers'. Skeletal evidence has, moreover, shown that most of those with distinctive signs of leprosy were buried not in the graveyards of 'leper' hospitals but in other cemeteries, again suggesting that society was more accepting of the disease than has commonly been assumed.

timeline

1927 The Leonard Wood Memorial, an institute for the eradication of leprosy, is founded in the USA, with a fund of $2 million.

1931 A patient at Carville – Stanley Stein, known as the Carville Crusader – produces the first issue of what is later known as The Star. Initially an in-house newspaper, it later attracts the attention of campaigners elsewhere.

1941 Promin, a sulphone drug, is introduced as a treatment for leprosy (via injections).

1945 A second drug, dapsone (administered orally), is tested, and by the 1950s is widely used. By the 1960s the causative bacterium begins developing resistance to dapsone.

1948 The US Public Health Service officially recognizes the name 'Hansen's disease' as a replacement for the term 'leprosy'.

1960 The World Health Organization (WHO) recommends the abolition of compulsory isolation of those suffering from leprosy.

1971 Scientists succeed in growing large quantities of Mycobacterium leprae in the nine-banded armadillo – the first real opportunity for studying the micro-organism since its discovery in 1873 by Hansen. It still has not been cultivated in vitro.

Care of sufferers was also probably more compassionate than popular opinion would suggest. Many responses to the disease were dictated by theology rather than medicine. In Christian societies, the concept of *Christus quasi leprous*, for example, was a reminder that Christ had been like a 'leper' in his suffering. Cures and preventatives to heal both soul and body ranged from prayer and confession to the adoption of a healthy diet, herbal baths, blood-letting and ointments (either soothing or caustic) for the skin.

'Leprosy is, perhaps, the most terrible disease that afflicts the human race. It is hideously disfiguring, destructive to the tissues and organs in an unusual degree, and is hopelessly incurable, the fate of its victims being, indeed, the most deplorable that the strongest imagination can conceive ... '

BRITISH MEDICAL JOURNAL (1887)

Between the 11th and 14th centuries leprosy appears to have been at its peak in Europe, but over the next few centuries, for reasons that are still not understood, it slowly retreated. In England, few new leprosaria were built after the 14th century, and by 1400 a number of hospitals had already been abandoned, while some were later used to house the elderly or those suffering from other diseases, such as plague or the pox. How and why the disease petered out and why leprosaria fell into disuse for leprosy patients may be accounted for by a combination of epidemiological, religious and socio-economic changes. Like many puzzles in the history of disease, the reasons for this decline will continue to give rise to lively debates, if few definitive answers.

LEPROSY RUMBLES ON IN EUROPE:
HEREDITARY OR CONTAGIOUS?

Leprosy was still endemic in Scandinavia in the mid-19th century, with around 3000 people known to have the disease in Norway when Hansen made his discovery of its causative agent. The first scientific study of leprosy was undertaken by the Norwegian dermatologist Daniel Danielssen (1815–94) – sometimes referred to as the 'father of leprology' – with his friend Carl Boeck (1805–75), working in the St Jørgens Hospital in Bergen. In 1847 they produced a remarkable book entitled *Om Spedalskhed* ('On Leprosy').

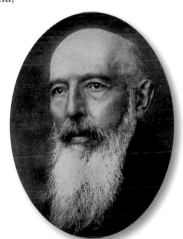

Gerhard Henrik Armauer Hansen, discoverer of the causative agent of leprosy.

1981 The WHO recommends a multi-drug therapy (MDT) regimen, combining dapsone, rifampicin and clofazimine.

1996 Japan passes an Act to Abolish the Leprosy Prevention Law, which ends compulsory isolation in leprosaria in Japan.

1999 The WHO, in collaboration with other agencies, launches the Global Alliance for Leprosy Elimination.

2000 The International Leprosy Association sets up a Global Project on the History of Leprosy, based at the Wellcome Unit for the History of Medicine, Oxford, UK. As part of this project, the oral histories of people who were for many years confined to leprosy colonies are being recorded.

2006 Following the dramatic decline in the number of cases of leprosy over the previous two decades, the WHO launches a Global Strategy for Further Reducing the Leprosy Burden and Sustaining Leprosy Control Activities, which continues to emphasize early case detection, treatment with MDT, overcoming the stigma and ameliorating the social and psychological consequences of leprosy.

Danielssen was, however, convinced that the disease was an inherited disorder. In order to prove his point, in 1856 he injected himself and some of his assistants repeatedly with 'leprous material' that he had extracted from the nodules of patients. They did not contract leprosy, and so Danielssen stuck to his theory that the disease was not a contagious one.

In 1873 Hansen (Danielssen's son-in-law) took two biopsies from the skin of the nose of one of his patients, and examined them under the microscope. There he saw large numbers of rod-shaped bodies. Convinced that he had found the causative agent of leprosy, Hansen tried a number of experiments with animals to confirm its infectious nature and to determine whether the rod-shaped bacilli (later called *Mycobacterium leprae*, or Hansen's bacillus) caused leprosy – though without success.

FATHER DAMIEN

In 1873 a Belgian priest and missionary named Joseph de Veuster (1840–89) – more widely known as Father Damien – went to the island of Molokai, Hawaii, to help in the leprosy colony at Kalawao. The first patients had been shipped there in 1866 when King Kamehameha V instituted an Act to Prevent the Spread of Leprosy and forced all those with the disease to be secluded on the island.

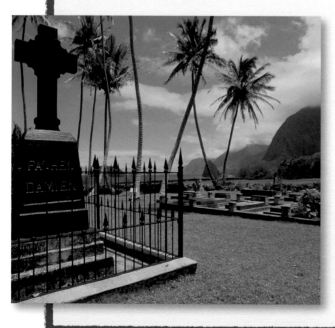

What Father Damien found, on arrival, was heartbreaking. There were some 800 leprosy sufferers housed in the most degrading conditions:

> 'Nearly all the lepers were prostrated on their beds, in damp grass huts, their constitutions badly broken down. The smell of their bodies, mixed with the exhalation from their sores, was simply disgusting and unbearable for a newcomer. Many times in fulfilling my priestly duties in their huts, I have had to close my nostrils and run outside for fresh air ... At that time the progress of the disease was fearful, the rate of mortality high ... '

Father Damien did what he could to help the people in the colony, serving as both priest and physician, and in a short time he had transformed their lives.

Sadly, he contracted leprosy himself, and died in 1889. Father Damien became an international figure, his example serving as an inspiration for others. His death from leprosy, however, reinforced the mistaken notion that the disease was highly contagious.

Father Damien's grave on the island of Molokai, Hawaii, a monument to a tireless crusader against leprosy.

One experiment though was to cost Hansen his job. Frustrated at his inability to use an animal model to confirm the infectious nature of the disease, in 1879 he inoculated leprous material from a patient with lepromatous (multibacillary) leprosy, the most aggressive chronic form, into the cornea of a 33-year-old female patient, Karl Nielsdatter, who was suffering from the tuberculoid (paucibacillary) or milder form – without harm, but without her consent. The case ended in court, and Hansen was banned from ever practising medicine again. He continued as medical officer for leprosy in Norway, but his days of clinical research were over. The bacillus that Hansen had first observed under the microscope continued to frustrate scientists for another five generations as they unsuccessfully attempted to grow it in a test tube or to infect experimental animals.

THE 'SEPARATING SICKNESS'

Although leprosy persisted in only a few areas of Europe in the 19th and early 20th centuries, the question of segregation of the infected raised many sensitive and conflicting issues. Because of the fear among a growing number of people that the disease was highly contagious and might become a global epidemic, leprosy colonies for the infected began to proliferate throughout the world, most commonly on off-shore islands. On the island of Molokai, Hawaii, where a colony was set up in 1866, the local name for the disease had become *mai ho'okawale*, the 'separating sickness'. Missionaries such as Father Damien went to leprosy colonies to offer care for the diseased and disfigured sufferers (see Father Damien, left). The Mission to Lepers in India (now more sensitively called The Leprosy Mission) was founded in 1873, the year of Hansen's discovery of the leprosy bacillus, with the aim of investigating the disease in British India, establishing a number of leprosaria, and bringing physical and spiritual relief to sufferers who had been shunned by society.

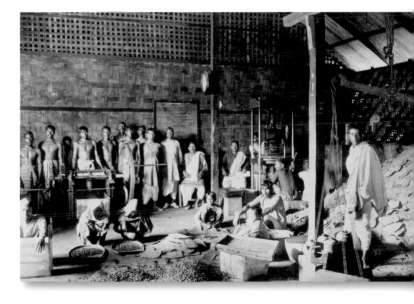

A chaulmoogra oil factory at Prasana Kumar Sen, Chittagong, in what is now Bangladesh, photographed in 1921. Chaulmoogra oil was one of the early treatments for leprosy.

From the mid-19th to the mid-20th century, efforts to contain, control or treat leprosy across the world varied widely, often with tensions between religious and medical approaches, indigenous practices and 'colonial' or 'state' interventions, and with arguments for and against enforced isolation, depending on whether the disease was viewed as highly contagious or completely non-contagious.

PIONEERING TREATMENTS

In 1915 Sir Leonard Rogers (1868–1962), a British doctor working in India and one of the founders of The British Empire Leprosy Relief Association (BELRA), pioneered a preparation for intravenous injection based on the active agents of

THE STORY OF CARVILLE

In the United States there has only ever been one leprosarium on the mainland, at Carville in Louisiana. Leprosy probably reached the Americas via European settlers and enslaved Africans. In Louisiana in the 19th century, leprosy was known as *la maladie que tu nommes pas* – 'the disease you do not name'. In 1894 five men and two women leprosy sufferers were taken to a former sugar plantation on the Mississippi River, establishing the Louisiana Leper Home at Carville.

Carville was slowly transformed from a 'swampy hell-hole' into a beautiful estate. The history of its patients and carers, the Sisters of Charity, is especially moving – there are many stories of sadness and separation, rejection and despair, tolerance and understanding, love and determination. Although in principle it was designated 'a place of refuge, not reproach; a place of treatment and research, not detention', Carville, like many leprosaria of the 19th and first half of the 20th century, imposed strict segregation and isolation policies. Carville encapsulates all that is both sad and good in the history of leprosy.

A number of new therapies were pioneered at Carville, and it became the focus of a transformation of attitudes towards the disease. Up until 1952 patients were not allowed to marry, and those already married were not permitted to live with non-patient spouses. Patients could not vote in elections, and outgoing post was sterilized. When patients were discharged they were handed a certificate that labelled them 'Public Health Service Leper' with, under reason for discharge, the comment: *'No longer a menace to public health'*.

The Louisiana Leper Home, photographed in 1955.

Beginning in the 1930s, one patient, Stanley Stein, did much to campaign for change and to raise awareness of the plight of leprosy sufferers. He began a newspaper, *The Star*, to help change perceptions of the disease. It was through the insistence of patients and staff at Carville that in 1948 the name Hansen's disease officially replaced the name leprosy.

After patients at Carville began to be treated successfully with the new drug dapsone in 1945, they started to envisage a life beyond the fence that separated them from society, adopting as their theme tune one of the hit songs of the time, 'Don't Fence Me In'. In 1948 the barbed-wire fence was removed. For those cured of the disease and trying to find a life elsewhere, the stigma of leprosy was, however, ever present. *No One Must Ever Know*, the title of a memoir published in 1959 by a former patient, Betty Martin, reflects the difficulty she and her fellow sufferers had in shaking off the past.

In 1986 the hospital at Carville was renamed the Gillis W. Long Hansen's Disease Center, and is now, from its new base in Baton Rouge, at the forefront of research into Hansen's disease.

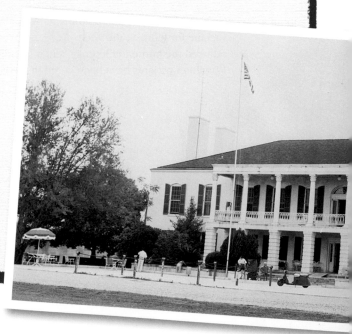

chaulmoogra oil, a traditional natural treatment used for centuries in Asia but with nauseating side effects when taken by mouth.

In 1941 a new drug called promin was tested on 22 patients at the leprosy hospital at Carville, Louisiana, with impressive results – described by one patient as a 'miracle' (see The Story of Carville, left). This was followed by dapsone – an even more effective treatment, which could be administered orally rather than by injections. Carville was also one of the centres to pioneer new techniques of reconstructive surgery. By the second half of the 20th century other drugs were available, and in the 1960s the World Health Organization (WHO) recommended the abolition of compulsory isolation of those suffering from leprosy – based on the scientific knowledge that the disease is not highly contagious and drug treatment was available. However, compulsory isolation continued in some countries, such as Japan, until the mid 1990s.

> 'Stigma shouldn't be seen as residing in an individual with a disease, but it resides in the society that has not found a way to be inclusive. We have a duty to diagnose and treat this stigma.'
>
> JOHN MANTON, THE INTERNATIONAL LEPROSY ASSOCIATION GLOBAL PROJECT ON THE HISTORY OF LEPROSY (2007)

LEPROSY TODAY

Scientists continue to try to unravel the immunology of leprosy, and its mode of transmission – possibly, but not always, involving inhalation of infected airborne droplets. They are also trying to understand the reasons for its exceptionally low infectivity level, and its long latency period. The disease is, as Hansen suspected, contagious, but of all the infectious diseases it is one of the hardest to catch. It would seem that 95 per cent of the population is naturally immune.

In the last few decades the World Health Organization (WHO) has been optimistic that there are sufficient drugs to eliminate leprosy. When cases of resistance to dapsone appeared in the 1960s, the WHO pushed for a multi-drug therapy (MDT) combining dapsone with clofazimine and rifampicin. Although there is as yet no vaccine for leprosy, the widespread use of MDT has dramatically reduced the burden of leprosy, and it is estimated that some 14 million patients have been cured in the last two decades.

Since 1995 the WHO has provided the drugs free of charge, and leprosy has now been eliminated from a number of countries where it was still a major problem in the mid-1980s. Leprosy is at present mostly concentrated in a number of countries in Africa, Asia and Latin America. Although there has been a decline in the global prevalence of leprosy, there are still over a quarter of a million new cases detected every year, as well as many more sufferers who have already been disabled by the disease and who are now beyond the hope of treatment. Some continue to feel the stigma of leprosy and do not come forward for early treatment. The disease is retreating, but it is far from being eradicated. It must not be forgotten.

SYPHILIS – the 'great pox' – struck Europe in the late 15th century,

and the impact was devastating. Many people in Italy, France, Spain, England and elsewhere became infected, primarily through sexual contact. The hideous symptoms induced horror and loathing, and in very many cases resulted in death. Over the next few centuries, syphilis became less lethal, but nevertheless remained a major cause of sickness and death for many people across the globe. Its causative organism, a bacterium called *Treponema pallidum*, was identified in the early 20th century, and since the mid-20th century antibiotics have proved highly effective against what was, until the advent of HIV/AIDS, the most dreaded of all sexually transmitted diseases.

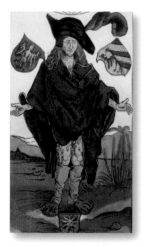

A late 15th-century syphilis sufferer, from a woodcut by Albrecht Dürer.

In 1530 an Italian physician, Girolamo Fracastoro (*c.*1476/8–1553), published a poem entitled *Syphilis sive morbus Gallicus* ('Syphilis, or the French Disease'). The poem tells the story of a swineherd named Syphilus who, for insulting the sun god Apollo, is punished with a horrible pestilence that brings out 'foul sores' on his body. The swineherd's name may be a combination of the Greek words for 'pigsty' and 'love'. Whatever its derivation, this was the first appearance of the word 'syphilis', although the disease had already been called by any number of different names since its eruption in Europe a few decades earlier.

NAMING THE DISEASE

The epidemic that hit the warring nations of Europe in the mid-1490s seemed to contemporaries to be a completely new and appalling affliction, one that caused gross pustules to erupt over the entire body, abscesses to eat into the bones and the flesh to fall off the face. Death was the outcome more often than not. It was said that the disease first appeared in 1495, after King Charles VIII of France (r.1483–98) laid siege to Naples (then under Spanish rule). When the city fell, the French army was struck by an unfamiliar and foul disease, forcing Charles to end his campaign. The French blamed the pestilence on the Neapolitans. But once the pox-ridden French army of soldiers and female camp followers disbanded and retreated to their homelands, they took the terrible scourge with them.

timeline

1492 *Christopher Columbus (1451–1506) becomes the first European to reach the islands of the West Indies.*

1495 *A 'new' disease called morbus gallicus erupts in Europe following the* French siege of Naples.

1497 *The Italian physician Nicolaus Leoniceno (1428–1524) writes one of the first treatises on syphilis, De epidemia quam vulgo morbum gallicum vocant ('On the epidemic* vulgarly called the French disease').

1530 *Girolamo Fracastoro (c.1476/8–1533) first uses the word 'syphilis' in his poem 'Syphilis sive morbus gallicus'.*

1746–7 *London's Lock Hospital for venereal cases opens near Hyde Park Corner.*

1879 *The German bacteriologist Albert Neisser (1855–1916) identifies the bacterium causing gonorrhoea.*

1905 *The German scientists Fritz Schaudinn (1871–1906) and Erich Hoffmann (1868–1959) isolate the syphilis bacterium, calling it Spirochaeta pallida, later renamed Treponema pallidum.*

1906 *Another German scientist, August von Wassermann (1866–1925), and his colleagues develop a blood test for syphilis, known as the 'Wassermann reaction'.*

1910 *The German bacteriologist Paul Ehrlich (1854–1915) and his Japanese colleague Sahachiro Hata (1873–1938) announce the discovery of the first 'magic bullet' – salvarsan – for syphilis.*

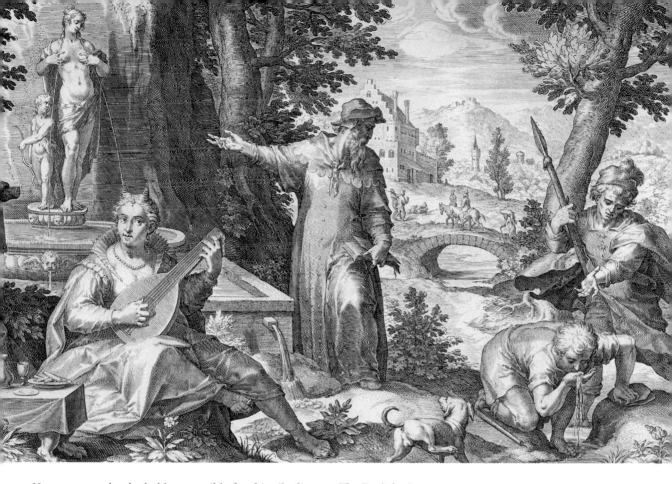

No one wanted to be held responsible for this vile disease. The English, Germans and Italians called it the *morbus gallicus* or the 'French disease'; the French preferred the 'disease of Naples' or the 'Spanish pox'; the Polish labelled it the 'Russian disease'; to the Turks it was the 'Christian disease'; and by the time it had spread to southern and eastern Asia in the mid-16th century, it was called the 'Chinese pox' by the Japanese and the 'Portuguese disease' in India and Japan. Despite being the most disowned affliction in history, two names stuck: *morbus gallicus*, the French disease, became the most common term in most of Europe, while to the French, it became known as *la grande vérole* – the 'great pox'.

This engraving from the late 1500s shows the shepherd Syphilus and the hunter Ilceus being warned by Girolamo Fracastoro against yielding to sexual temptation because of the danger of infection.

1927 The Austrian neurologist Julius von Wagner-Jauregg (1857–1940) wins the Nobel Prize for his malariatherapy treatment of syphilis.

1928 Alexander Fleming (1881–1955) discovers penicillin, though it is not widely used as a treatment until the 1940s when scientists recognize its therapeutic value.

1943 Penicillin begins to be manufactured in large quantities. It is effective against syphilis, gonorrhoea and a wide range of other bacterial infections.

1945 Alexander Fleming, Howard Florey (1090–1960) and Ernst Chain (1906–79) share the Nobel Prize for 'the discovery of penicillin and its curative effect in various infectious diseases'.

1950s The incidence of syphilis falls to an all-time low.

1980s HIV/AIDS becomes the most devastating sexually transmitted 'new' disease to emerge since the 1490s.

21st century With a worldwide resurgence of STIs (sexually transmitted infections), syphilis continues to cause concern.

29

The mystery of the origin of the 'great pox'

The name syphilis, coined by Fracastoro in 1530, was not widely adopted until the early 19th century, although his published Latin verse on the *morbus gallicus* was read by many and translated into several languages. But while each nation blamed somebody else for the terrible disease, physicians throughout Europe were anxious to discover why and from where this 'great pox' had actually arisen. Had it just struck the French army in Naples out of the blue – a thunderbolt from the Almighty, perhaps, to punish people for their sins (as Fracastoro's Apollo had cursed the swineherd)? Or, as many began to suspect, had the disease been brought from overseas – by sailors returning from the New World?

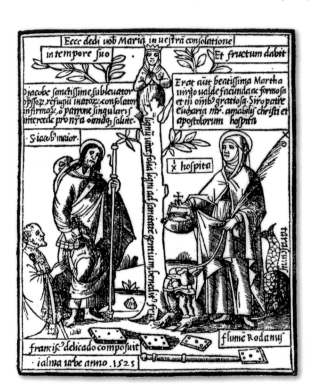

A depiction of the preparation of guaiacum, or 'holy wood', the remedy for syphilis advocated by German scholar and sufferer of the disease Ulrich von Hutten.

It is a question that has engaged some great minds over the past five centuries, and one that still perplexes historians and palaeopathologists. The traditional notion that the disease was brought back by Columbus and his crew appears to fit the chronology of a 'new' pestilence erupting in Europe in the late 15th century, and it is thought that some of Columbus's Spanish sailors, who were possibly infected in the New World, were sent to help defend Naples against the French, and passed the disease to the locals. For some, this 'Columbian' thesis has a certain poetic justice, since many lethal diseases (such as measles, smallpox, malaria and influenza) were taken across the Atlantic from the Old World to the New, wreaking havoc amongst the Native American populations, who had no immunity to such diseases.

Alternative hypotheses abound. There are those who believe (on the basis of supposedly 'syphilitic' evidence in pre-Columbian European skeletal remains) that the disease was endemic in Europe before 1492 and was, perhaps, confused with other disfiguring diseases, such as leprosy. Others have suggested that over the course of time syphilis evolved from a number of related diseases, such as yaws, pinta and bejel – which are primarily childhood diseases spread through the skin – to become a sexually transmitted infection of adults. Some adhere to the idea that one or several syphilitic infectious agents were present in both the Old and the New World, and that they mutated or fused to become more virulent in the late 15th century.

There are also medical historians who feel that it is impossible to make a correct retrospective analysis of a disease, especially one that has so many names and so many confusing and conflicting versions. Such diseases are therefore best left 'undiagnosed', according to these authorities, and their histories should be written from a contemporary rather than a retrospective point of view. But with the development of new techniques for analyzing skeletal remains, it is still possible that one day the dead will give up their secrets, and help to resolve the debate once and for all.

'ONE NIGHT WITH VENUS, AND A LIFETIME WITH MERCURY'

The association of the 'great pox' with loose women, prostitutes and 'general godlessness' was recognized from an early date. This gave rise to the use of yet a further term: *lues venerea* or venereal disease (from Venus, the Roman goddess of love). Another venereal disease, gonorrhoea (often known as 'the clap' or *chaude pisse* – 'hot piss'), had been around since ancient times and, when syphilis struck Europe, some thought that the two diseases were one and the same. The alarming and more serious symptoms of syphilis were, it was mooted, just one added complication caused by the same venereal poison spreading more widely around the body.

'[The physician] cared not even to behold it ... for truly when it first begun, it was so horrible to behold. They had boils that stood out like acorns, from whence issued such filthy stinking matter, that whosoever came within the scent, believed himself infected. The colour of these was a dark green, and the very aspect as shocking as the pain itself, which yet was as if the sick had lain upon a fire.'

ULRICH VON HUTTEN (1488–1523), A GERMAN SCHOLAR WHO SUFFERED FROM THE 'GREAT POX' AND DESCRIBED THE HORROR OF THE NEW DISEASE, AS WELL AS THE TORTURE OF MERCURY TREATMENT

The authorities in a number of countries were so appalled by the heightened escalation of venereal diseases (VD) that they attempted to control the levels of prostitution and casual sexual encounters. Henry VIII of England (r.1509–47) tried to close down the 'stews', or brothels, of London as well as communal bathhouses. (It has often been speculated that he himself suffered from syphilis, but this was probably not true.)

DR CONDOM

Folk etymology claims that the word 'condom' came from a certain Dr Condom who made the devices for Charles II, King of England (1660–85). It is more likely that the term originated from the Latin *condere*, 'to hide, suppress or conceal'. Condoms were used in ancient times (probably for ritual purposes), and over the centuries were made from anything from sheep's gut to tortoiseshell, leather or silk. In the 17th century, condoms were recommended as a prevention against the 'great pox', rather than as a contraceptive. The English gentry, eagerly awaiting their arrival in the post from France, called them 'French letters'. The French aristocracy returned the compliment, calling them *capotes anglaises* ('English overcoats'). The first rubber condoms came on to the market in 1855. With the introduction of antibiotics, venereal diseases were no longer perceived as a risk, and their use as a method of birth control declined with the advent of the contraceptive pill. However, condoms have made a comeback as a means of preventing the transmission of HIV.

Fifty to a hundred years after its initial spectacular appearance, the disease seemed to become less virulent and less lethal. It nevertheless caused agonizing long-term symptoms for its sufferers, as well as shameful sores, known as chancres. Syphilis has three stages. The primary stage begins with genital sores, usually at the site of contact. In the secondary stage these lesions heal, and several weeks later a rash appears, often accompanied by fever, aches and tiredness. The tertiary stage might occur after a long latent period in which the patient has few symptoms. This last stage, however, is the worst: abscesses crop up all over the body, and the disease may eat away the face, bones and internal organs. In some cases the disease can also invade the cardiovascular or nervous systems, leading to paralysis, blindness, insanity and eventual death. Children born to syphilitic mothers can also be infected in the womb: these so-called 'innocents' may be afflicted with various deformities, including blindness, deafness and characteristic 'peg-shaped' teeth.

Any number of treatments were touted as cures for this notorious disease. The ancient custom of bleeding was widely practised – to no avail. Rose's Balsamic Elixir offered, according to its vendors, to cure *the English Frenchify'd* by removing *all pains in three or four doses and making any man, tho' rotten as a Pear, to be as sound as a sucking lamb*. One of the most common treatments involved the use of mercury – hence the saying, *One night with Venus and a lifetime with Mercury*. Patients would be wrapped in blankets, left to sweat in a hot tub or by a fire and given mercury, either as a drink or as an ointment for their suppurating sores. It was said that the patient needed to produce at least three pints of saliva for the poison to be expelled from the body. In fact, the highly toxic mercury 'cure' caused as many complications as the disease itself.

MADNESS AND MALARIATHERAPY

'Though this be madness, yet there is method in't.'
Polonius, in William Shakespeare,
Hamlet, II.ii

Prior to the advent of antibiotics as a treatment for syphilis, an interesting idea came to the Austrian neurologist, Julius von Wagner-Jauregg (1857–1940). Many people with late-stage syphilis ended up in mental asylums suffering from 'general paralysis of the insane' (GPI), the name given to the form of mental illness caused by syphilis. In a psychiatric hospital in Vienna, Wagner-Jauregg noticed that patients who also came down with malaria seemed to show a marked improvement in their physical and mental health. It was likewise observed that when *Treponema pallidum* was cultured in a test tube, it could be killed by heat. What if, Wagner-Jauregg wondered, he gave his syphilitic patients a dose of malaria? Might the resulting high fever get rid of the syphilis germ?

The practice seemed to work, at least by slowing the progress of dementia and other symptoms of late-stage syphilis. Quinine was available to kill off the malarial parasites once the experimental treatment had been given. Wagner-Jauregg was awarded the Nobel Prize in 1927 for his novel 'discovery' of using one disease to fight another, and malariatherapy was given to thousands of GPI patients all over the world, until it was superseded by early treatment with penicillin.

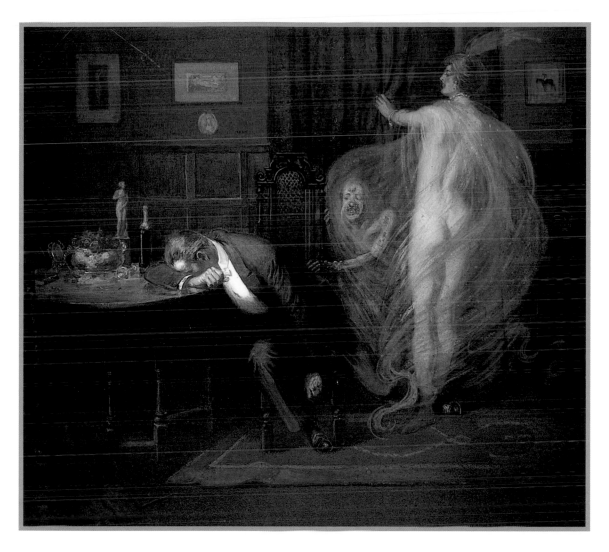

The German scholar Ulrich von Hutten (1488–1523) advocated a far more gentle remedy called guaiacum or 'holy wood', a decoction made from a tree native to the West Indies. Since it was presumed by some that the disease itself came from the New World, a local plant seemed an attractive remedy. Whether it worked or not is another matter, but it was certainly less dangerous than mercury.

A 'MAGIC BULLET'

Confusion over the differences and similarities of syphilis and gonorrhoea had long vexed physicians. In the mid-18th century, after conducting a gruesome experiment, the Scottish surgeon John Hunter (1728–93) claimed that they were the same disease. He inoculated an 'unknown individual' (possibly himself) with 'venereal matter' taken from a patient who had gonorrhoea. Hunter then watched to see the development of symptoms. During the following months, the signs of both 'the clap' and 'the pox', including the chancre of syphilis, were evident. It is

Rendered in gouache and watercolour, *Syphilis*, painted in 1910 by the artist Richard Cooper, was a graphic yet salutary reminder of the possible hidden dangers of sexual encounters.

quite likely that the 'donor' actually had both syphilis and gonorrhoea, deluding Hunter into thinking that the two were from the same poison.

Over the course of the 19th and early 20th centuries, much of the confusion about the cause of these two venereal diseases was cleared up. In 1879 the gonococcus germ causing gonorrhoea was identified, and in 1905 the German researchers Fritz Schaudinn (1871-1906) and Erich Hoffmann (1868-1959) found spiralling thread-like bacteria in syphilitic chancres. The causative organism of syphilis was subsequently given the name *Treponema pallidum* (meaning 'pale twisted thread'). In 1906 a new blood test was developed, known as the 'Wassermann reaction', which could easily identify those suffering from syphilis. The first sign of hope in the form of a treatment for syphilis came in 1910. Paul Ehrlich (1854-1915), a German medical scientist, had been studying over 600 different arsenical compounds in the search for a 'magic bullet', a chemical compound that would attack and kill a specific micro-organism. Number 606, which he called salvarsan, did just that – or almost. It was initially hailed as a remarkable drug – but it was still fairly toxic and had some unpleasant side effects. A modified compound, neosalvarsan, was produced, but it was not until the introduction of penicillin in the 1940s that a real 'wonder cure' was available for both syphilis and gonorrhoea.

The Tuskegee Syphilis Study

The Tuskegee Syphilis Study in Macon County, Alabama, was one of the most infamous medical experiments ever carried out. Some 400 poor black male share-croppers who had latent syphilis (but were told they had 'bad blood') were tracked and left untreated over a period of years from 1932 to 1972 so that the US Public Health Service could monitor the progress and effects of the disease. In 1997 President Bill Clinton formally apologized for this 'outrage to our commitment to integrity and equality for all our citizens', though by then many of those in the study, as well as their wives and children, had already died.

GUARD AGAINST VD

The First and Second World Wars saw a sharp rise in venereal diseases, as well as a real fear that soldiers returning from the theatres of war would spread the infections far and wide, as they had done in the late 15th century. The policies for dealing with the threat were quite different in each of the wars, and differed also from one country to another.

In the First World War, soldiers who contracted syphilis or 'the clap' lost their pay. Propaganda material warned the Allies that '*A German bullet is cleaner than a whore*', and closing down brothels made sense to the American military at this time on the grounds that '*to drain a red-light district and destroy thereby a breeding place of syphilis and gonorrhoea is as logical as it is to drain a swamp and thereby a breeding place of malaria and yellow fever*'. Although condoms were available as a preventative, these were strongly discouraged on the grounds that they would simply encourage licentious behaviour.

By the Second World War, there was less emphasis on the stigma and shame of VD and more concern for public health, family and social welfare. Campaigns aimed at servicemen began to promote ways to avoid the infection or seek treatment for it. Condoms were encouraged. Posters reminded soldiers to: '*Guard against VD. Keep straight - keep sober. You owe it to yourself, your comrades, your efficiency*'.

From VD to AIDS

In the second half of the 20th century, a more open policy towards syphilis was established in many countries, with free VD clinics, posters to spread the message of prevention and penicillin for those who needed it. The incidence of syphilis fell and, although it remained a dreaded disease, there was hope that it could be stamped out entirely. The recent HIV/AIDS epidemic (see pages 192–201) has overshadowed the older fears of syphilis. Syphilis does, however, still remain a persistent, albeit treatable, sexually transmitted infection (STI) in many parts of the world, with over 30,000 new cases reported every year in the USA, and many times that number in the developing world, with some 60 per cent of all deaths from syphilis being recorded in Africa. People with syphilis are also at greater risk of becoming infected with HIV. The incidence of gonorrhoea is even higher, and a newly emerging bacterial STI, chlamydia, is thought to be the most prevalent infectious disease in the USA after the common cold. It is the AIDS virus, however, with its devastating global impact, that looms largest in the public-health arena of the 21st century.

In retrospect, the emergence of the scourge of the 'great pox' in the 1490s bears frightening parallels with the escalation of AIDS in the late 20th and early 21st centuries. The two diseases, while quite different from a pathological and immunological perspective, both share similar pathways of transmission, both have long dormant periods during which patients are infectious but show few symptoms, and both have generated huge debates about their origin, and how best to tackle treatment in the light of the associated moral issues.

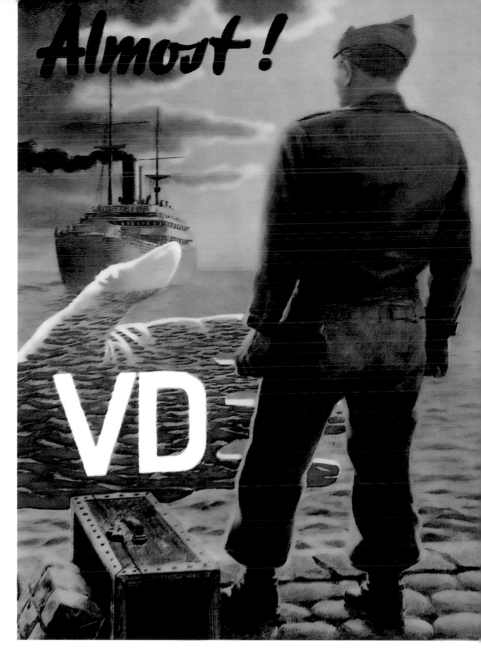

The dangers of venereal diseases were brought to the awareness of the American public by posters such as the one above from 1946.

Typhus is an acute infectious disease that is transmitted by *Pediculus humanus corporis* –

or, as it is more commonly known, the body louse. For centuries typhus was especially prevalent where there was overcrowding and poor standards of hygiene, causing horrible suffering and innumerable deaths. There are many graphic descriptions of epidemics during wars and famines, and on a number of occasions the disease has even changed the course of human history. However, by the end of the Second World War a combination of vaccination, insecticides and antibiotics had led to a decline in the incidence of typhus. It is now relatively uncommon, but does still occur in parts of Asia, Africa and Central and South America.

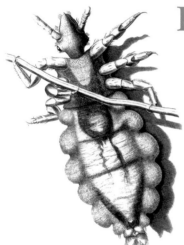

The body louse, carrier of typhus. The human body can play host to three types of louse – the body louse, the head louse and the pubic or crab louse.

In 1577 a Catholic bookbinder called Rowland Jenks was tried in Oxford, England, for distributing 'popish' books. His trial attracted considerable interest both from the citizens of the town and the dons of the university. The courtroom was crowded, stuffy and, above all, smelly. Jenks got off lightly. He was found guilty, had his ears cut off, and lived another 30 or so years. Many of the people who attended the trial, however, later sickened and died from a horrible 'spotted fever'. It is estimated that some 500 people, including 100 members of Oxford University, died during this episode, one of the many so-called 'Black Assizes' that occurred in England during the 16th century.

These Black Assizes occurred despite courtrooms being decked with aromatic herbs in the belief that it was the bad smells of the prisoners that caused contagion. Sweet-smelling scents, as well as the 'refreshing' vapours of garlic and vinegar, were thought to be the best way for the judges, jury and spectators to preserve their health and prevent 'jail fever' spreading from the felons in the dock to the assembled company.

BODY LICE

Historians suspect that the Oxford outbreak, like many similar outbreaks of 'jail fever', was typhus – a disease that we now know is spread by body lice, or, more precisely, their infected faeces. Body lice live and lay their eggs in the warm clothes of humans (preferring woollen or cotton underwear to silk). They do

timeline

1489–90 *During the Spanish siege of Granada – the last Moorish stronghold in Spain – typhus kills 17,000 Spanish soldiers. This is the first*

clear evidence of a typhus epidemic during wartime in Europe.

1494 *French troops in Italy lose 30,000 soldiers to typhus.*

1618–48 *During the Thirty Years' War in Europe, typhus is a major problem.*

1643 *Both the Parliamentarian and Royalist armies in the English Civil War are ravaged by typhus, which spreads through England, turning*

the country into 'one huge hospital'.

1812 *Napoleon's 'Grande Armée' is seriously depleted by typhus and other diseases*

during the French invasion of Russia.

1845–9 *Typhus – 'famine fever' – kills many people during the 'Great Hunger' in Ireland.*

1854–6 *In the Crimean War nearly twice as many soldiers die from diseases such as typhus as die from their wounds.*

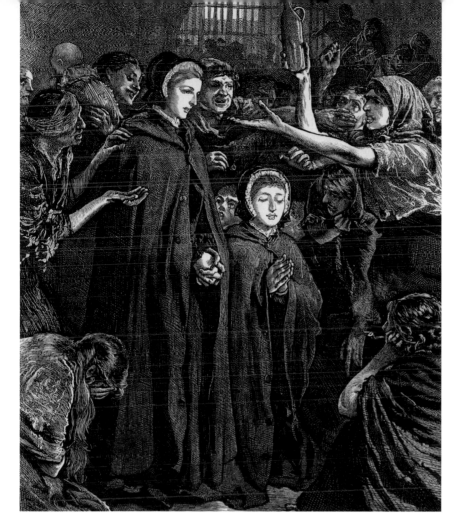

Prison reformers visiting women prisoners in Newgate Prison in 1813. Typhus frequently broke out in the filthy conditions of prisons. In the early part of the 18th century, for every prisoner hanged at Tyburn, four would die of 'jail fever' at Newgate Prison before they could be executed.

not jump, hop or fly, but every now and again crawl out of the clothes on to the skin for a quick nip of blood. If the lice suck blood from a person suffering from typhus, they become infected and ultimately die from damage to their digestive organs. But – and this is the critical part – if they first move to another person (deserting the feverish or dead host) and then defecate, their infected excrement can easily be rubbed into the slightest scratch or wound, including those made by the louse itself. It is also possible for someone to be infected by sniffing or breathing in dried louse faeces in clothing or bedding; the typhus organism then enters the body via the mucous membranes in the nose or mouth. Once infected

1909 *The body louse is found to be the vector that transmits typhus.*

1914–22 *Typhus kills several million during the First World War on the Eastern Front and subsequently in the Soviet Union and eastern Europe.*

1937 *The first typhus vaccine is produced.*

1943–4 *During the latter part of the Second World War, DDT is used for the first time to delouse soldiers.*

1940s *Antibiotics prove effective against the organism causing typhus.*

21st century *Although now rare, typhus is still endemic in the mountainous regions of Mexico, in Central and South America, in central and* *eastern Africa and in many countries in Asia. Epidemics may occur during war and famine.*

with typhus, victims become feverish, even delirious; they experience an intense headache, with pains in the muscles and joints, and exhibit a vivid rash of bright red spots which resemble flea bites. They also emit a vile stench – giving further credence to the formerly popular idea that bad smells cause disease. Death rates in untreated cases range from 10 to 40 per cent, increasing with age. Death results from toxaemia (the accumulation of toxic substances in the blood).

A 'HAZY' DISEASE

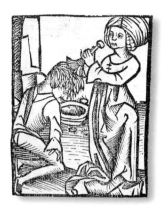

A woman brushes lice from a sufferer's head into a bowl in this illustration of delousing from 1499.

The term 'typhus' was first used in the 18th century. It is derived from the Greek word *typhos*, meaning 'smoky' or 'hazy', one of the characteristic symptoms of the disease being the stupor or dullness of mind experienced by its victims. It was not until the mid-19th century, however, that typhus was clearly differentiated from typhoid (see pages 54–61) and a number of other fevers. There are many accounts in the preceding centuries of foul and fatal epidemics variously known as 'spotted fever' in English, *fleckfieber* in German (after its characteristic rash), or *tabardillo* in Spanish (meaning 'red cloak'). The Veronese physician Girolamo Fracastoro (*c.*1476/8–1553) described the spots that appear on the arms and torso of the infected as *lenticulae* ('small lentils'), *puncticulae* ('small pricks') or *petechiae* ('flea bites'). The disease was also named after the circumstances in which it broke out – hence it was known as 'jail fever', 'ship fever', 'famine fever' and 'camp fever'.

The close association of typhus with conditions of poor hygiene, overcrowding, cold, hunger and – above all – unwashed bodies and clothes, singled it out as a classic disease of dirt and distress. It plagued prisoners, seafarers, beggars, slum dwellers and soldiers, and, in Europe from the late 15th century when the disease first made its appearance, it repeatedly devastated armies. Typhus – along with other pestilences such as dysentery (the 'bloody flux'), relapsing fever, scurvy and typhoid – was an almost invariable accompaniment to warfare, and such diseases accounted for far more losses than the actual fighting.

A MISERABLE MOB

One of the most striking epidemics of 'camp fever' occurred in 1812. That summer the French emperor Napoleon (1769–1821), with his 'Grande Armée' numbering more than half a million men, embarked on the ill-fated invasion of Russia. During the course of the advance many of his troops sickened or died of typhus and dysentery, and roughly constructed hospitals had to be erected en route for the wounded and the victims of disease. By mid-September, following the Battle of Borodino, Napoleon reached Moscow with a depleted army of only 90,000 men. But the Russians were one step ahead of him. Taking with them most of the supplies and provisions, they had abandoned the city and put it to the torch. Napoleon entered a city that was silent, empty and smouldering. Despondent and

'Typhus fever spread among the civilians, who were not only afflicted by the terrible scourge of our passing armies, but also became the victims of a murderous contagion … Wherever we went, the inhabitants were filled with terror and refused to quarter the soldiers.'

A FRENCH SOLDIER RECALLS THE RETREAT FROM MOSCOW, 1812

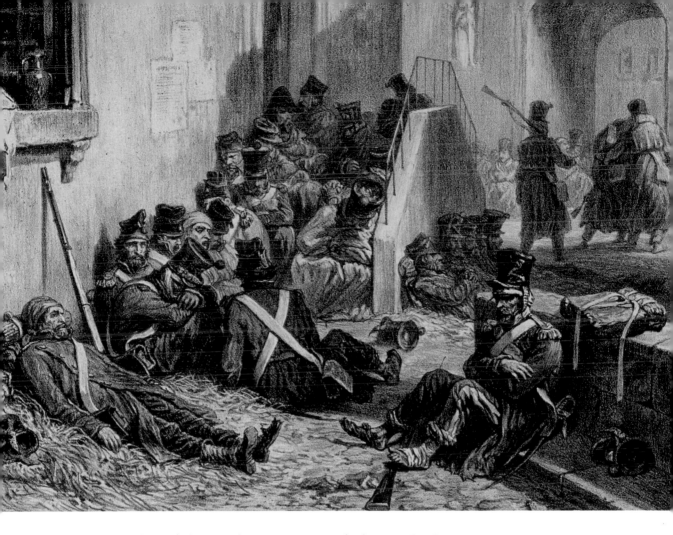

wretched, the Grande Armée began its long retreat west as the ferocious Russian winter began to close in.

It was a bedraggled mob who started out on the long cold trek back to France. The hospitals set up on the outward march were by now in a deplorable condition – crowded, filthy, smelly and filled with unwashed, starving, diseased, frostbitten and emaciated men. They could hardly handle any more sick and dying soldiers. Horse meat became the staple diet of desperate soldiers – they even gnawed at leather or drank their own urine, for want of victuals. Some simply froze to death. By mid-December, Napoleon had just 30,000 of his original 600,000-strong Grande Armée left alive – and only a thousand of these were ever again fit for duty. The majority of men in this catastrophic campaign had succumbed to typhus or extreme cold and hunger, and Napoleon's dream of a vast French empire extending through Russia to India had come to a staggering halt.

FAMINE FEVER
Over the next few years, carried by the louse-ridden remnants of the Grande Armée and the equally infested Russian cavalry who pursued them, typhus

An early 19th-century engraving shows soldiers lying in the street exhibiting the listless behaviour which accompanies typhus.

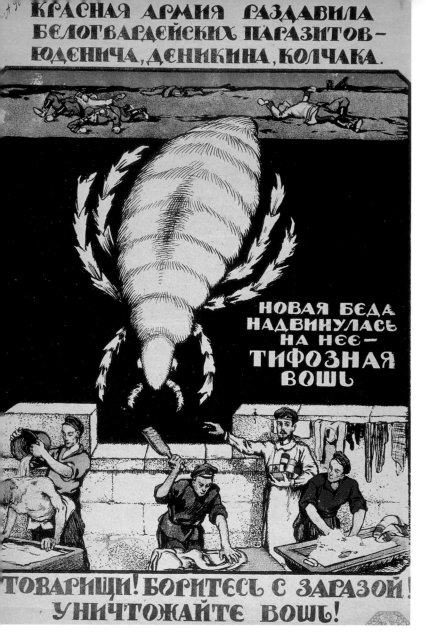

КРАСНАЯ АРМИЯ РАЗДАВИЛА
БЕЛОГВАРДЕЙСКИХ ПАРАЗИТОВ-
ЮДЕНИЧА, ДЕНИКИНА, КОЛЧАКА.

НОВАЯ БЕДА
НАДВИНУЛАСЬ
НА НЕЕ-
ТИФОЗНАЯ
ВОШЬ

ТОВАРИЩИ! БОРИТЕСЬ С ЗАРАЗОЙ!
УНИЧТОЖАЙТЕ ВОШЬ!

A communist propaganda poster, c.1921, exhorts Red soldiers to defeat a new enemy in the form of the typhus louse. Soldiers are seen washing themselves and their clothes vigorously.

spread far and wide across Europe. In 1815–19, the period immediately after the Napoleonic Wars, a combination of severe cold weather, widespread crop failure and the uprooting of starving peasants sparked another major epidemic in Europe, and many thousands perished.

Some decades later, Ireland was gripped by a terrible famine when a fungal blight destroyed the potato crop – the staple diet of the Irish peasantry. During the 'Great Hunger' of 1845–9 around a million people died – some from direct starvation but the overwhelming majority from famine-related diseases such as typhus, relapsing fever, scurvy and dysentery. Typhus was spread rapidly by bands of roving and ravenous beggars. Many of those still alive emigrated in desperation to England, Scotland, Canada and the United States, but great numbers fell sick in transit on what became known as the 'coffin ships'. The population of Ireland fell from possibly as many as 9 million to 6.5 million, and it was said that in some parts of the country the only living things left were the rats and dogs devouring the bodies of the dead. The 'Irish fever' spread to the urban slums of England, and in North America raged amongst the immigrant population but for some reason did not spread further.

THE BODY LOUSE REVEALED

The first breakthrough in the understanding of the epidemiology and ecology of typhus occurred in the United States. It had generally been assumed that typhus and typhoid were varieties of the same fever, until, in the winter of 1835–6 the physician William Wood Gerhard (1809–72) studied an outbreak of typhus amongst recent Irish immigrants living in a slum in Philadelphia. In 1829 the French physician Pierre Louis (1787–1872) had coined the word 'typhoid' (meaning 'like typhus'), and Gerhard, who had previously worked in both Britain and France, had developed a hunch while he was in Paris that typhoid (common in France) was different from typhus (common in England and Ireland). Other leading physicians contributed to the debate, and by the 1860s most agreed that typhus and typhoid were distinct entities. A key feature showed up at autopsies: typhoid victims had inflamed lesions in their small intestines, but these were absent from typhus victims (see pages 54–61).

It took another 70 years or so before the final clue as to the cause of typhus came to light. In 1909–10 Charles Nicolle (1866–1936), the French director of the Institut Pasteur in Tunis, North Africa, showed that it was the body louse – *Pediculus humanus corporis* – that was the main vector for the disease. He observed that patients who were stripped of their clothing, shaved and washed before entering the hospital in Tunis did not go on to infect others. Summing up his conclusions when he won the Nobel Prize in 1928, he recalled: *'It could only be the body louse. It was the louse'.*

Nicolle's findings were substantiated by two other scientists – the American pathologist Howard Taylor Ricketts (1871–1910) and the Polish zoologist Stanislas J.M. von Prowazek (1875–1915), both of whom died while investigating the cause of typhus. In 1916 the Brazilian scientist Henrique da Rocha Lima (1879–1956) named the causative agent *Rickettsia prowazekii* in honour of their discoveries. Since then a number of other so-called rickettsial diseases have been identified – the disease-causing agents are now thought to be types of bacteria, and are carried by lice, ticks, mites, fleas and other arthropods. Once the role of the body louse in the transmission of typhus was recognized, many of the patterns of past epidemics made sense: insanitary, crowded conditions, cold winters, thick layers of unwashed clothes, humans huddled together – all were ideal environments for the spread of typhus. The discovery of the role of the louse also provided a vital key to preventing the disease: delousing troops on active service.

AMERICAN LICE – RIFE BUT NICE?

A curiosity about the history of typhus is its relative absence from North America in the past even though it was a common disease in Central and South America. Certainly body lice were rife in the USA in the past but, at times when outbreaks of typhus might have been expected, they failed to materialize.

During the American Civil War of 1861–5, for example, one commentator described the Confederates in a Union prison camp:

'Prisoners are permitted to lounge about in their filth, with no other duty to perform seemingly than to amuse themselves by slaughtering the vermin crawling about their filthy persons.'

The conditions were perfect for an outbreak, but for some reason it just didn't happen. One historian has suggested that maybe American body lice were different from their European cousins and less likely to transmit typhus.

German soldiers on the Western Front removing lice from their clothes during the First World War. This basic hygiene measure became a regular, daily occurrence once the role of the lice in the transmission of disease was understood.

Two 'lousy' world wars
Typhus did, nonetheless, ravage Europe during the First and Second World Wars. In both conflicts it seemed to have a very marked predilection for the Eastern Front. In 1914 typhus (like the war) erupted in Serbia, and within the first six months over 150,000 people had died of the disease. Russia, too, was hit exceptionally hard, in spite of efforts to control the disease. Between 1917 and 1922 there were an estimated 25 to 30 million cases of typhus and 3 million deaths in eastern Europe and what, by the end of the period, had become the Soviet Union. This experience led the Soviet leader

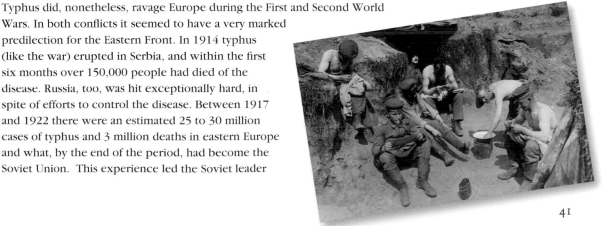

'Swords and lances, arrows, machine guns, and even high explosives have had far less power over the fates of nations than the typhus louse, the plague flea, and the yellow-fever mosquito.'

HANS ZINSSER, *RATS, LICE AND HISTORY* (1934)

Vladimir Ilyich Lenin (1870–1924) to declare: *'Either socialism will defeat the louse, or the louse will defeat socialism.'*

On the Western Front in the First World War strict measures were taken to prevent a catastrophic outbreak of typhus – and here an understanding of the vector and the mode of transmission certainly paid off. Mobile laboratories, laundries and delousing stations were set up, and soldiers and prisoners of war were bathed, disinfected and shaved. Bodies and clothing were deloused, a process involving steam treatment, fumigation and rubbing with anti-lice powders – getting rid of lice in the soldiers' underclothes became one of the daily rituals of life.

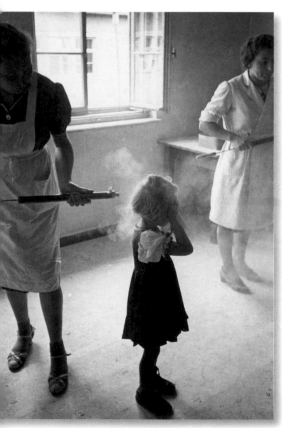

Fumigation with the insecticide DDT was a widely used measure for treating lice. Here a German child refugee is treated at a UNICEF camp in 1948.

Despite determined efforts, and almost no outbreaks of epidemic typhus on the Western Front, another louse-borne disease – which became known as 'trench fever' – tormented and incapacitated more than a million soldiers. 'Trench fever' was a mild infection also spread by the body louse. Although it did not cause huge fatalities, the irritation from the louse was an ever-present nuisance even with the delousing measures, and soldiers often tried to rid themselves of infestation by stubbing their burning cigarette ends on to the lice. Trench fever caused a greater loss of manpower during the war than did any other malady except influenza (see pages 172–183).

Between the First World War and the end of the Second World War there were two medical advances that became vital in preventing an escalation of typhus, especially amongst the Allied troops: a vaccine and an insecticide. In 1937 Herald R. Cox (1907–86) of the US Public Health Service produced a vaccine that, though not fully effective in preventing typhus, did at least reduce the virulence of the disease for those military personnel to whom it was administered in the last few years of the Second World War. Previous attempts to produce a vaccine had been based on grinding up the guts or faeces of infected lice. The 'Cox vaccine' – based on culturing *rickettsiae* in the yolks of hens' eggs – was the first effective and commercially viable vaccine for typhus.

Over the next few years the powerful insecticide DDT (dichloro-diphenyl-trichloroethane) was given its first airing. A typhus epidemic in recently liberated Naples, Italy, in the winter of 1943–4 was brought to a halt with the use of DDT. So effective was the new insecticide that long queues of people formed at disinfecting stations eager to be given a thorough delousing. DDT, which could be used as a powder, was administered through 'blowing machines'. No longer

NIT-PICKING

When most people think of lice today they think of head lice (*Pediculus humanus capitis*) and their tiny eggs, known as nits. Fortunately, head lice do not carry typhus or any other infectious disease. They are about 3 millimetres (0.12 in) long, grip tightly on to the hairs of the head and feed on human blood.

Head-lice infestations – so common today among younger schoolchildren – date back thousands of years, as the many ancient nit combs found by archaeologists attest. The Roman naturalist Pliny the Elder (AD 23–79), who died during the eruption of Vesuvius, suggested bathing in viper broth as a cure, while Montezuma (1466–1520), the Aztec emperor, paid people to pick nits off his subjects. He then had the nits dried and saved them in his treasury.

In the Middle Ages, etiquette lessons were given to young members of the nobility as to when and how to dispose of one's lice. It was very much frowned upon to scratch or attempt to remove one's lice while in company, except in the most intimate circles. Nicholas Culpeper (1616–54), the English herbalist, recommended tobacco juice to kill lice on children's heads.

Samuel Pepys (1633–1703) recorded in his diary on 23 January 1669:

> *When all comes to all she [Pepys's wife] finds that I am lousy having found in my head and body above twenty lice little and great, which I wonder at, being more than I have had I believe these twenty years.'*

Pepys changed his clothes and cut his hair short, *'so shall be rid of them'*. He also found nits in his newly purchased wig, which, he wrote, *'vexed me cruelly'.*

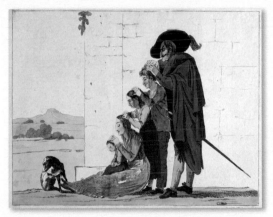

In former times, almost everyone needed to have their parasites removed – including small children. In this historical print, even the dog seems to be joining in the grooming session.

did soldiers have to undress and have their underwear deloused – the blowing machines could direct DDT straight to the lice and zap them on the spot.

Typhus did, however, continue to be a severe problem in the Nazi concentration camps, in spite of strict delousing measures for all POWs. The Jewish teenager Anne Frank (1929-45), who left a diary of her life and experiences, died in March 1945 in the Bergen-Belsen concentration camp, probably from a combination of typhus fever, hunger and maltreatment. Serious epidemics of typhus again struck the Eastern Front, while its relative, 'scrub typhus' or tsutsugamushi (a rickettsial disease spread by mites) caused many casualties in the Pacific theatre of war.

By the late 1940s broad-spectrum antibiotics were proving effective against the rickettsia that cause typhus. Globally typhus is now fairly rare, but there are pockets of the disease in some colder and more poverty-stricken areas of the Andes of South America, the Himalayas of Asia and parts of Africa.

CHOLERA is an extremely unpleasant and potentially fatal disease caused by the bacterium *Vibrio cholerae*. The symptoms are hideous: victims are convulsed with pain, and suffer violent vomiting and uncontrollable watery diarrhoea. Many, if their severe dehydration is not treated, turn blue and die within a short time.

In the 19th century, pandemics of cholera spread out from the Ganges Delta in the Indian subcontinent, killing millions of people around the world. In the latter part of that century, scientists were able to show that cholera is spread when food or water becomes contaminated with faecal matter containing cholera bacteria. Improvements in sanitation have made cholera uncommon in the Western world, but it still poses a threat to many people in parts of Asia, Africa and South America.

In October 1831 a local newspaper in the port of Sunderland in northeast England warned its readers of a dangerous new epidemic heading their way: Asiatic cholera. Its early symptoms, according to the *Sunderland Herald*, included:

> *'a sick stomach … vomiting or purging of a liquid like rice-water … the face becomes sharp and shrunken, the eyes sink and look wild, the lips, face and … whole surface of the body a leaden, blue, purple, [or] black.'*

The reporter noted that there was, as yet, no specific treatment for the disease, but reassured readers that:

> *'the greatest confidence may be expressed in the intelligence and enthusiasm of the doctors … who will surely find a method of cure.'*

Sunderland was hit by cholera in the following months. It went on to attack many other towns in the British Isles, killing over 5000 people in London alone in 1832. It was rife in Asia and Europe, and reached New York City, from where it spread across the whole American continent. This was Asiatic cholera's first visitation to the western hemisphere and, despite the Sunderland newspaper's optimism, there was no cure.

timeline

1st millennium BC Ancient Sanskrit, Chinese and Greek texts describe a cholera-like diarrhoeal disease.

AD 1543 Portuguese explorers report cholera in India.

c.1817–23 The first cholera pandemic: the disease spreads from its cradle in the Ganges-Brahmaputra Delta through Asia but does not reach Europe or the Americas.

c.1826–37 The second pandemic: the disease devastates Asia, North Africa and Europe, reaching England in 1831 and the Americas in 1832.

1842 In his 'Report of an Inquiry into the Sanitary Conditions of the Labouring Population of Great Britain', Edwin Chadwick (1800–90) recommends improvements in sewerage, water supply and drainage.

c.1846–63 The third pandemic: the disease again spreads from India across much of the globe. 1854 is one of the worst years on record.

1849 John Snow (1813–58) publishes On the Mode of Communication of Cholera, after 50,000 people in England die of the disease.

1851–2 The first International Sanitary Conference is held in Paris, with its principal focus on cholera. More such conferences follow.

44

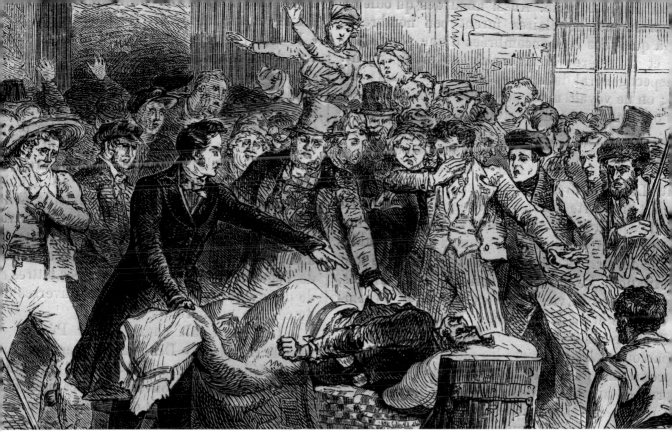

TRACKING CHOLERA PANDEMICS IN TIME AND SPACE

The word 'cholera' is derived from the Greek *khol* meaning 'bile', and *rhein*, 'to flow'. The word (or the fuller Latin term *cholera morbus*) had been used since ancient times to describe any sporadic diarrhoeal affliction. However, the devastating and unstoppable diarrhoea that characterized the Asiatic cholera was unlike anything that had been experienced before. Indeed, we now know that its watery contents contain bits of the body's gut as well as swarms of cholera bacteria, and it is rapid dehydration that leads to the shrunken features and the blueish tinge, accompanied by shock and, finally, death.

It is hard to say for sure whether the cholera pandemics that erupted and spread over the globe in the 19th century were different from earlier episodes of *cholera*

A depiction of the cholera epidemic of Paris, which reached the capital in the spring of 1832. The outbreak claimed the lives of 18,000 people in Paris and more than 100,000 in France as a whole.

1854 *John Snow has the handle of the Broad Street pump in London removed to prove that cholera is transmitted through drinking water that is contaminated with raw sewage.*

1854 *The Italian scientist Filippo Pacini (1812–83) is the first to observe the cholera bacillus; in 1879 he proposes intravenous injections of saline solution as a treatment. His ideas are overlooked.*

c.1865–75 *The fourth pandemic: perhaps the most widespread of them all, spreads from India to affect large parts of the world, including Europe, much of Africa, and the Americas.*

1881–96 *The fifth pandemic: the first in which cholera was identified with certainty as the true cause.*

1883–4 *The German bacteriologist Robert Koch (1843–1910)*

identifies in Egypt and India the cause of cholera – a comma-shaped bacterium known as Vibrio cholerae.

1885 *The Spanish physician Jaime Ferrán (1851–1929) tries out a vaccine against cholera,*

first testing it on himself and then inoculating 30,000 people.

1899–1923 *The sixth pandemic: cholera spreads from India across Asia and into eastern and southern Europe.*

It is especially severe in India – where nearly 1 million die in 1900 alone – and also in Russia during the First World War and the 1917 Revolution.

(continued ...)

'Sur ... We aint got no priviz, no dust bins, no drains, no water-splies, and no drain or suer in the hole place. The Suer Company, in Greek Street, Soho Square, all great, rich powerfool men take no notice watsomdever of our complaints. The Stenche of a Gulley-hole is disgustin. We all of us suffer, and numbers are ill, and if the Cholera comes Lord help us.'

AN APPEAL PRINTED IN *THE TIMES* OF LONDON IN 1849, AS CHOLERA SPREAD THROUGH ENGLAND

morbus. Contemporaries, and historians since, have generally agreed that the origin of the great pandemics of cholera lay in the populous Ganges–Brahmaputra Delta in India (where the disease had probably been endemic for centuries) - hence, the adoption in the West of the term 'Asiatic cholera'. The first pandemic (and there have been at least six more since) began to spread from its natural heartland in 1817 right across Asia. It did not, however, continue to move any further west, and by 1823 it had petered out: many mysteries still surround the sudden eruption and cessation of these pandemics.

It was the second and subsequent pandemics of the 19th century that engulfed nearly all the populated regions of the world. When in the 1830s the disease struck Moscow in Russia, Hamburg in Germany, Sunderland and London in England, Paris in France, Quebec in Canada and New York City in the USA, Asiatic cholera was well and truly on the world map. Carrying a mortality rate of at least 50 per cent, and conveyed unwittingly over land and sea by traders, soldiers, sailors, pilgrims, refugees and migrants, each pandemic (lasting from five to 30 years) followed a somewhat different trajectory. But all who found themselves in the path of the dreaded disease were terrified that they would be its next victim.

THE STENCH AND SQUALOR OF THE SLUMS

Cholera affected young and old, rich and poor, but its striking epidemiological characteristic in the 19th century was its devastating impact on centres of pilgrimage such as the Ganges and Mecca, and on the stinking slums of the rapidly expanding industrial towns of Europe and North America. The shock of the disease - its sudden onslaught and the haste with which death followed - was matched by its foul symptoms. Vomit and profuse diarrhoea produced a sickening and humiliating stench, and when cholera struck the burgeoning towns of Europe and the USA it added one more intolerable smell to the noxious vapours already

timeline

1905 *The Vibrio El Tor strain of cholera is isolated from the intestines of six Muslim pilgrims returning from Mecca and housed in the El Tor quarantine station on the Sinai Peninsula.*

1961–present *The seventh pandemic: the longest ever, and this time originating in Indonesia and largely featuring the El Tor strain. Cholera engulfs most of Asia, the Middle East,*

Russia and parts of southern Europe. It also spreads to West Africa and South America.

1970s *Scientists use oral rehydration therapy (ORT) to reduce cholera mortality in the refugee camps during and after the 1971 Indo–Pakistan War.*

1978 *The WHO creates the diarrhoeal disease control programme to popularize the use of ORT.*

1993 *Another new strain of cholera emerges in Asia, called V. cholerae O139 Bengal.*

2005 *Fifty-two countries report 131,943 cases and 2272 deaths from cholera. The real figure is likely to be higher, and cholera remains a serious disease in Asia, South America and Africa, and is*

particularly likely to flare up in times of war, famine and natural disaster. It has also been observed that the cholera organism can live outside the human body in aquatic environments.

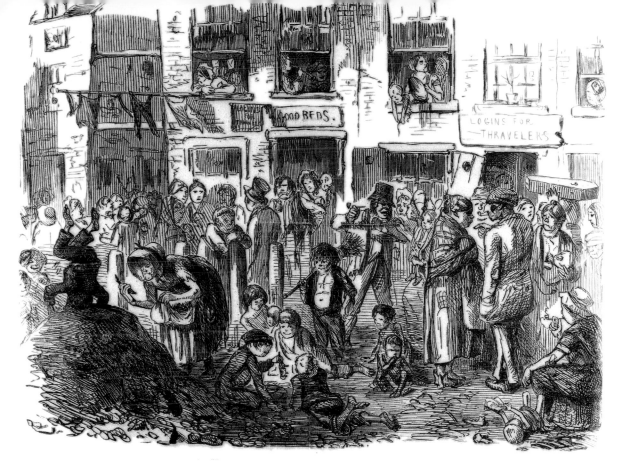

oozing from dung-fouled streets, festering tenements, unwashed bodies, belching factories, stinking slaughterhouses, putrid rivers, overflowing cesspools and open sewers that were so often features of everyday life.

The doctors who sought to understand and deal with cholera were totally confused as to how and why this 'new' disease was spreading. Furious debates ensued. The miasmatists (or anti-contagionists) were convinced that, like other epidemic fevers that afflicted the poor, cholera's root lay in the stench and squalor of the slums. Edwin Chadwick (1800–90), the English social reformer, wrote:

> 'All smell is, if it be intense, immediate, acute disease; and eventually we may say that, by depressing the system and rendering it susceptible to the action of other causes, all smell is disease.'

William Farr (1807–83), the English medical statistician, said that lethal miasmas were like a mad dog prowling forth from the city's cesspools and sewers. Chadwick, Farr and others in Europe and the USA, including Lemuel Shattuck (1793–1859) in Boston, amplified their arguments with 'sanitary' or 'effluvia' maps and vital statistics that showed a direct correlation between the filthiest, most overcrowded or poorest parts of the cities and the highest mortality rates. In Bethnal Green in London, the average age of death was 16 years in the mid-19th century. In the more 'salubrious' areas, it was 45 years. Infant mortality rates in the worst parts of London, Liverpool, Manchester, Paris, New York and elsewhere were

The Court of King Cholera as this 19th century engraving was entitled. The squalid, insanitary conditions that existed in parts of London and other places were a breeding ground for cholera. Words cannot adequately evoke the stenches that assaulted the noses of our 19th-century forebears.

THE GONG HOUSE

A single privy – variously known as the gong house, bog house, place of easement or temple of convenience – was often shared by as many as 40 people in Victorian cities. Night-soil men (known in Medieval times as gong-fermors) collected the contents of privies from some houses and dung heaps – usually at night. Human excrement was sold and recycled as fertilizer for farmers' fields. Privies in poor districts were rarely emptied, however, and invariably seeped into underground pits or cesspools, from where they eventually contaminated water supplies.

In the early 19th century in London, water closets began to be installed in the houses of the rich. Unfortunately, without a functioning sewerage system to connect to the WCs, their contents often made their way back into the drinking

A man in Highland dress, *seated on a latrine with his legs thrust down the holes in the board, relieves himself in a 'bog house' in this engraving from 1745.*

water supplies, making matters even worse.

Thomas Crapper and others later designed new toilets with fancy names such as 'Niagara Falls', 'Waterloo', 'Deluge', 'Rapido' and 'Tornado'. The first paying public toilet in Victorian London – which cost a penny – was at the Great Exhibition in 1851. Toilet paper was invented in the 1860s.

The pure gatherers

One of the worst jobs in Victorian England was that of 'pure-finder'. 'Pure', or decomposing dog dung, was used in 'purifying' or softening leather, and men and women gathered it as a final resort rather than going into the workhouse. A bucketful of 'pure' bought a day's lodging and food.

shocking – as many as one in three or four babies dying before their first birthday. Life expectancy was very low – little more than 20 to 30 years among the working classes. Cleaning up the poverty and squalor, washing the 'Great Unwashed' and sorting out the stenches and foul sanitation of urban and industrial areas were high on the agenda of the 19th-century miasmatists and social reformers.

Their opponents – the contagionists – observed the path of Asiatic cholera as it tracked its way from east to west, from ports to inland towns, via ships, river boats, canals, wagon trains and (later) railways. The contagionists believed that the disease must be transmitted by some poison passed from person to person. The only way to prevent the disease spreading, they argued, was through strict quarantine measures. However, this posed a threat to the commercial activities of the industrializing nations, and international sanitary conferences were set up to debate the question.

There were others who saw cholera as just one aspect of the moral and physical degradation of the working classes. Wherever there was rottenness, drunkenness and uncleanliness, there poverty and disease struck most viciously and – they argued – deservedly. Countering such arguments, humanitarians tried to convince their contemporaries that the poor were diseased not because of their immoral state of mind or body but because they were living and working in conditions of appalling filth, hunger and wretchedness. Cholera, with its spectacularly ghastly effects, was evidence not of moral justice but of human injustice.

In his 1845 book, *The Condition of the Working Classes in England*, Friedrich Engels (1820–95), the German political theorist, described a typical urban scene in Manchester. Everywhere he went he met *'pale, lank, narrow-chested, hollow-eyed ghosts'* cooped up in houses that were mere *'kennels to sleep and die in'*:

> *'Passing along a rough bank, among stakes and washing lines, one penetrates into the chaos of small one-storied, one-roomed huts, in most of which there is no artificial floor; kitchen, living and sleeping-room all in one ...'*

Engels went on to note the piles of residue and offal, and the constant disgusting stench. Others depicted the miserable conditions of the hordes of people who were crammed into basement rooms through which the effluent from outside privies oozed. Such conditions aroused horror and indignation in Engels and other sympathetic observers.

The diseases that afflicted the poor in such slums were numerous – typhus, typhoid, smallpox, tuberculosis, measles, dysentery, infantile diarrhoea, diphtheria, scarlet fever, rickets, whooping cough, bronchitis and pneumonia, to name a few. Many people also met their end in accidents, especially in factories and mines. Some were poisoned by industrial toxins and adulterated food, or exhausted by hard labour and hunger. But it was cholera, with its sudden and dramatic impact, that prompted the greatest concern and confusion. What was its cause and how was it transmitted? As the debates rumbled on, one man found the answer – or thought he had.

TURNING OFF THE CHOLERA

In 1849 the satirical magazine *Punch* published a cartoon entitled 'Mistaking cause for effect', in which a young boy turns to his little friend and comments: 'I say, Tommy, I'm blow'd if there isn't a man a turning on the cholera'. In 1854 a British doctor, John Snow (1813–58), attempted to 'turn off the cholera' by requesting the removal of the handle of the Broad Street pump in Soho, London.

Snow had witnessed the horrors of the second cholera pandemic in a village near Newcastle-upon-Tyne in northeast England late in 1831, shortly after its initial outbreak in Sunderland. He later practised in the bustling but squalid Golden Square area of Soho, where he became convinced that cholera might be caused by

A satirical cartoon entitled 'Mistaking cause for effect', from an 1849 edition of Punch. The original caption below the illustration read: 'I say, Tommy, I'm blow'd if there isn't a man a turning on the cholera'. Many towns in England at the time did not provide piped water to houses. People queued, drew and paid for their water from street stand-pipes, and cholera-contaminated water from such pipes killed many.

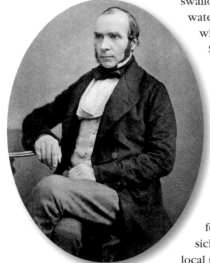

swallowing '*some as-yet-unidentified*' infective particle in sewage-contaminated water. The River Thames was, as Snow observed, in effect an open sewer into which excrement was discharged. In 1849, with cholera once more raging, Snow published the first account of his 'waterborne' theory. Cholera continued to strike, killing perhaps some 50,000 in Britain between 1848 and 1850, and recurring with a vengeance in the following decade. The year 1854 was one of the worst years in the global history of cholera.

In the oppressively hot August of that year, the baby daughter of Thomas and Sarah Lewis of 40 Broad Street, Soho, London, fell ill with vomiting and green watery stools that emitted 'a pungent smell'. Sarah, desperately trying to cope with her baby's soiled nappies, washed them in a bucket and threw some of the water into a cesspool in the basement at the front of their house. The following day their upstairs neighbours fell ill, and a few days later whole families in the surrounding area began to sicken – often dying together in their dark, squalid rooms. Within ten days, 500 local residents were dead – 10 per cent of the area's population.

John Snow, photographed in 1856. This young, teetotal and vegetarian doctor played a major role in the discovery of the waterborne nature of cholera after observing fatalities around the Broad Street pump in Soho, London, in 1854.

John Snow inspected with meticulous detail the drinking habits of the victims of this outbreak. He noted that most of those who caught cholera were drawing their drinking water from the Broad Street pump – which was right outside No. 40 Broad Street. In a nearby workhouse and brewery, both of which had their own private water supplies, there were almost no casualties. On 7 September 1854, two weeks after the local outbreak began, Snow persuaded the authorities to remove the Broad Street pump's handle. Cholera abated.

Where the miasmatists had been convinced that all smell was disease, Snow was now able to pinpoint, in the case of cholera, one particularly noxious source of disease – foul water, not foul air. And while the contagionists had provided a strong case for the infectious nature of the disease, Snow showed that cholera (which affected the intestines rather than the lungs) was not directly transmitted through airborne particles, but by drinking contaminated water. The cycle of cholera was clear, but more subtle than hitherto suspected: what came out one end was flushed into the cesspools or rivers, and the infective particles then made their way back into the pumped drinking water and the gastro-intestinal tracts of its victims.

When John Snow showed Reverend Henry Whitehead (1826–96) his now famous 'ghost' map of the cholera deaths and the location of the water pumps in the Golden Square area, drawn up in the autumn of 1854, he too became convinced by Snow's theory. Whitehead, a young curate who had tirelessly worked to mitigate the worst effects of the outbreak, conducted his own bit of detective work and discovered in the death registers the tragic record of the little baby, who, he subsequently concluded, was the first case and 'cause' of the transmission of cholera. The cause of her death was given as follows:

> *'At 40 Broad Street, 2 September, a daughter, aged five months, exhaustion after an attack of diarrhoea four days previous to death.'*

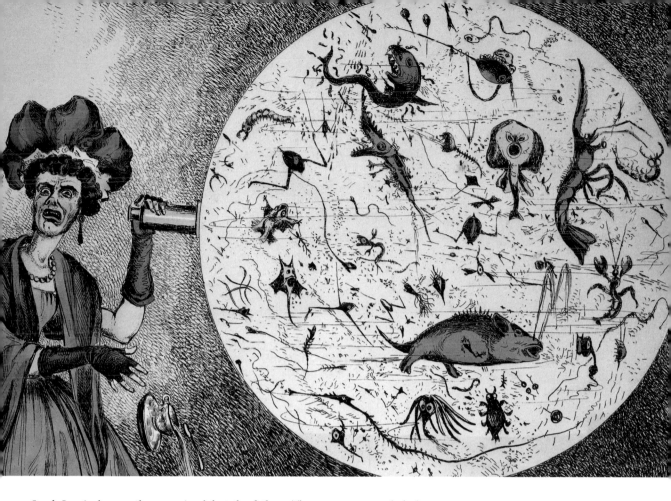

Sarah Lewis, her mother, survived, but the father, Thomas, contracted cholera and died two weeks later. Sarah continued to throw contaminated excreta – this time her husband's – into the cesspool but, fortunately for others, the Broad Street pump had been temporarily turned off.

Today, next to the site of the pump in Broad Street (now Broadwick Street), is the John Snow Pub, which commemorates the significance of Snow's discovery.

DYING FOR A DRINK

What in retrospect could have been a 'magic' medical breakthrough was not immediately appreciated, however. Indeed, some (including Snow) thought that by the time the Broad Street pump had been removed, cholera in Soho was already on the wane. Many others expressed scepticism – wasn't this just a coincidence? But, although Snow's clever medical detective work did not in itself lead to a widespread acceptance of his waterborne theory, there were other forces at work that continued to convince 'sanitarians' in many parts of the Western world that the populous towns, as well as the countryside, needed a big clean-up. The 'Great Stink' of London in the summer of 1858, when the House of Commons had to break off its proceedings and soak the curtains in chloride of lime to cover up the stench, showed that the time was ripe for drastic sanitary reform.

Although darkly humorous, this satirical engraving left no one in doubt about what was generally thought to be present in the foul, sewage-laden water of the 19th-century River Thames. The original caption read: 'Microcosm dedicated to the London Water Companies; brought forth all monstrous, all prodigious things, hydras and gorgons, and chimeras dire. A Monster Soup, commonly called Thames Water, being a correct representation of that precious stuff doled out to us!'

It was not until the 1880s that the critical piece of the cholera puzzle, which had eluded Snow and others, was finally fitted into place. The fifth cholera pandemic of 1881–96 spread westward from the Indian subcontinent just like the previous ones had done and, although it did not reach the shores of Great Britain, its severity elsewhere prompted scientists to investigate its cause. German and French bacteriologists had already put forward the so-called 'germ theory' of disease in the 1860s and 1870s, but the 'germ' causing cholera still remained a mystery. This was despite the fact that in 1854 an Italian, Filippo Pacini (1812–83), had observed the microbes that cause cholera in the excreta and intestinal contents of victims. Unfortunately, his valuable work had been overlooked by other scientists.

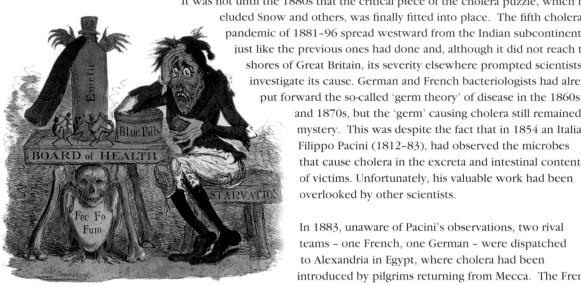

Entitled 'A cholera patient', this early 19th-century etching shows a cholera victim experimenting with remedies. Cholera became one of the most feared and terrible scourges to emerge in western Europe after bubonic plague.

In 1883, unaware of Pacini's observations, two rival teams – one French, one German – were dispatched to Alexandria in Egypt, where cholera had been introduced by pilgrims returning from Mecca. The French 'Pasteurians' took cholera-contaminated waste and attempted to reproduce the disease in animals. As cholera has no mammalian host outside the human body, their efforts failed, and when one of their team succumbed to cholera they returned to France. The German team, headed by the famous bacteriologist Robert Koch (1843–1910), proceeded down a different route. They performed autopsies on ten cholera victims and there, in the intestines, they identified under the microscope a short, curved, 'comma-shaped' bacillus.

Koch confirmed his findings the following year in the teeming, cholera-infested suburbs of Calcutta, India, where he found the same cholera bacillus (*Vibrio cholerae*) in both the local drinking water and the stools of victims. John Snow had been right – although it is claimed that Koch did not know of his work any more than he was aware of Pacini's. Cholera was, indeed, a waterborne disease, communicated mainly by polluted water and transmitted through the faecal-oral route. But now scientists could 'see' the swarms of bacteria that invaded and multiplied in the guts and gushed out with the watery diarrhoea of its victims. A vaccine, albeit only partially effective against cholera, was developed in the late 19th century. More significantly, Koch's confirmation of the mode of communication of cholera gave a belated and much needed impetus to the authorities to put in place measures for disease prevention and control.

'We prefer to take our chances with cholera and the rest than to be bullied into health.'

THE TIMES OF LONDON (1854), IN RESPONSE TO EDWIN CHADWICK'S PROPOSAL TO PUMP CLEAN WATER FROM SURREY INTO CENTRAL LONDON

EFFLUENCE AND AFFLUENCE

Many people, when asked to name the greatest medical breakthroughs of the past, think of such discoveries as the germ theory, anaesthesia, penicillin or vaccination. But in a recent UK poll of doctors and the public, it was in fact sanitation that topped the list of the greatest 15 medical milestones since the

1840s. Turning on the cholera had been easy. Turning it off was more problematic, but improvements in sanitation over the course of the second half of the 19th century and the 20th century in the industrialized world eventually achieved radical gains for the lot of the poor, as well as the rich. In other parts of the globe, the story has been very different. Beginning in the 1960s, a seventh pandemic of cholera (of a new strain known as El Tor) erupted, this time in Indonesia, and spread to many parts of Asia, Africa and South America. Easily and rapidly conveyed by air, land and sea, cholera has taken a huge toll on people living in squalid slums with little access to safe water, and on those forced into overcrowded and foetid refugee camps during natural or man-made crises.

A SIMPLE SOLUTION?

Improvements in sanitation and the provision of safe water are still desperately needed in much of the developing world. There is now, however, one cheap and simple method of treating those who are infected with cholera: oral rehydration therapy (ORT). Originally suggested in the early 19th century and used intravenously from the early 20th century, a simple solution of clean water, salt and sugar – promoted in the 1970s as an oral therapy – can drastically reduce the mortality rate of cholera, from 50–60 per cent in untreated cases to as little as 1 per cent for those given ORT. The cholera bacteria produce and secrete toxins that trick the cells of the intestines into expelling prodigious quantities of water. Dehydration and the resulting loss of essential water and salts lead to rapid death. Antibiotics can help reduce the numbers of *Vibrio cholerae* in the intestines and shorten the period of communicability, but ORT, by replacing the lost fluid and salts, can change cholera from a life-threatening condition to a disease that can be quickly treated at home.

ORT is also invaluable for those dehydrated by other diarrhoeal diseases that afflict many parts of the world. Diarrhoeal and faecal–orally transmitted diseases together account for millions of deaths in the world today. In the 1980s nearly 5 million children under the age of five died each year from diarrhoea. By the 21st century diarrhoea as a cause of death in young children had fallen from 33 per cent of deaths to 18 per cent, and it is estimated that some 50 million lives have been saved over the past 25 years thanks to ORT.

Today, the greatest challenge is how to reach the poorest sections of the population with this life-saving intervention and avoid the 2 million or so preventable deaths from cholera and diarrhoeal diseases every year. 'Sanitation and health for all' remains an ultimate goal for the 21st century.

A COCKTAIL OF CHOLERA

One of Robert Koch's sceptical colleagues, the Munich hygienist Dr Max von Pettenkofer (1818–1901), decided to test Koch's theory that cholera was caused by a germ. He asked Koch to send him his cholera vibrios and put them to the test:

'Herr Doctor Pettenkofer presents his compliments to Herr Doctor Professor Koch and thanks him for the flask containing the so-called cholera vibrios ... Herr Doctor Pettenkofer has now drunk the entire contents and is happy to inform Herr Doctor Professor Koch that he remains in his usual good health.'

Remarkably, Pettenkofer survived his cocktail, which contained billions of cholera germs – enough to infect a whole army. He may have been one of the lucky ones to survive this deadly disease, perhaps he had an excess of 'bile' (stomach acid) which can kill the germs before they do their damage.

TYPHOID fever is one of those unpleasant diseases

that are spread when food or water becomes contaminated with human faeces – a mode of transmission known as the faecal–oral route. The causative agent is a bacterium, *Salmonella typhi*, and this can spread rapidly in areas of poor sanitation and inadequate hygiene. Typhoid causes a range of symptoms, including abdominal pain, blinding headache, a rash and a high fever. If left untreated, it can be fatal in about 10 to 20 per cent of cases. The disease has undoubtedly been around for centuries, but looking back it is difficult to differentiate typhoid fever from many other 'fevers' of the past. Improvements in public health, water supply and food hygiene have helped reduce its incidence in the industrialized world. Today, there are also antibiotics and vaccines for typhoid but, in some parts of the world, it continues to claim many lives, including those of a million or so children every year.

In London during the long, hot summer of 1858 the stench of untreated sewage floating in the River Thames was so horrendous that it was becoming almost impossible for members of the House of Commons to conduct their business. The windows were draped with curtains soaked in chloride of lime. But even that was not enough. The smell was sickening. Politicians choked and retched and threatened to leave London. It was, moreover, generally believed that the very smell itself was the cause of the deadly fevers that continually plagued the city. This 'Great Stink' would, it was feared, lead to further outbreaks of pestilence. One writer at the time of the Great Stink remarked:

> 'Stench so foul, we may well believe, had never before ascended to pollute this lower air. Never before, at least, had a stink risen to the height of an historic event.'

Queen Victoria (1819-1901) was on the throne - in the 21st year of her reign and deeply in love with her husband, Prince Albert (1819-61). There had, a few years earlier, been a fever scare at their royal castle at Windsor - but it had come to nothing. Britain was moving into the new age of flush toilets and industrial innovation. In 1851 Prince Albert had masterminded the Great Exhibition at

timeline

1829 *The French physician Pierre Louis (1787–1872) coins the term 'typhoid' (meaning 'like typhus'). Scientists begin to draw a distinction between typhoid and typhus.*

1858 *The Great Stink of London raises fears of an outbreak of fever.*

1860s *By the 1860s, most scientists and physicians agree that typhus and typhoid are distinct entities.*

1861 *Prince Albert dies of a 'bowel fever' – possibly typhoid.*

1870s *Scientists show that food, water and certain articles such as handkerchiefs and towels convey the typhoid infection.*

1870s onwards *Public-health measures in Europe and the USA eventually lead to improvements in sanitary practices and water supply.*

1884 *Scientists including Georg Gaffky (1850–1918) isolate and culture the typhoid bacillus.*

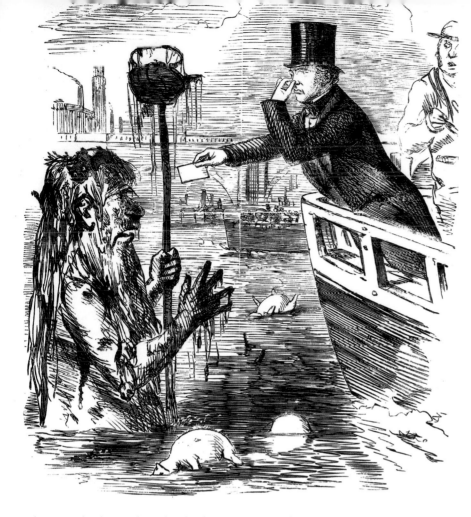

the Crystal Palace, where for the first time visitors had enjoyed an opportunity to 'spend a penny' in one of the latest attractions of the Industrial Revolution – the paying public toilet. Back home, Prince Albert had tried to sort out 53 overflowing cesspools at Windsor Castle, but whenever the Thames rose and saturated the grounds with raw royal sewage, the royal gardeners had simply raked up the filth and shovelled it back into the river.

Three years after the Great Stink, Prince Albert was fighting for his life. He was running a high fever and was violently sick, while on his torso there appeared

1896 *The diagnostic Widal test is introduced.*

1898 *Development of a typhoid vaccine gets under way.*

1906 *The case of Mary Mallon ('Typhoid Mary') as a healthy carrier of typhoid begins.*

1914–18 *Mandatory typhoid vaccination introduced for*

British troops in the First World War. When the USA joins the war in 1917, American troops are also vaccinated.

1933 *The bacterial agent of typhoid is named as Salmonella typhi, joining a large family of bacilli named after Daniel Elmer Salmon (1850–1914).*

1948 *Introduction of chloramphenicol, leading to a significant reduction in mortality for typhoid patients.*

1964 *Five hundred cases of typhoid fever in Aberdeen, Scotland, are traced to tins of corned beef imported from Argentina. After processing under sterile conditions,*

the tins had been cooled in a sewage-laden river where microscopic cracks in the seams of the cans permitted contamination.

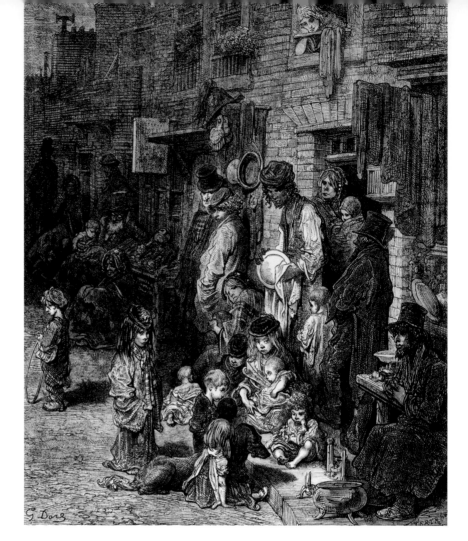

The overcrowded and squalid conditions that once prevailed in many places – such as here at Whitechapel in the East End of London in 1872 – were a breeding ground for all manner of contagious diseases, such as typhoid. The infectious agent for typhoid, the bacillus *Salmonella typhi*, is named after Daniel Elmer Salmon (1850–1914) – not the fish of the same name.

a few rose-coloured spots. The royal physicians, Sir James Clark (1788–1870) and Sir William Jenner (1815–98), were in constant attendance. They diagnosed a 'bowel fever' (probably typhoid), but they could do little for him. On 14 December 1861, following a crisis the day before, Prince Albert died, aged only 42. Queen Victoria was inconsolable, and dressed in black for the rest of her long life. To the public she became the 'Widow of Windsor'.

FOUL AND FATAL FEVERS

London in the middle of the 19th century was not so different – in terms of its poor sanitation – from other major European and American cities of the period. It was also not so very different in this respect from many of today's rapidly expanding cities in Asia, South America and Africa. In London the Great Stink alerted physicians and the government to the appalling state of squalor and sanitation in both the towns and the countryside. Fevers, it seemed, accounted for a huge proportion of all deaths – especially amongst the poor. But, as Prince Albert's death showed, fevers could attack anyone. So what caused these fevers, and were they all from the same source?

There were many febrile diseases at the time. Some, like smallpox (see pages 128–39) and yellow fever (see pages 146–51), were reasonably well recognized and defined (if not understood), but many others were lumped together or described by their feverish symptoms and fatal effects rather than by their causative agents. For many physicians the overpowering stench of their environs suggested that the real cause of most fevers must lie in the noxious vapours or 'miasmas' emitted by the stinking ordure, stagnant marshes, overflowing cesspools, raw sewage and foul industrial waste that contaminated the fields, streets and water of both towns and countryside. *'All smell is disease'*, claimed Edwin Chadwick (1800–90), the pioneering English campaigner for improvements in sanitary conditions. 'Effluvia' that arose from the sick and poisoned the air were also blamed for the contagions.

> '**To get into them [the worst slums in London]** you have to penetrate courts reeking with poisonous and malodorous gases arising from accumulations of sewage and refuse scattered in all directions and often flowing beneath your feet … you have to grope your way along dark and filthy passages swarming with vermin … '
>
> ANDREW MEARN, *THE BITTER CRY OF OUTCAST LONDON* (1883)

The 'miasmatic theory' of disease was so in vogue with many scientists throughout much of the 18th and early 19th centuries that the term 'mal'aria' (from the Italian *mala aria*, 'bad air') began to be used as a catch-all description of the cause of disease. In 1827 John MacCulloch (1773–1835) wrote an influential book entitled *Malaria: An essay on the production and propagation of this poison and on the nature and localities of the places by which it is produced*. The book is not simply a description of the mosquito-borne disease we now call malaria. In it MacCulloch, like others of his time, sets out to show that any number of diseases – in all sorts of 'poisonous' localities – are caused by 'mal'aria', or foul air.

Two diseases that became especially muddled and mired in this 'miasmic mess' were typhoid and typhus – both clearly associated with filth, poverty, poor sanitation and, above all, poisonous stenches.

TYPHOID – LIKE TYPHUS?

In 1829 the French physician Pierre Louis (1787–1872) coined the term 'typhoid' – meaning 'like typhus' (from the Greek *eidos*, 'like'). The disease Louis called typhoid was common in Paris, and appeared to some scientists to be different from typhus, which was especially common in England and Ireland. Louis did not draw any conclusions about the real difference between typhoid and typhus. (To make matters even more confusing, 'paratyphoid' was identified in 1902 as a separate but milder disease that was 'like typhoid'.)

The last moments of Prince Albert. He is thought by most medical historians to have died from typhoid fever. Some, however, have challenged this theory, suggesting instead that Albert died either from Crohn's disease or cancer of the stomach. The debate highlights one of the difficulties of making retrospective diagnoses.

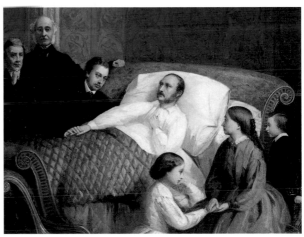

It took another 50 or more years before the real culprits were tracked down and a distinction between typhoid and typhus was conclusively drawn on scientific grounds. Three Williams - the American physician William Wood Gerhard (1809-72), the British royal physician William Jenner (1815-98), who attended Prince Albert and who himself contracted both typhoid and typhus, and the British epidemiologist William Budd (1811-80) - all played a crucial role in coming up with an answer to the puzzle.

William Budd, in particular, was intrigued by the Great Stink of 1858 and the dire predictions that the overpowering stench would lead to a huge rise in mortality. But when in 1873 he examined the reports for sickness and death in the years 1858-9 he noted:

> *'Strange to relate, the results showed, not only a death-rate below the average, but ... a remarkable diminution in the prevalence of fever, diarrhoea, and the other forms of the disease commonly ascribed to putrid exhalations.'*

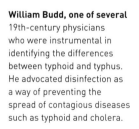

Budd - like John Snow in his investigations of cholera in London (see pages 44-53) - had begun to suspect that it was not the smells that caused disease, but something in contaminated water. He was finally proved right in the early 1880s when the typhoid bacillus was identified and cultured by a group of German scientists. This was one of the first discoveries of a bacterial agent as a cause of disease. It took a while longer for the cause of typhus (transmitted by the body louse) to be elucidated (see pages 36-43).

William Budd, one of several 19th-century physicians who were instrumental in identifying the differences between typhoid and typhus. He advocated disinfection as a way of preventing the spread of contagious diseases such as typhoid and cholera.

Towards the end of the 19th century the germ theory of disease - first put forward by Louis Pasteur (1822-95) in the middle of the century - was becoming more widely accepted, although even in the 1890s Charles Creighton (1847-1927), in his two-volume *History of Epidemics in Britain* (1891-4), still adhered to the miasmatic theory of disease. But by 1900 over 20 micro-organisms had been identified as the cause of specific diseases, and the germ theory had become firmly established. Typhoid had its own distinct identity and also a diagnostic test - the Widal test, developed by Fernard Widal (1862-1929) in 1896. This was too late to say for sure whether Prince Albert had died from typhoid, but in time to sort out a new puzzle - the case of 'Typhoid Mary' (see box, right).

A HUMAN RESERVOIR AND THE HEALTHY CARRIER

In the early 20th century it was recognized that typhoid is transmitted by the faecal-oral route: the bacterium responsible can move from the gut of an infected individual into the faeces or urine, which can then contaminate water and food and so enter the mouth of the next victim. In principle, the typhoid cycle is one of the simplest. There is no other reservoir except for humans, and breaking the cycle should be possible by strict hygiene - for example, washing hands before handling food, providing pure water supplies, keeping faecal-feeding flies away from food, and ensuring that what comes out of humans does not go back in through the drinking water.

THE TALE OF TYPHOID MARY

'The Most Harmless and yet Most Dangerous Woman in America'
HEADLINE FROM AN AMERICAN MAGAZINE, 1909

In the summer of 1906 Henry Warren, a New York banker, was enjoying a vacation with his family in Oyster Bay, Long Island. They felt especially fortunate to have as their cook a young Irishwoman, Mary Mallon (c. 1869–1938). Mary Mallon, a large, somewhat uncommunicative person, could produce dishes to die for. Her 'peaches on ice' were a particular speciality. But something that summer prompted Mary to move on and find employment elsewhere.

Then, for the Warren family, disaster struck. Within a few weeks of Mary's departure, six of the 11 members of the household came down with typhoid. It was a terrible shock – surely this was an affliction of the filthy slums, not the clean summer residences of the rich? Warren called in the New York sanitary engineer George Soper (1870–1948) to investigate.

As chance would have it, Soper had read Koch's paper on healthy carriers of typhoid fever (see page 60). Once he had ruled out various other possibilities, he began to suspect the Warrens' former cook. Soper tracked her down to New York. He also looked into her employment record: she was esteemed as an excellent cook – but wherever she had been, cases of typhoid – including some deaths – had followed. He decided it was time to check her out:

'I was as diplomatic as possible, but I had to say I suspected her of making people sick and that I wanted specimens of her urine, faeces and blood. It did not take Mary long to react to this suggestion. She seized a carving fork and advanced in my direction. I passed rapidly down the long narrow hall, through the tall iron gate, out through the area and so to the sidewalk. I felt rather lucky to escape.'

Soper's next attempt was met by *'a volley of imprecations from the head of the stairs'*. He called in reinforcements – the public-health inspector Dr S. Josephine Baker (1873–1945) and five New York policemen. But Mary Mallon had disappeared.

After a three-hour search, she was discovered in an outdoor closet, and was dragged out kicking and cursing. Her stools proved positive – they were teeming with typhoid bacilli. She was, as Soper suspected, a healthy carrier of typhoid.

Mary Mallon spent the next three years of her life at the Riverside Hospital, an isolation hospital on North Brother Island in New York's East River. In 1910, after a public outcry, she was released – on condition that she had her gall bladder removed (*Salmonella typhi* appears to concentrate in the gall bladder) or stopped working as a cook. She did neither, and then the health authorities lost track of her.

In 1915 an outbreak of typhoid erupted in the Sloane Maternity Hospital in Manhattan. Investigations revealed that the hospital's cook, Mrs Brown, was in fact none other than 'Typhoid Mary'. She was sent once more to North Brother Island, and here she spent the rest of her life in the company of her dog until her death in 1938.

But there was one more intriguing mystery about the infectious nature of typhoid. In 1873 William Budd had already made an important observation when he noted:

The precise date at which the fever patient ceases to give fever to others is not easy to define. But I have seen so many in which fever had broken out in a family living in a previously healthy neighbourhood soon after the arrival of a convalescent, that I am quite sure that patients so

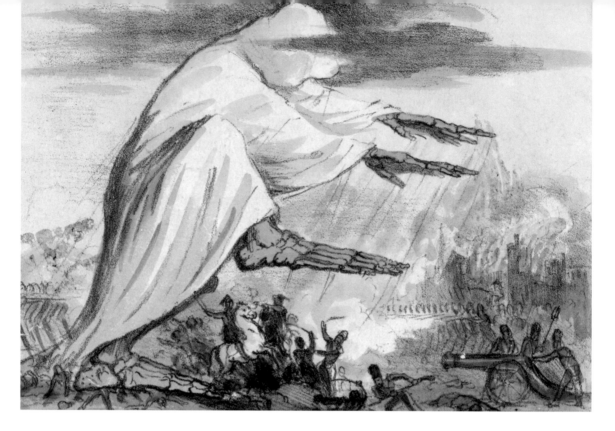

far recovered cannot always be safely allowed to mix with others without precaution.'

In 1902 the German bacteriologist Robert Koch (1843–1910) also proposed that convalescing patients could still shed the bacterium in their faeces and so act as a source of infection even after they had recovered from the disease. In an era when there was no treatment, the key question was how long such survivors could continue to be a source of infection.

The answer – possibly a lifetime – came with the famous investigation and incarceration in New York in the early decades of the 20th century of the Irish cook Mary Mallon – known to posterity as 'Typhoid Mary' (see The Tale of Typhoid Mary, page 59). Wherever Mary went typhoid was sure to follow. The story of Mary Mallon showed that in a small number of cases – perhaps 2 or 3 per cent of those who contract typhoid and then fully recover – subjects can remain carriers of a potentially life-threatening disease for the rest of their lives.

Sanitation and vaccination

The horrors of the so-called 'filth' diseases of the 19th century – such as typhoid, dysentery, typhus and cholera – eventually led to huge campaigns to clean up the deplorable state of many cities. In Europe there were a number of public-health acts and a massive drive to separate water contaminated with sewage from drinking water. The USA followed suit. Even seemingly small and simple measures – hand washing, boiling drinking water, protecting food from flies, improved handling of food and milk, the provision of dustbins with lids – may well have had a substantial impact. In the industrial nations typhoid declined significantly in the early 20th century.

However, the disease remained a serious threat in times of war. Troops in the Second Boer War (1899–1901) in South Africa were seriously affected by typhoid. In the Spanish–American War of 1898 there were over 20,000 cases of typhoid and 1500 deaths among a total of 100,000 US troops. Walter Reed (1851–1902) – head of the army's typhoid commission – inspected army camps in the USA where typhoid was rampant, and found the state of sanitation to be appalling. He also demonstrated the role that flies could play in moving improperly treated waste matter to the mess tents. To make his point, he sprinkled lime into the filthy latrines, then watched as flies trailed their lime-covered feet over the men's food.

In the late 19th and early 20th centuries, a number of scientists began to work on the possibility of developing a vaccine for typhoid. By the time of the First World War there was a vaccine available, and both the American and British commands ordered mandatory typhoid immunization as well as better military sanitation – measures that may well have prevented many cases of typhoid in the trenches. Post-revolutionary Russia, however, was racked by serious outbreaks of typhoid in the 1920s.

A typhoid vaccine was also used extensively during the Second World War, and with the introduction in 1948 of an effective drug – chloramphenicol – there was for the first time a treatment for typhoid, although by this time the disease was already on its way out in some parts of the world.

TYPHOID TODAY

There have been a small number of typhoid outbreaks in Europe and the USA in the last few decades (including an alarming epidemic in Aberdeen, Scotland, in the early summer of 1964 – attributed to cans of corned beef imported from Argentina). But for the most part typhoid is a disease of the past in the developed world. It does, however, remain a huge problem in the poorer countries, and is endemic through most of Central and South America, as well as much of Africa and Asia. Worldwide, the annual incidence of cases is estimated at about 17 million, with approximately 600,000 deaths a year.

Although there are drugs and improved vaccines, one particularly worrying development is that typhoid strains are becoming resistant to some of the key antibiotics in several areas of the world. Improvements in sanitation and public health, which have proved so effective in eliminating the disease from most developed countries in the past century, are urgently needed to prevent the incidence of typhoid and many other water- and food-borne diseases in the developing world, where supplies of clean water and effective sewerage are by no means the norm. As the African proverb has it, *Filthy water cannot be washed'*.

One of the key figures in the development of an anti-typhoid vaccination was the British scientist Sir Almroth Wright (1861–1947), known by his critics as 'Sir Almost Wright', or even 'Sir Always Wrong' – and caricatured as Sir Colenso Ridgeon in George Bernard Shaw's 1906 play *The Doctor's Dilemma*.

TUBERCULOSIS – or TB – is a chronic bacterial

infection that has probably plagued humankind since antiquity. It can be transmitted by both humans (via *Mycobacterium tuberculosis*) and cattle (via *Mycobacterium bovis*), and may affect almost any tissue or organ of the body. Identifying many of the past forms of tuberculosis can be confusing. The great variety of names – such as scrofula, phthisis, consumption, graveyard cough and the White Death – mirrors the myriad symptoms of this varied and deadly disease. The most common form is pulmonary tuberculosis, which affects the lungs and is spread from person to person through airborne droplets. This form of tuberculosis became one of the greatest scourges of the industrial towns and cities of the 19th and early 20th centuries. Despite the development of an effective cure in the 1950s, there has more recently been an alarming resurgence of tuberculosis, including drug-resistant TB, and in 1993 the World Health Organization declared TB a global emergency.

In 1924 the German novelist Thomas Mann published what many believe to be his masterpiece, *The Magic Mountain*. The novel is an evocative depiction of life and death in a TB sanatorium in the Swiss Alps at the turn of the 20th century.

'The highest of the sanatoriums is the Schatzalp – you can't see it from here. They have to bring their bodies down on bob-sleds in the winter, because the roads are blocked.

"Their bodies? Oh, I see. Imagine!" said Hans Castorp. And suddenly he burst out laughing, a violent, irrepressible laugh, which shook him all over and distorted his face, that was stiff with the cold wind, until it almost hurt.'

Tuberculosis - as Castorp soon discovers - is no laughing matter. It is not laughter that distorts the faces of those racked by the terminal stages of TB, but the violent, bloody cough, the breathlessness, the pain, the night sweats, the slow, insidious wasting and decay of young tormented bodies. Castorp, whose failing health obliges him to stay in the sanatorium for seven years, comes to understand *'that one must go through the deep experience of sickness and death to arrive at a higher sanity and health'.*

While the history of tuberculosis may conjure up images of health-restoring sanatoria and pale-faced, slender, love-sick men and women, below the 'Magic Mountain', in the squalor and filth of overcrowded slums across the world, lies the grim reality of a disease that over the course of the last few hundred years has destroyed the lives of millions, and which today once again ranks as one of the most devastating infectious diseases in the world.

PHTHISIS AND THE MYSTERIES OF ANTIQUITY

When, where and how humans were first infected with tuberculosis is a mystery. It is likely to have been around for at least 3000 years in its varied forms. Ancient Egyptian paintings show hump-backed figures typical of those with spinal TB. Scars on the lungs of mummies reveal signs of the pulmonary variety of the disease. Clay tablets in Mesopotamia dating from the seventh century BC describe lists of ailments, including one in which the patient coughs continually. *'What he coughs up is thick and frequently bloody,'* says the tablet. *'His breathing sounds like a flute. His hand is cold, his feet are warm. He sweats easily, and his heart activity is disturbed'.*

> ### 'I know the colour of that blood! It is arterial blood. I cannot be deceived ... That drop of blood is my death warrant. I must die.'
> JOHN KEATS, IN 1820, A YEAR BEFORE HIS DEATH AT THE AGE OF 25

A hillside tuberculosis sanatorium in the warm climate of Puerto Rico, photographed in 1922.

Röntgen (1845-1923) discovers X-rays, enabling physicians to screen for TB.

1921 The BCG vaccine is developed.

1944 Discovery of streptomycin, the first antibiotic effective against TB.

1950s Irish-born physician John Crofton (b.1912) develops the 'Edinburgh method', which combines three drugs to treat TB, with excellent results.

1980s TB seems to be declining in the Western world.

1990s TB re-emerges as a major public-health concern, along with HIV/

AIDS and multi-drug resistant strains of TB.

1993 The World Health Organization (WHO) declares TB a global emergency.

2006 The WHO launches a new 'Stop TB' programme.

Whether the human form of the disease evolved from an animal form (bovine tuberculosis) – possibly through the consumption of infected dairy products after people began to domesticate animals – or whether humans gave it to their herds is a much debated question. But certainly by the time of the Greek physicians Hippocrates (*c.*460–*c.*370 BC) and Galen (AD 129–*c.*210), pulmonary tuberculosis – or 'phthisis' as it was known (meaning 'dwindling' or 'wasting away') – is clearly recognizable. The Greeks ascribed the disease to 'evil airs'. The Romans recommended bathing in human urine, drinking elephants' blood or devouring wolves' livers. The Arabs treated the disease with asses' milk and powdered crab shells. Some ancient and early Medieval doctors advised the patient to seek a change of air – a practice revived in the 19th and 20th centuries.

VARIETIES OF TUBERCULOSIS

Most people appear to have a natural resistance to TB: only one in ten of those infected develop the active form of the disease. Pulmonary tuberculosis, which progressively destroys the lungs, is the most common form of TB, and once a person begins to show active symptoms – coughing up blood, night sweats, wasting and general debility – it can soon prove fatal. Tuberculosis can also affect other parts of the body. In the Middle Ages a disease known as scrofula may have been the glandular form of the disease. The word 'scrofula' is the diminutive of the Latin *scrofa*, meaning 'a breeding sow' – the puffy appearance of someone with swollen lymph glands in the neck apparently resembled a 'little pig'. This form of tuberculosis was also known as the 'King's Evil' (see The Royal Touch, left).

The King's Evil and scrofula were amongst any number of names once used to describe the various forms of tuberculosis. While for many centuries phthisis remained the term applied by physicians to pulmonary tuberculosis, the popular equivalent was 'consumption', a word that aptly captured the way victims seemed to be literally consumed by the disease, becoming pale, weak and emaciated. 'Galloping consumption' and 'graveyard cough' signalled imminent death. *Lupus vulgaris*, 'the common wolf', was the name given to tuberculosis of the skin, which causes horrible disfigurement, especially of the face. Tuberculosis of the spine became known as Pott's disease, after Percival Pott (1714–88); and tuberculosis of the cortex of the adrenal glands was named Addison's disease after

THE ROYAL TOUCH

For centuries, French and English kings and queens claimed to be able to cure those suffering from scrofula or the 'King's Evil' by the Royal Touch. They believed this power was vouchsafed by God only to the true line of kings, and ceremonies involving the Royal Touch were used to legitimate those who acceded to the throne. But why scrofula should have been singled out for royal attention is a mystery.

In England, Edward the Confessor 'touched' numerous people during his reign (1042–66). Charles II (r. 1660–85) is said to have 'laid hands' on nearly 100,000 subjects. At his coronation in 1722, Louis XV of France touched over 2000 scrofula victims. In England, the last person to receive the Royal Touch in Queen Anne's reign (1702–14) was the young Samuel Johnson (1709–84) who went on to become a great literary figure (although it is not certain that Johnson, or anyone else, was really 'cured'). The practice died out in England in the 18th century, but continued in France until 1825, when Charles X gave the last performance.

An English gold touchpiece from the 1550s, given at ceremonies of the Royal Touch.

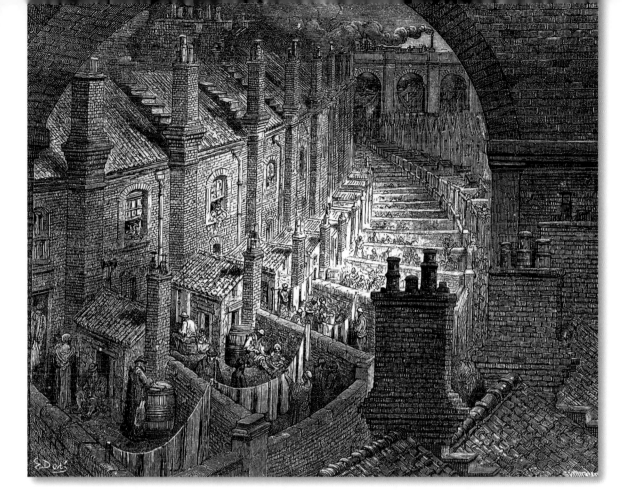

another English physician, Thomas Addison (1793–1860). The range of names used in the Medieval and early modern period makes it difficult to conclude with any certainty the full impact of the disease. In the London Bills of Mortality in the 17th century, however, even during the terrible plague year of 1665, *'consumption and tissick [phthisis]'* claimed the lives of 4808 Londoners, third only to plague and fevers, while another 86 died from the 'King's Evil'.

NAMING AND IDENTIFYING THE DISEASE

In his treatise of 1689, *Phthisiologia*, the British physician Richard Morton (1637–98) first applied the word 'tubercle' – from the Latin *tuberculum*, the diminutive of tuber, meaning 'lump' or 'bump' – to the tiny nodules of inflamed tissue he found in the lungs of patients who had died of phthisis. In 1816 the French physician René Théophile Hyacinthe Laënnec (1781–1826) – who himself probably died of tuberculosis – invented a device that made it possible to diagnose the disease in those who were still alive. This was the stethoscope, and with it doctors could listen to the amplified sounds of breathing, the noise of blood gurgling round the heart,

London's overcrowded Victorian slums provided the perfect environment for tuberculosis to be transmitted from person to person, leading to a vast increase in the disease in the 19th century.

'In the future struggle against this dreadful plague of the human race, one will no longer have to contend with an indefinite something, but with an actual parasite.'

ROBERT KOCH (1843–1910)

65

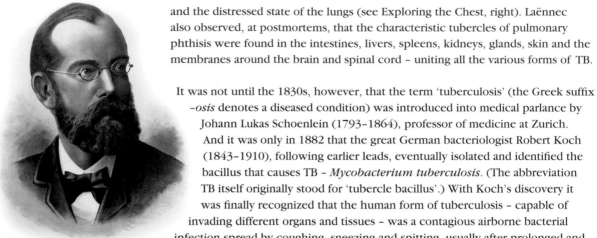

Robert Koch in about 1887.
As well as discovering the
bacillus responsible for
tuberculosis, Koch carried
out important work on
the identification of other
diseases including anthrax
and cholera. He was awarded
the Nobel Prize for Physiology
or Medicine in 1905.

and the distressed state of the lungs (see Exploring the Chest, right). Laënnec also observed, at postmortems, that the characteristic tubercles of pulmonary phthisis were found in the intestines, livers, spleens, kidneys, glands, skin and the membranes around the brain and spinal cord – uniting all the various forms of TB.

It was not until the 1830s, however, that the term 'tuberculosis' (the Greek suffix -*osis* denotes a diseased condition) was introduced into medical parlance by Johann Lukas Schoenlein (1793–1864), professor of medicine at Zurich. And it was only in 1882 that the great German bacteriologist Robert Koch (1843–1910), following earlier leads, eventually isolated and identified the bacillus that causes TB – *Mycobacterium tuberculosis*. (The abbreviation TB itself originally stood for 'tubercle bacillus'.) With Koch's discovery it was finally recognized that the human form of tuberculosis – capable of invading different organs and tissues – was a contagious airborne bacterial infection spread by coughing, sneezing and spitting, usually after prolonged and close contact with an infected person. Bovine tuberculosis was later shown to be transmitted to humans through infected cows' milk and meat.

THE WHITE DEATH

In the 19th century and the first half of the 20th century, tuberculosis – especially the pulmonary variety – probably killed millions of people. It became known as the White Death or the White Plague, referring to the characteristic pallor of its victims, and was, though in a very different way, as devastating as the Black Death of half a millennium earlier. For unlike bubonic plague, the White Death did not come and go in epidemic waves. It was ever present, sapping the energy and destroying the lives of young men and women, and even children, across the globe. The poet John Keats (1795–1821) lost his mother and his brother to tuberculosis. In his 'Ode to a Nightingale' he refers to the symptoms of the disease, the '*weariness, the fever, and the fret*', and yearns to escape a world '*Where youth grows pale, and spectre-thin, and dies*'. When in 1820, the year he published his great poem, he saw blood on his handkerchief, he knew that he too had contracted the disease and did not have long to live.

'One [doctor] sniffed at what I spat out, the second tapped where I spat it from, the third poked about and listened how I spat it. One said I was going to die, the second that I was dying and the third that I was dead … All this has affected the Preludes, and God knows when you will get them.'

FRÉDÉRIC CHOPIN (1810–49), IN A LETTER SHORTLY BEFORE HIS DEATH (POSSIBLY FROM TB, ALTHOUGH RECENTLY IT HAS BEEN SUGGESTED HE MAY HAVE DIED FROM CYSTIC FIBROSIS)

Characters suffering from 'consumption' make frequent appearances in the novels, plays and operas of the period. Among the notable ones are: Mimi in Puccini's *La Bohème*, Violetta in Verdi's *La Traviata* (inspired by the fate of Marguerite Gautier in *La Dame aux Camélias* by Alexandre Dumas), Fantine in Victor Hugo's *Les Misérables*, and Smike in Charles Dickens's *Nicholas Nickleby*. TB was, as one scholar has written, '*once responsible for no less than one in seven deaths – and a good many more if novels and operas are included*'.

A SLOW AND SILENT KILLER

John Keats, like others racked with the early stages of consumption in the 19th century, sought refuge in 'healthier' climes, away from the polluted city. For some it was already too late. After Keats died in Rome in 1821, aged only 25, his apartment at the foot of the Spanish Steps was fumigated and his furniture burnt in the hope that this would destroy whatever it was that caused this mysterious, deadly infection. But for many a change of air was not an option, and it was in the filthy and crowded slums and factories of Europe and North America that this slow and silent killer had its greatest impact.

Tuberculosis, along with a host of other 'crowd' diseases, wiped out generation after generation of people in the prime of life – depriving children of parents, families of breadwinners, lovers of sweethearts. Life expectancy among the labouring classes was little over 30 years in some industrial towns, and tuberculosis ranked high as a cause of death in the mid-19th century. Even in the early 20th century, TB still killed more people worldwide than any other infection. In many cities during this period, autopsies suggested that a high proportion of the urban population were, at some point in their lives, infected with the bacillus – with perhaps 10 per cent going on to develop the active form of the disease, and 80 per cent of those ultimately dying from tuberculosis.

'NO SPITTING, PLEASE'

Koch's discovery in 1882 of the tubercle bacillus and the infectious nature of the disease quashed some of the older theories about its cause: some had suggested a hereditary 'consumptive disposition', others blamed the 'indigent' habits of the poor or the 'sorrowful passions' of young lovers. The fact that Koch showed TB to be an infectious bacterial disease in many ways confirmed what had been suspected and observed all along: the disease hit hardest at those whose lives were blighted by poverty and poor nutrition, and worked in badly ventilated, overcrowded, cold, damp or dusty conditions.

Tuberculosis in the late 19th and early 20th centuries figured largely as a disease of the urban poor. It became clear that the bacilli spread rapidly and easily when people lived or worked in close proximity, breathing in one another's airborne particles from coughs, sneezes and sputum. Those most likely to succumb to the symptoms were people with little resistance to fight off the infection. Isolating the infected and giving them the opportunity to rest became the preferred way of dealing with the disease, for which there was as yet no cure.

EXPLORING THE CHEST

The word stethoscope derives from the Greek word *stethos*, 'chest', and *skopein*, 'to look at'. It was invented in 1816 by a rather embarrassed French physician, René Théophile Hyacinthe Laënnec (1781–1826). Laënnec had wanted to listen to the heart of a young, somewhat plump, female patient, but felt it inappropriate to do anything as intimate as putting his head so close to her bosom. So he rolled up his notebook and put one end on the young lady's chest and the other to his ear. *Voilà!* He could clearly hear not only the sounds of her heart, but also her breathing. Soon after this the stethoscope became a hollow tube of wood, and later many new designs were created, including the flexible form that became one of the physician's most useful diagnostic aids.

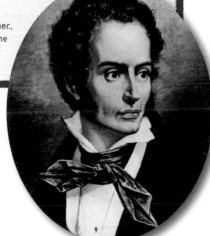

A portrait of René Théophile Hyacinthe Laënnec, the inventor of the stethoscope.

The old idea of seeking 'healthy airs' – whether in spas, by the seaside or in the mountains – gave rise to an expansion of institutionalized sanatoria. And it was not just the wealthy 'lungers' who benefited; the 'contagious' poor were also encouraged or even pressurized to enter one of the state- or charity-run sanatoria. By the 1930s in Britain there were 420 sanatoria with 30,000 beds in hilly or rural settings, offering 'cool and fresh air' for diseased lungs. In the USA the sanatoria movement – including the world-renowned Adirondack Cottage Sanatorium at Saranac Lake, New York – also took off in the early 20th century. Rest, sun, fresh air, rich food and moderate exercise were part of the daily routine. Because of their warm and dry climates, California, New Mexico and Arizona became known as the 'Land of the New Lungs'.

Public-health campaigns went further by instructing people on how to avoid contracting or spreading tuberculosis. One clear directive was 'no spitting in public places', and spittoons were provided to try to limit the spread of airborne bacilli. In New York City spitting became a punishable offence, and by 1916 nearly 200 American cities had rules in force against spitting in public.

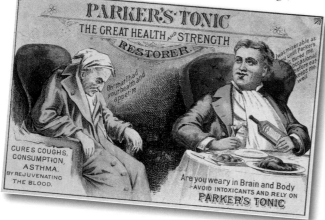

A highly graphic trade card extolling the virtues of Parker's Tonic as a means of curing a variety of diseases including consumption – an earlier name for TB.

The discovery of X-rays in 1895 by Wilhelm Röntgen (1845–1923), professor of physics at the University of Würzburg in Bavaria, enabled doctors to get a clearer picture of the lungs of tuberculous sufferers. In the early 20th century TB became a notifiable disease in a number of countries, and from the 1920s mass X-ray screenings were undertaken to detect those likely to be infectious.

A VACCINE AND THREE DRUGS

While many of these measures were designed to prevent tuberculosis from escalating out of control, the search for an effective vaccine or therapeutic drug was far more problematic. Koch himself was convinced that he had found a glycerine extract to treat tuberculosis, which he called 'tuberculin'. He kept his remedy secret for a while but, when he announced his exciting 'cure' in 1890, it failed to live up to its promise (though it was subsequently used as a valuable diagnostic test for both humans and cattle).

Development of a TB vaccine was eventually achieved in 1921 by two French scientists – Albert Calmette (1863–1933) and Camille Guérin (1872–1961) – and called BCG (Bacillus Calmette-Guérin). This vaccine – one of the major medical breakthroughs of the early 20th century – was widely used in many countries after the Second World War, although it was less popular in the USA. It was followed in the mid-1940s by the discovery of the first antibiotic effective against TB – streptomycin. Selman Waksman (1888–1973), a Ukrainian-born American, found the compound in a mould growing in the throats of chickens that had been reared in a heavily manured field. Two other drugs – para-amino-salicylic acid

(PAS) and isoniazid – were subsequently combined with streptomycin as a way of preventing resistance to any single drug. This triple therapy, developed by Sir John Crofton (b.1912) and his team in Edinburgh in the 1950s, became known as the Edinburgh method. It proved spectacularly successful in treating TB and over the following decades saved millions of lives globally. Pasteurization of milk and keeping cattle herds free of TB, with the aim of reducing the incidence of bovine tuberculosis, also became important in the postwar era. With a vaccine to prevent TB and powerful antibiotics to treat anyone who contracted it, there was by the mid-20th century tremendous optimism that this disease could be eliminated, and by the early 1960s many sanatoria had already closed. Indeed, over the next few decades the incidence of tuberculosis fell dramatically, to a point in the 1980s when it was no longer considered a public-health threat in the West.

THE DECLINING INCIDENCE OF TB

As historians have looked back at the changing death rates of TB over the previous century and a half, they have noticed that (notwithstanding the huge toll exacted by TB until well into the 20th century) the downward trend of mortality from TB had begun long before the introduction of these 'magic bullets', and some time before Koch's discovery of its causative agent. Indeed, three-quarters of the reduction had occurred before the BCG vaccine or antibiotics were introduced.

The reasons for this change have puzzled historians. If vaccination and therapeutic medicine played no role in the earlier stages of the decline of TB, what else might have helped? Some have argued that improved nutrition was a key factor, enabling people to cope better with the infection. Others have pointed to broader public-health measures, including the isolation and care of the sick in hospitals and sanatoria, along with a concerted effort to prevent the spread of infection and to provide supportive health-care measures for chronic sufferers. Social and economic improvements – better housing and working conditions for the poor – are yet other factors likely

'An X-ray will show it before you know it.' 'People queue for a free chest X-ray to check for tuberculosis at this mobile clinic, photographed in Maple Valley, Washington, USA, In 1948.

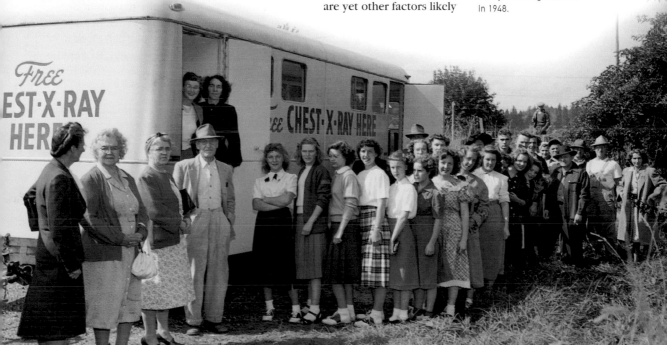

to have contributed to the downward trend. Or, possibly, there was a decline in the virulence of the disease over the course of the 19th and 20th centuries.

Tuberculosis is a disease with many complex pathways and manifestations, and it is likely that some combination of these factors was responsible for the decline, a trend that was then accelerated with the introduction and widespread use of screening, vaccination and antibiotic treatment. Whatever the exact chain of events, the decline of TB in the northern hemisphere was hailed as a huge victory, and by the 1980s the White Plague had become in the Western world a thing of the past. In some countries, vaccination was no longer even seen as necessary.

'I cannot so properly say that he died of one disease, for there were many that had consented, and laid their heads together to bring him to his end. He was dropsical, he was consumptive, he was surfeited, was gouty, and, as some say, he had a tang of the pox in his bowels. Yet the captain of all these men of death that came against him to take him away, was the consumption, for it was that that brought him down to the grave.'

JOHN BUNYAN (1628–88), *THE LIFE AND DEATH OF MR BADMAN* (1680)

THE DISEASE THAT NEVER WENT AWAY

The declining incidence of tuberculosis in the West is only one part of the global story. Beyond western Europe and the USA lay a world where TB was slowly, silently and needlessly destroying millions of lives. In the poorer countries of Africa, Asia and South America, TB became an increasingly serious problem over the course of the 20th century, and around the world it has recently shown a terrifying resurgence. It has turned out to be the disease that never went away.

It took another major epidemiological tragedy to bring TB back onto the international health agenda – HIV/AIDS (see pages 192–201). In the mid-1980s cases of TB in the USA began to surface in inner city areas amongst the homeless, drug users and prison inmates, as well as amongst foreign-born individuals. In eastern Europe and the former USSR following the fall of communism, cases of TB soared in the wake of social and economic dislocation, wars and ethnic conflict. In western Europe, in cities like London, TB cases also began to rise amongst immigrant and refugee populations. But it was the AIDS epidemic, coupled with the emergence of multi-drug resistant (MDR) strains of TB, that catapulted the disease back into the limelight. The most alarming development was the phenomenon of parallel epidemics of AIDS and TB in the developing world, especially in Africa and Southeast Asia.

The combination of HIV/AIDS and multi-drug resistant TB is proving a lethal synergy that makes both diseases more deadly, as each speeds the other's progress. For adults with a latent TB infection who are also infected with HIV, the risk of developing clinical symptoms of TB rises from around 10 to 50 per cent. In some parts of sub-Saharan Africa, between 10 and 15 per cent of the adult population are infected with both HIV and TB, and the number of annual TB

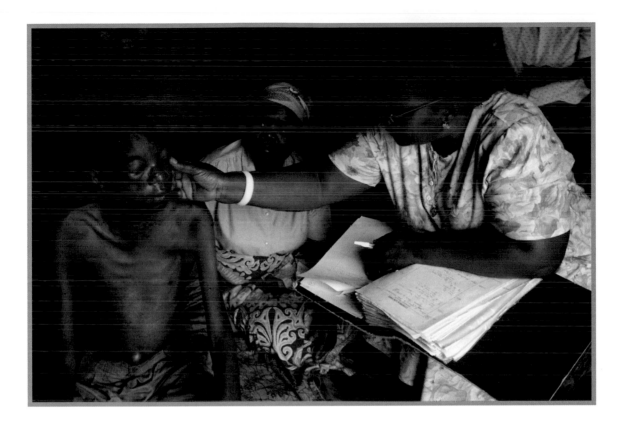

cases has risen up to tenfold since the 1980s. These statistics have shocked international health officials, and in 1993 the World Health Organization (WHO) declared TB a global emergency.

In the mid-1990s, the 'Stop TB' campaign was introduced, and a method of monitoring drug treatment, known as DOTS ('directly observed therapy with short-course antibiotics') became the internationally recommended strategy for TB control – one of the great problems of treating TB is making sure that patients take the correct combination of drugs every day for some months. Although DOTS has been successful in parts of the world, the current TB figures give rise to great concern. TB is now one of the greatest single infectious killers in the world. An estimated 2 billion people – nearly one-third of the world's population – are infected with TB bacilli, 8 to 10 million become ill, 1.5 to 2 million die each year, and every second of every day someone in the world is newly infected. Almost 9 million new TB cases were reported in 2005, with the majority in Africa and six Asian countries – Bangladesh, China, India, Indonesia, Pakistan and the Philippines.

The link between TB, poverty and malnutrition – as well as diseases like HIV/AIDS that suppress the immune system – is clear. With the hope of more effective drugs and vaccines, a new 'Stop TB' campaign, launched in 2006 by the WHO, aims to reverse the increase in TB over the coming decade. Meanwhile, the disease that never went away remains a major global health problem in the 21st century.

A volunteer from a Catholic homecare project tends a patient suffering with both TB and AIDS in Ndola, Zambia. This is possibly the first time in history that two concurrent pandemics have caused such high mortality rates. Globally, over 11 million people are infected with both TB and HIV.

PUERPERAL FEVER was for several

centuries the most common cause of maternal death following childbirth, reaching epidemic proportions in the lying-in hospitals of Europe and the United States in the 19th century. *Streptococcus pyogenes*, the bacterium responsible for puerperal fever, was discovered in 1879, but it was not until the 1930s, following the introduction of the sulphonamides and then penicillin, that puerperal fever – also called childbed fever – ceased to be a major problem in developed countries. However, streptococcal infection still remains a serious threat for mothers and babies in parts of the world with limited health facilities.

In 1797 Mary Wollstonecraft (1759-97), pioneering feminist and author of *A Vindication of the Rights of Women*, gave birth to her second child at home with the assistance of a midwife from the Westminster Lying-in Hospital in London. On Wednesday, 20 August a healthy baby daughter was born. Following some difficulties with the placenta, Mary was attended by a doctor from the hospital. A few days later she developed a 'shivering fit', followed by a high fever and agonizing abdominal pain. She died on Sunday, 10 September, aged 38. Her daughter, also Mary, later married the poet Shelley, and achieved enduring fame in her own right with the novel *Frankenstein*. Her mother was just one of countless women who, several days after the joy of giving birth, died of puerperal fever.

A FEMALE EVENT

Puerperal fever was first identified as a specific disease in the 18th century - its name being derived from the Latin *puer*, 'boy', and *parere*, 'to bring forth'. The term 'puerperium' was used to denote the period immediately following childbirth - the 'lying-in' or 'confinement'. Puerperal fever had probably been a cause of maternal mortality for centuries, but it was not until the 18th and 19th centuries that it captured the attention of the medical profession.

Giving birth had always been an ordeal, a risky time for both mother and child. With no anaesthetics apart from opiates and alcohol, no antibiotics and little in

timeline

1800 The British chemist Humphry Davy (1778–1829) experiments with laughing gas (nitrous oxide), to which he becomes addicted. Others later develop the use of anaesthetics for operations and to help alleviate the pain of childbirth.

1844 The American dentist Horace Wells (1815–48) uses nitrous oxide as an anaesthetic while extracting a tooth.

1846 William Morton (1819–68) conducts the first operation using ether at Massachusetts General Hospital, Boston.

1846 The Scottish surgeon Robert Liston (1794–1847) becomes the first European to operate using anaesthesia.

1846 In Vienna Ignaz Semmelweis (1818–65) begins to investigate the cause of high mortality from puerperal fever in hospitals and concludes that hand-washing is vital to prevent the spread of infection.

1847 The Scottish physician James Young Simpson (1811–70) gives chloroform (pleasanter and more potent than ether) for the first time to a woman in labour.

1853 John Snow (1813–58) administers chloroform to Queen Victoria during the birth of her eighth child. Queen Victoria describes the effects as 'soothing, quieting and delightful beyond measure'.

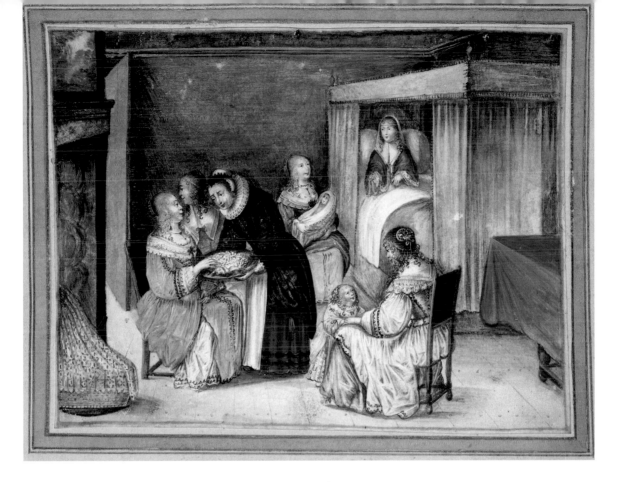

the way of antiseptics, the risk of infection was high. In the Middle Ages and early modern period, most mothers gave birth at home – sometimes alone, sometimes with a group of other women or 'gossips', and occasionally with the assistance of the local (untrained but often experienced) midwife. It was an exclusively female event.

Only in the case of difficult deliveries would a male practitioner be summoned. Fathers and siblings would huddle outside the birth chamber in hushed silence, listening to the screams of the mother, and anxiously awaiting the first cries of the new baby.

In a 17th-century Dutch birth room a maid hands round sweets to 'gossips' – females who attend the birth.

1854–6 During the Crimean War, Florence Nightingale (1820–1910) emphasizes the importance of cleanliness in hospitals.

1865 Joseph Lister (1827–1912) uses carbolic acid as an antiseptic in the course of treating a fractured tibia poking through the skin of an 11-year-old boy.

1871 Joseph Lister operates on a 15-centimetre (6-in) abscess under Queen Victoria's armpit using his carbolic spray. Thirty years later, Lister claims: 'I am the only man who has ever stuck a knife into the queen'.

1879 Louis Pasteur (1822–95) describes the micro-organisms responsible for puerperal fever.

1935 Introduction of sulphonamides, effective against the bacteria responsible for puerperal fever.

1940s–50s With the introduction of penicillin, cases of puerperal fever eventually fall.

21st century In the Western world, there is less than a 1 in 10,000 risk of mothers dying during pregnancy and childbirth.

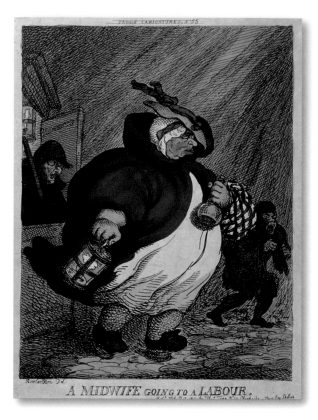

An early 19th-century cartoon depicting a midwife on her way to a labour in the early hours of the morning.

HOTBEDS OF INFECTION

The late 17th and early 18th centuries witnessed the beginnings of lying-in hospitals. These hospitals, often run as charitable institutions, offered poor women a comfortable and safe place to give birth, providing them with free food, warmth and shelter. The delivery was handled by skilled medical accoucheurs (male midwives). Ironically, it was these very maternity hospitals that gave rise to some of the worst outbreaks of puerperal fever.

In some of the larger lying-in hospitals, 5 to 20 per cent of mothers died from puerperal fever, and in the smaller hospitals severe outbreaks might see off as many as 70 to 100 per cent of lying-in women. In the early 19th century, the risk of dying from puerperal fever in Queen Charlotte's Maternity Hospital in London – one of the most prestigious of its kind – was 17 times as high as it was for a woman delivered at home in the worst slums of the East End of the city. The lying-in hospitals soon gained a reputation as 'slaughterhouses' or 'necropolises'.

The more enlightened physicians tried fumigating the wards and the women's clothing, and recommended regular washing and good ventilation. Various concoctions of herbs were tried to help the mothers once infection set in. Purging, venesection (copious bleeding using a lancet) or applying leeches to the mother's abdomen were also popular – but did nothing to stem the tide of death. Doctors grappled with the question as to why so many mothers were dying under their care. Was it a miasma or poison in the atmosphere of the hospitals? Was it some noxious influence that seeped out of soiled bedclothes, or the invasion of the womb by putrid matter? Or was it some inherent complication of pregnancy, labour and birth?

'Epidemics of puerperal fever are to women as war is to men. Like war, they cut down the healthiest, bravest, and most essential part of the population; like war, they strike their victims in the prime of their lives ...'

JACQUES-FRANÇOIS-ÉDOUARD HERVIEUX (1818–95)

DEATH IN THE HANDS OF DOCTORS AND MIDWIVES

Only a small proportion of mothers actually gave birth in these charitable institutions, and epidemics of puerperal fever could also happen outside the hospitals. The disease seemed to affect indiscriminately the rich and the poor, the robust and the weak, younger mothers and older mothers, and could follow both normal and abnormal labours. As doctors began to look more closely at the outbreaks, however, they came up with findings that were uncomfortable for their own profession. It became clear that there was some kind of link between women who contracted puerperal fever and certain birth attendants – whether midwives or doctors – who came to be seen as 'harbingers of death'. One of the first to point out this connection was Alexander Gordon (1752-99), following an epidemic of puerperal fever in 1789-92 in Aberdeen, Scotland. By 1795 Gordon had come to a disturbing conclusion:

> *'It is a disagreeable declaration for me to mention,'* he confessed, *'that I myself was the means of carrying the infection to a great number of women.'*

One doctor in Philadelphia, Dr Rutter, was so distressed at the number of cases of puerperal fever in his practice that he became fastidious about washing, shaving and changing his clothes, and even made sure he used a fresh pencil to take notes while attending a new case. Yet, despite his efforts, the disease seemed to follow him wherever he went and, in the end, like others in such a situation, he was forced to give up his practice.

FROM CORPSES TO CONFINEMENTS

In 1843 Oliver Wendell Holmes (1809-94), a young physician and poet in Boston, documented a number of cases which, he believed, illustrated the 'contagious' nature of puerperal fever, its links with another infection – erysipelas – and the possibility that the infection was carried by doctors from corpses to confinements. His observations were reprinted in 1855 as a pamphlet, *Puerperal Fever as a Private Pestilence*, in which he wrote the following:

> *'In view of these facts, it does appear a singular coincidence that one man or woman should have ten, twenty, thirty, or seventy cases of this rare disease, following his or her footsteps with the keenness of a beagle through the streets and lanes of a crowded city, while the scores that cross the same paths on the same errands know it only by name.'*

Holmes cited one distinguished doctor who removed the pelvic organs at the postmortem of a patient who had died of puerperal fever. He then put them in his coat pocket before going on to deliver a number of women – all of whom subsequently died. Such practices, Holmes argued, were criminal, and should be banished. He also recommended that anyone attending an autopsy, or a case of puerperal fever or erysipelas, should take sensible precautions to avoid conveying the contagion to a midwifery case.

'TO DO THE SICK NO HARM'

'Cur'd yesterday of my Disease, I died last night of my Physician.'
Matthew Prior, 1714

Doctors, nurses, midwives and other health workers do all they can to cure diseases and save lives. In the Hippocratic writings of the fifth century BC physicians are reminded: *'As to diseases, make a habit of two things – to help, or at least to do no harm'*. Florence Nightingale (1820–1910) reiterated the point: *'It may seem a strange principle to enunciate as the very first requirement in a Hospital that it should do the sick no harm'*. But as in the story of the great puerperal epidemics of the 19th century, in which doctors and nurses were unwittingly responsible for spreading the infection, there can be times when things go horribly wrong.

Today, there is a worrying upward trend of 'hospital-acquired super-bugs', including MRSA (Methicillin-resistant *Staphylococcus aureus*) and *Clostridium difficile*. Ignaz Semmelweis (see next page) and Florence Nightingale would be seriously concerned. Hand washing using anti-bacterial soaps, the use of masks and other basic preventive measures to stop cross-infections in hospitals remain as critical today as they were in the past.

'I make my confession that God only knows the number of women whom I have consigned prematurely to the grave.'

IGNAZ SEMMELWEIS (1818–65)

Wash your hands

It is the Hungarian physician Ignaz Semmelweis (1818–65) who has gone down in history for making the critical connection between corpses and confinements. In 1846 Semmelweis was an assistant in Vienna's famous teaching hospital, the Allgemeines Krankenhaus. There were two obstetrical clinics in the hospital, and expectant mothers were randomly allocated to either one. The one where Semmelweis worked was used for teaching male medical students, the other for training female midwives. Semmelweis discovered that cases of puerperal fever and mortality rates were far higher in the clinic with the medical students. When a good friend, who was professor of forensic medicine, died, Semmelweis read the autopsy report. His friend had been nicked by a knife while conducting an autopsy, and the report suggested that he had died from the same disease as women who died in childbirth. Semmelweis had a sudden insight. He scrutinized the practices of the doctors in his clinic and observed that they would often go straight from assisting with autopsies to carrying out vaginal examinations of women in labour – without washing their hands or changing their clothes. There had to be a connection.

Semmelweis, unaware of Holmes's paper, put forward his 'cadaveric theory', suggesting that infectious particles from patients who had died of, or were infected with, the fever were conveyed to healthy lying-in women on the hands of the students. He insisted that the students and physicians washed their hands and scrubbed their nails in a bowl of chloride of lime placed at the entrance to the ward, so that '*not the faintest trace of cadaver aroma*' would be left. Cases of puerperal fever on the ward fell dramatically.

This simple and effective method for preventing the spread of puerperal fever was not taken up more widely, however, and mortality from puerperal fever in many countries actually rose in the following years. It was not until some 20 years after his death in 1865 in a lunatic asylum that the significance of Semmelweis's findings was widely realized, and he became hailed as an unsung hero. In the meantime, there had been two further breakthroughs.

Germs and antisepsis

The discovery of the causal agent of puerperal fever is usually credited to Louis Pasteur (1822–95), who in 1879 described the bacterial micro-organisms responsible as *microbes en chapelet* ('microbes like a rosary'). His finding was confirmed by others, and the bacterium causing puerperal fever was

THE FLESH-EATING BUG

In the mid-19th century the USA was struck by a frightening and mysterious epidemic.

A contemporary wrote:

'No language can give an adequate description of the revolting aspects of this form of the epidemic in many individuals ... the flesh would drop off from the limb, or the whole member presenting the disgusting spectacle of a livid mass of putrefaction ... '

This was probably necrotizing fasciitis, formerly known as 'hospital gangrene' – the scourge of hospitals in the pre-antibiotic era. It is now commonly called the 'flesh-eating bug' but, fortunately, it is quite rare. It is caused by the group of bacteria (group-A streptococci) that cause puerperal fever.

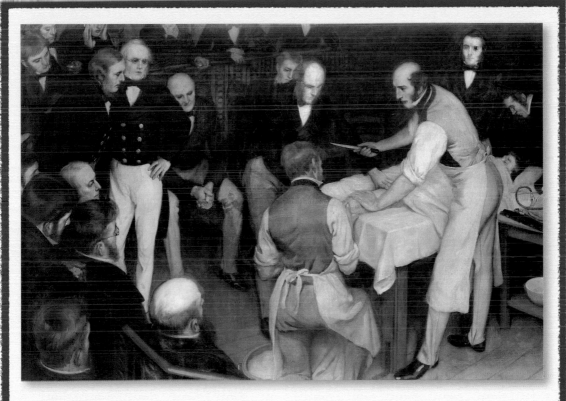

Robert Liston performing an operation. Many of his operations were carried out without anaesthetic, but in 1846 he also performed the first operation in Europe on a patient who was under an anaesthetic.

THE FASTEST OPERATOR

Before the advent of anaesthetics, patients about to undergo an operation were heavily dosed with rum or opium and forcibly held down or strapped to the operating table. The pre-eminent skill for a surgeon was speed. The Scottish surgeon Robert Liston (1794–1847) was the fastest cutter in the pre-anaesthetic era. It was said that, when he operated, the gleam of the knife was followed so quickly by the sound of the bone being sawn as to make the two actions seem almost simultaneous. With students packing the gallery of the operating theatre, pocket-watches in hand, Liston would stride across the bloodstained floor, often in Wellington boots, and call, *'Time me, gentlemen, time me'*.

Once when he amputated a patient's leg in his usual time of two and a half minutes, his flashing knife also removed the man's testicles. The patient apparently died later of hospital gangrene. During the operation Liston, in addition, inadvertently cut off the fingers of his young assistant, who later also died of hospital gangrene. He managed, too, to slash through the coat tails of a distinguished spectating surgeon, who, fearing the knife had pierced his vitals, dropped dead from fright. It is said that Liston performed the only operation in the history of medicine with a 300 per cent mortality rate.

James Young Simpson (1811–70), who first used chloroform as an anaesthetic for women in labour in 1847, noted the similarity between hospital gangrene (or 'surgical fever') and puerperal fever.

'All that would be needful would be to purify the surface of the skin of the part to be operated upon by means of some efficient antiseptic, to have my own hands, and those of my assistants, and also the instruments, similarly purified; and then the operation might be performed without the antiseptic spray ... and no one would rejoice more than myself to be able to dispense with it.'

JOSEPH LISTER, 1875

subsequently named *Streptococcus pyogenes* (from the Greek *streptos*, 'twisted like a chain', *coccus*, meaning a 'berry' and *pyogenes*, translated as 'pus-producing'). Pasteur's great discoveries in the understanding of germ theory were matched by those of Joseph Lister (1827–1912) in the field of antisepsis and asepsis in surgery. Lister is best remembered for his carbolic acid spray (of 1871), his insistence that instruments, dressings and gowns be sterilized, and his emphasis on scrupulous cleanliness. His methods were not widely adopted by obstetricians in lying-in hospitals until the 1880s, but, once their significance was recognized, puerperal fever was seen as eminently preventable.

The strong smell of disinfectant began to pervade some maternity wards. In the best-managed hospitals, everybody and everything – from the mothers in labour to the doctors and midwives (in their clean caps, gowns, masks and gloves), and all the instruments used to assist the birth – were washed down with soap and hot water or doused in disinfectant or sterilized in heated autoclaves. Those suffering from puerperal fever were isolated. The effect in some hospitals, especially in continental Europe, was startling.

Antisepsis was a major breakthrough in preventing thousands of needless deaths. But in many maternity hospitals in the USA and Britain, birth attendants continued to practise without the necessary preventive measures. In the USA, where many deliveries took place in hospitals, one-quarter of a million mothers died in childbirth in the 1920s. Even by the 1930s there were still no masks, gloves or sterilized instruments in Queen Charlotte's Maternity Hospital, London. It has since been shown that wearing a mask is one of the most effective preventive measures, as the streptococcal bug is transmitted primarily by carriers via respiratory droplets exhaled onto patients.

An operation using the Lister carbolic acid spray, 1882. The surgeons' hands, instruments, towels and other equipment are constantly in the cloud of spray, thus ensuring antiseptic conditions.

In the early 20th century, the majority of women in Europe continued to give birth at home. In Scandinavia, Belgium and the Netherlands home deliveries were attended by midwives strictly trained and fully aware of the vital importance of preventing the spread of puerperal fever – while in some other countries midwives attending home births might have little awareness of simple antiseptic practices. In Great Britain in the first half of the 1930s the risk of women dying from puerperal fever was as high as it had been in the 1860s. It took another medical revolution to radically bring down maternal mortality across the Western world.

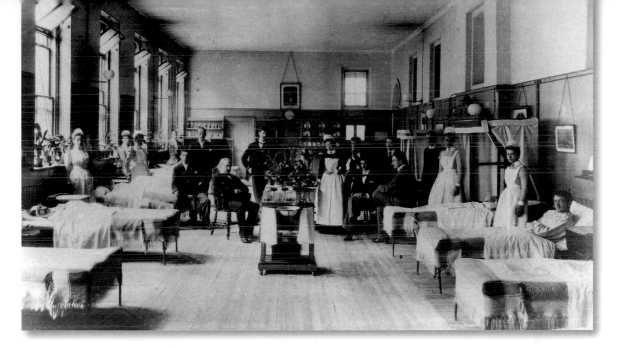

A NEW ERA: ANTIBIOTICS

The introduction of anti-bacterial drugs was the greatest advance for the treatment of bacterial infections in the history of medicine. The first drugs to be used for puerperal fever, in the late 1930s, were the sulphonamides. These proved highly effective against group-A streptococcal infection, and mortality from puerperal fever dropped dramatically. With the availability of penicillin in the mid-1940s, a new era dawned. Penicillin was more active and less toxic than the sulphonamides, and could also treat a rarer cause of puerperal fever, *Staphylococcus aureus*. Mothers in labour could at last be reasonably optimistic that they would live to see their newborn infants grow up.

By the 1950s puerperal fever in the Western world was no longer a life-threatening disorder, and its very name now has an old-fashioned ring about it. Maternal mortality – from all causes – has continued to fall sharply over the second half of the 20th century, and death in childbirth is now the exception rather than the half-expected outcome.

THE CONTINUING TRAGEDY OF DEATH IN CHILDBIRTH

Sadly, this is not the case in many of the poorer countries of the world, where mothers often give birth in the harshest conditions and without any means to prevent or treat infections. Puerperal sepsis (a term now used to cover a number of causal infectious agents) constantly threatens the life of mothers and babies, especially in Africa and parts of Asia. At least half a million mothers still die every year in pregnancy; 99 per cent of these deaths are in the developing world, and 25 per cent are from infections. The World Health Organization (WHO) has made a commitment, as part of its Millennium Development Goals, to reduce maternal mortality. But the number of mothers and babies dying from preventable infections and complications of pregnancy remains one of the greatest tragedies of the modern world.

Joseph Lister, by then Baron Lister, seen seated front left with members of his staff in Victoria Ward, King's College Hospital, London. The photograph was taken in 1893.

ENCEPHALITIS LETHARGICA

– or the 'sleepy sickness' – is a mysterious affliction that spread as a pandemic around the globe from about 1916–27. Sufferers experienced a range of bizarre symptoms and devastating after-effects. The disease attacked the brain, leaving its worst-affected victims motionless and speechless. About one-third died during the acute stages of the disease, but thousands of others were left in a somnolent state that subsequently progressed to a condition known as parkinsonism. There are still a few sporadic cases of encephalitis lethargica (possibly following a bacterial infection), but why it hit the world with such force in the early 20th century remains a puzzle.

One of the first physicians to describe – and the first to name – encephalitis lethargica was Baron Constantin von Economo (1876-1931), a Romanian-born neurologist working in Vienna, Austria:

> 'Some died within a few weeks, others lingered for weeks or months, falling into periods of deep sleep punctuated by comas … The most affected surviving patients … sit motionless, aware of their surroundings, but lethargic and unresponsive, like extinct volcanoes.'

Von Economo observed his first cases of this mysterious disease in the wards of the Psychiatric Clinic in Vienna in the winter of 1916-17, while the European powers were mired in the horrors of the First World War. Other similar but equally ill-defined cases had been noted in France in the winter of 1915-16, and it is likely that earlier cases had occurred in Central Europe some two or three years previously.

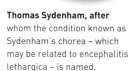

Thomas Sydenham, after whom the condition known as Sydenham's chorea – which may be related to encephalitis lethargica – is named.

Soon after von Economo's description, the disease appears to have spread in waves across the world. It was described in Australia in late 1917, in England in early 1918 (where it was at first attributed to botulism - a severe form of food poisoning) and in North America by late 1918 to early 1919. It continued to take

timeline

1529 One of a number of mysterious outbreaks of 'sweating sickness' in England – this one characterized by somnolence as well as sweating.

1580s Europe is swept by a serious febrile and lethargic illness, which leads to neurological complications.

1673–5 An unusual epidemic occurs in London; it is described by Thomas Sydenham (1624–89) as 'febris comatosa'. Symptoms include sleepiness and hiccoughs.

1712 In Germany there is a strange outbreak of a 'sleepy sickness', in which the afflicted also show signs of morbid changes in the structure of the brain.

1890–1 A mysterious and severe somnolent illness known as 'nona' occurs in northern Italy, following an influenza pandemic in 1889–90.

1916–17 In Vienna, Constantin von Economo (1876–1931) observes patients with a mysterious condition, which he names encephalitis lethargica.

c.1916–27 Encephalitis lethargica spreads in waves across most of the world, but by the 1930s has disappeared as quickly as it had arrived.

its toll during the 1920s, and in 1929 there were 6351 cases and 3580 deaths worldwide. By the 1930s the pandemic had seemingly come to an end – almost as quickly as it had arrived.

The symptoms of those stricken were so varied and so complex that the medical establishment had no idea whether they were dealing with one disease or a thousand different ones. One feature, however, seemed to unify all those affected – lethargy (*encephalitis lethargica*, derived from the Greek, means 'inflammation of the brain that makes you tired'). In spite of various speculations at the time, its cause was a mystery.

THE BAFFLING NATURE OF ENCEPHALITIS LETHARGICA

In the period 1916–27 anywhere between 1 and 5 million people, of all ages but especially young adults, were affected by encephalitis lethargica. Possibly as many as one-third died quickly after the acute phase, either in a 'deep sleep' or in a state of insomnia. Those who survived displayed a baffling range of peculiar symptoms – sore throats, headache, fever followed by severe lethargy, tremors, hiccoughs, tics, twitching and disturbances of eye movement (including 'oculogyric crises', in which the eyeballs are fixed in one position for a period of time). Some of those who were afflicted by the complaint recovered after a few days or weeks, but many others became lethargic and unresponsive, and unable to interact with or share in the world around them.

'Young people ... now appear senile, emaciated, bent, with a demented "greasy face", dripping mouth and trembling chin, and drag themselves along with a hesitating gait. To look at these people of twenty and thirty years of age is most terrible for the physician.'

FROM THE 1931 ENGLISH TRANSLATION OF CONSTANTIN VON ECONOMO'S MONOGRAPH *ENCEPHALITIS LETHARGICA* (2ND EDITION, 1929)

Many of the long-term survivors were affected, some time after the original infection, by a condition known as post-encephalitic parkinsonism, similar in presentation but unrelated in origin, to Parkinson's disease. Many experienced severe neurological problems, psychotic episodes and behavioural disturbances, and some were confined to institutions, where they existed like living statues, unaware of their surroundings or the passage of the years.

Late 1960s Some survivors of encephalitis lethargica, subsequently affected by parkinsonism, are treated with the drug L-dopa.

1973 *Oliver Sacks (b.1933) publishes* Awakenings, *in which he describes the effect of L-dopa on those who had been institutionalized and 'asleep' for nearly half a century.*

1980s The American researchers R.T. Ravenholt and W.H. Foege suggest, on the basis of its chronology and geographical distribution, that encephalitis lethargica may have been related to the influenza pandemic of 1918–19.

21st century Scientists currently investigating occasional cases of encephalitis lethargica suggest it may occur when the body's immune system, triggered by a throat infection (possibly streptococcal), attacks the nervous system and the brain.

L-DOPA AND THE AWAKENINGS

In the 1960s a new drug, L-dopa, seemed to offer exciting possibilities as a treatment for those suffering from Parkinson's disease. Oliver Sacks (b.1933), a British neurologist working at the Beth Abraham Hospital in New York, was among the first to try out this drug on a group of patients with post-encephalitic parkinsonism, who, as Sacks put it, had been *'frozen and hidden for decades – profoundly isolated – half-forgetting, half-dreaming of the world they had once lived in'.*

In his 1973 book *Awakenings* (which was made into a feature film in 1990), Sacks recounts the moving stories of some of his patients – their amazing and miraculous 'awakenings' when first treated with L-dopa in the spring of 1969, and then the subsequent bizarre effects when the drug failed to live up to expectations.

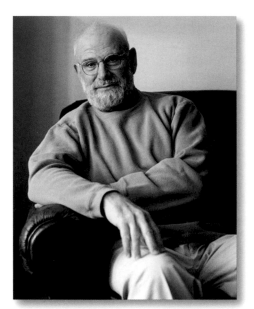

One patient, known as Rose R., who had been struck by a virulent form of encephalitis lethargica in 1926, had been in the hospital since 1935. In 1969 she 'came joyously to life' after being given L-dopa. But she was entirely engrossed in her memories of the 1920s, seeing herself still as a flapper girl, in love with the music of Gershwin. But then, as L-dopa proved less and less effective, her mood began to veer from elation to anxiety. The world of 1969, into which she awoke, was not real. *'Is 1926 now?'* she asked. In the end, Rose – a Sleeping Beauty whose 'awakening' was too unbearable for her – wanted never to be woken again.

Another patient, Leonard L., made a miraculous recovery after he was first given L-dopa. But it became harder and harder to find an optimal dose to keep him awake and to stop him from regressing. When, some years later, ailing and very frail, he was given a final dose of L-dopa, his 'awakening' response was to question why he should be 'resurrected' when it was already too late.

Oliver Sacks, the British neurologist, seen here in 2001, was one of the first to use L-dopa to treat patients suffering from post-encephalitic parkinsonism. In his book *Awakenings*, he writes: *'The central theme – falling asleep, being turned to stone; being awakened, decades later, to a world no longer one's own – has an immediate power to grip the imagination. This is the stuff that dreams, nightmares and legends are made of – and yet it actually happened'.*

WAS ENCEPHALITIS LETHARGICA RELATED TO INFLUENZA?

With the current fear of a major pandemic of human influenza following outbreaks of bird flu, a number of researchers have recently looked back at the historical records to try to determine what caused the pandemic of encephalitis lethargica. It has generally been suspected that it was a viral disease, and its timing and worldwide distribution have suggested that it might have been related to the devastating influenza pandemic of 1918–19 (see pages 172–183).

One idea is that encephalitis lethargica is a type of post-viral syndrome afflicting influenza sufferers, and some have pointed to its similarity to complications following previous influenza epidemics, including the mysterious outbreak of a severe somnolent illness known as 'nona' that occurred in northern Italy following an influenza pandemic in 1889–90.

THE DANCING MANIA

There have been a number of neurological conditions in the past as mysterious as encephalitis lethargica. Some began with manic dancing, followed by stupor, death or permanent tremors in the survivors.

In the 1370s in the Rhine basin of Germany and the Low Countries, there was an epidemic of what was known as St Vitus' dance. It involved groups of people joining hands and dancing wildly for hours in a delirium, until they fell exhausted to the ground.

In the 17th century Thomas Sydenham (1624–89) applied the name 'St Vitus' dance' to what is now known as Sydenham's chorea. This is characterized by rapid unco-ordinated jerking movements, motor weakness and behavioural disorders, possibly occurring as a latent effect of a streptococcal infection following rheumatic fever. It has been suggested that this condition might be related to encephalitis lethargica.

Manic dancing, such as in this scene by Brueghel, has been attributed to several different infections.

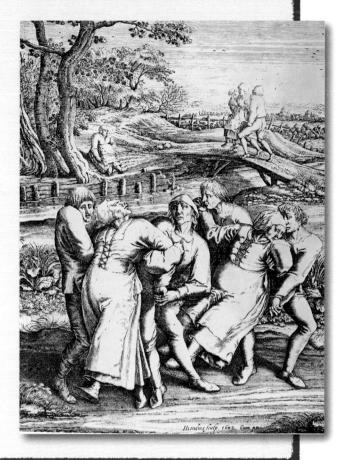

However, the onset of the epidemic of encephalitis lethargica seems to have preceded the influenza pandemic, and it continued to rage for at least ten years after the influenza pandemic had receded. Recently some scientists have re-examined the evidence and have suggested that encephalitis lethargica is a bacterial disease rather than a viral disease, in which the body's immune system reacts violently to an infection (possibly streptococcal) by attacking the nerve cells of the brain. Even if this line of inquiry proves to be correct, it does not tell us why the disease erupted so violently, and why it then, after a decade, apparently almost disappeared.

For those who died or suffered a lifetime of frozen 'sleep', any retrospective diagnosis is too late. Today there are still occasional cases in young people of what appears to be encephalitis lethargica, so understanding the causes of the disease and finding an effective treatment are still critical – especially as it is impossible to say if or when at some time in the future there will be another sudden violent eruption of this mysterious disease.

MALARIA is a life-threatening parasitic disease transmitted from person to person

by the bite of an infective female *Anopheles* mosquito. It is one of the most significant health problems in the world today, affecting some 300–500 million people across the globe, and killing between 1 million and 3 million, mostly infants and children, every year.

Malaria is one of the oldest recorded diseases in human history, and in the past it ranged from Archangel in the Russian Arctic to Australia and Argentina in the southern hemisphere. Today the disease is largely confined to around 100 countries in the tropical and sub-tropical regions of Africa, Asia and Latin America, where it causes immense suffering in some of the poorest areas of the world. Scientists and international health organizations are now giving much-needed attention to malaria as a serious global health problem, with increased commitment and funding to find effective drugs and a vaccine, as well as the promotion of insecticide-treated bed nets.

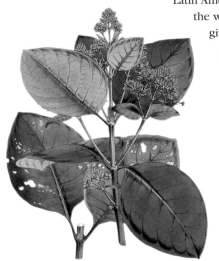

The cinchona plant, source of the anti-malarial drug quinine. Quinine is still added to 'Indian tonic water' today.

In 1937 the American malariologist Lewis Hackett (1884-1962) articulated the complex and variable nature of malaria: *'Everything about malaria is so moulded and altered by local conditions that it becomes a thousand different diseases and epidemiological puzzles. Like chess, it is played with a few pieces, but is capable of an infinite variety of situations.'*

The pieces involved in this deadly game comprise the mosquito, the parasite that causes the disease, and the human host. However, there are in fact 60 species of the mosquito genus *Anopheles* capable of transmitting malaria, and four species of the protozoan parasite that infect humans: *Plasmodium falciparum* (the deadliest form), *P. vivax*, *P. ovale* and *P. malariae*. This multiplicity results in a wide range of possible variations in the local pattern of disease transmission and clinical symptoms.

timeline

2700 BC *The Chinese medical classic, Nei Ching, contains a description of what may be malaria.*

4th century BC *Hippocrates describes malarial symptoms and classifies fevers* as quotidian (daily), tertian (occurring every other day) and quartan (occurring every third day).

323 BC *Alexander the Great dies, possibly from malaria.*

168 BC *The medicinal value of qinghaosu – sweet wormwood (Artemisia annua) is mentioned in a Chinese book of recipes (as a remedy for haemorrhoids).*

AD 1630s *The Spanish bring back cinchona bark from South America.*

1740 *The word 'malaria', from the Italian word mal'aria, is first introduced to the English language by Horace Walpole* (1717–97), 4th earl of Orford.

1820 *Quinine is isolated from cinchona bark.*

1877 *Patrick Manson (1844–1922) discovers that the filarial worms that cause lymphatic filariasis are transmitted by mosquitoes.*

1880 *Charles Louis Alphonse Laveran (1845–1922), a French army surgeon working in Algeria, first recognizes malaria parasites in the blood of a soldier.*

LIFE CYCLE AND SYMPTOMS

When a female mosquito carrying plasmodium parasites bites a human being, the parasites are injected into the blood. The parasites then rapidly enter cells in the liver and change into new forms that invade red blood cells. Every 48 or 72 hours (depending on the species), the parasites complete a cycle of multiplication in the red blood cells and then burst out, inducing the periodic fevers that characterize the disease. Any female mosquito biting an infected person becomes infected itself, so continuing the cycle.

The clinical course of malaria is characterized by a range of symptoms. These can include alternate bouts of hot and cold sweats, high fever, headache, malaise, and aches and pains. Malaria can be mild, chronic or fatal. In severe cases the disease may lead to chronic anaemia, and complications such as coma and cerebral malaria can be fatal. The fatality rate among untreated children and non-immune adults may be 10–40 per cent or higher. Pregnant women with malaria are subject to miscarriages and often give birth to underweight babies, many of whom die. Even for those who survive their early episodes of malaria, the disease can still be severely debilitating, and chronic malaria is inextricably linked to poverty.

THE STENCH OF THE SWAMP

The role of the mosquito and its parasite in transmitting malaria was not unravelled until the late 19th century. In previous centuries people ascribed the disease to a range of factors and called it by a host of different names, including 'ague', 'tertian fever', 'quartan fever', 'malignant fever', 'marsh fever', 'swamp fever', 'autumnal fever', 'Roman fever' or 'the shakes'.

' ... the large quantity of stagnating waters engenders such noxious and pestilential vapours as spread sickness and frequent death on the inhabitants ... the sickly countenances of them plainly discovering the unwholesome air they breath in.'

EDWARD HASTED (1797–1801), DESCRIBING THE MARSHES OF SOUTHEAST ENGLAND

In many parts of the world people noticed that the disease was found near foul-smelling stagnant marshes and swamps. This led to the idea that the disease was caused by poisonous or noxious vapours emanating from the marshes.

1889 The Italian scientists Ettore Marchiafava (1847–1935) and Angelo Celli (1857–1914) identify parasites under the microscope and give the organism its generic name, Plasmodium. Other Italian scientists distinguish three different forms of the plasmodium – P. vivax, P. falciparum and P. malariae.

1897 In India Ronald Ross (1857–1932) discovers malaria parasites in mosquitoes, and in the following year he elucidates the life cycle of malaria in birds.

1898 The Italian scientists Giovanni Battista Grassi (1854–1925), Amico Bignami (1862–1929) and Giuseppe Bastianelli (1862–1959) show experimentally that malaria is transmitted to humans by Anopheles mosquitoes.

1912–15 In the USA 1 million cases of malaria occur every year among a population of 25 million in the 12 southern states.

1922–3 One of Europe's most devastating malaria epidemics in the modern era spreads across Russia from the central Volga basin and reaches as far north as the Arctic Circle, with an estimated 7–12 million people infected and thousands of deaths.

Late 1920s–1940s Development of first new synthetic anti-malarial drugs, including atebrine in 1928 and chloroquine, synthesized in Germany in the 1930s and developed after the Second World War.

(continued ...)

85

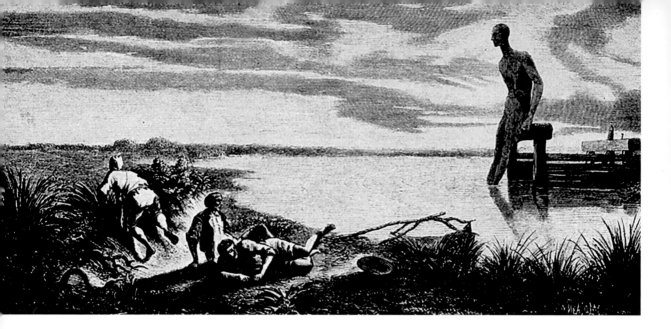

The Ghost of the Swamp.
This allegorical engraving from the mid-19th century linked the rank conditions found near stagnant water and marshes with malaria. The Italians in the 16th century gave the disease the name *mal'aria*, literally meaning 'foul air'.

MALARIA IN THE ANCIENT AND EARLY MODERN WORLDS

In the past malaria had a much wider distribution than it does today and was, for example, a common disease around the Mediterranean basin from ancient times to the mid-20th century. Some scholars have even speculated that the disease played a role in the decline of both ancient Greece and the Roman empire.

The exact chronology and geographical distribution of the disease in ancient times are currently the subject of historical investigation, but the existence of genetic traits that confer some protection against malaria, such as sickle-cell anaemia and thalassaemia, indicate a long evolutionary history, and it is likely that malaria has plagued humans for more than 6000 years. In the early modern period, in areas of Italy such as the Po Valley, the Pontine Marshes, the Roman Campagna and the Mezzogiorno region of the south, malaria was a serious problem with major social and economic consequences until its final eradication in the mid-20th century. One 19th-century Italian writer described its impact:

> *'Malaria penetrates your bones with the bread that you eat and every time you open your mouth to speak, whilst walking along the stifling streets choked with dust and sunlight, when you feel your knees buckling*

timeline

1939 The Swiss chemist Paul Müller (1899–1965) synthesizes and discovers the insecticidal properties of DDT, which is used towards the end of the Second World War for destroying body lice in typhus epidemics, and by

the late 1940s in malaria and yellow-fever control programmes.

1940s Malaria is a major cause of sickness and death in the Second World War.

1950s Malaria is virtually eradicated from the USA, recorded cases declining from around 5000 in 1949 to 97 in 1958. A more substantial decline in cases had occurred in the period 1938–42, even

prior to the intensive use of DDT from the late 1940s.

1955 The World Health Organization (WHO) launches the Global Malaria Eradication Programme. By 1969 it is acknowledged

that it has failed to reach its goal.

1970s The Chinese rediscover the ancient remedy Artemisia annua as an effective anti-malarial drug.

1970s onwards Malaria resurges dramatically in many sub-tropical and tropical areas.

1975 WHO declares that Europe is free of malaria.

1980s onwards A few episodes of locally acquired malaria in the USA are reported as well as around 1600 imported cases every year in the USA and 2000 a year in the UK.

under you, or you slump on the pack saddle of an ambling mule, head hung low … For malaria seizes the inhabitants in the empty lanes or strikes them down by the sun-bleached house door, shaking with fever in their overcoats, with all the blankets in the house heaped on their shoulders … '

Between the 17th and 19th centuries, another form of malaria appears to have become endemic in parts of the temperate world. Capable of being transmitted in areas where average summer temperatures are over 16° C (61° F), *P. vivax* is generally known as the 'benign' or milder form of the disease. Yet historical accounts from northern Europe suggest that even this form of the disease was anything but mild. In the marshes of Kent and Essex and the eastern fenland counties of England, where the disease was endemic in some localities up until the early 20th century, one in three babies died before their first birthday – with malaria adding to the high death toll.

FROM THE OLD TO THE NEW WORLD

Although some have suggested that malaria was already present in the Americas prior to 1492, it is more likely that travellers from northern Europe carried the *P. vivax* parasite to the New World after that date. The local mosquitoes would have become infected, passing on the disease in turn to the indigenous populations and early colonists. In New England in the 17th century the disease was popularly known as the 'Kentish ague'.

Travel and trade between the Americas and southern Europe – and the importation of slaves from Africa – brought the more deadly *P. falciparum* parasite to the sub-tropical and tropical parts of the New World.

POPPY JUICE Opium has been used for medicinal and recreational purposes since ancient times. In the 19th century much of the opium used in Britain came from India, and it came as a surprise to some to discover that in the marshy Fens of eastern England – where malaria was formerly endemic – the locals actually grew their own opium poppies. Opium was said to prevent the shivering fits of 'the ague', and the local beer was laced with it, while infants were dosed with poppy-head tea.

In 1864 a doctor reported that *'there was not a labourer's house in which the bottle of opiate was not to be seen … it is also sold in pills or penny sticks, and a well-accustomed shop will serve 300 or 400 customers with the article on a Saturday night'*. Opium-eating infants were described as *'wasted … shrank up into little old men … wizened like monkeys'*. As a result of both malaria and narcotic poisoning, the infant mortality rate in the Fens was very high.

1990s *Artemisinin and its derivatives are found to be effective in treating drug-resistant malaria.*

1997 *International agencies establish the Multilateral Initiative on Malaria (MIM).*

1998 *The WHO launches its Roll Back Malaria programme with the aim of halving the burden of malaria by 2010.*

2000 *The United Nations and its member states endorse their commitment to*

key Millennium Development Goals – a set of global goals (that include reducing the burden of malaria) to lift millions of people out of extreme poverty.

2001 *Establishment of the Global Fund to Fight AIDS, Tuberculosis and Malaria (GFATM), an international financing initiative aimed at ending the 5.6 million deaths every year from the world's three*

leading infectious diseases.

2002 *The complete genome sequence of Plasmodium falciparum is announced.*

2003 *The complete genome sequence of*

the Anopheles gambiae mosquito is announced.

2007 *Malaria is estimated to kill between 1 and 3 million per annum world-wide, and seriously affect the health and lives of millions*

of others, especially in sub-Saharan Africa.

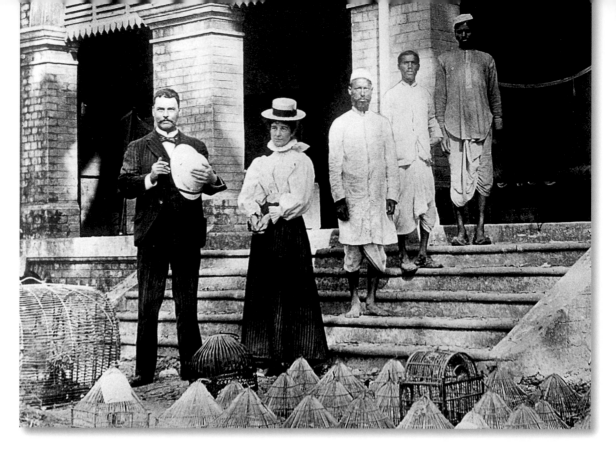

Ronald Ross, photographed with his wife and some laboratory assistants on the steps of his laboratory in Calcutta, India, in 1898. The cages in the foreground are for malarial birds, which he studied to unravel the malaria-mosquito life cycle. Ross was scrupulous in using a bed net to avoid getting malaria – advice that still holds good today.

The southern regions of North America and parts of South and Central America became severely affected, and malaria had also reached the Mississippi Valley by the 19th century. In southern Illinois, during the summer of 1865, one doctor noted that *'every man, woman and child … at least within my range shook with the ague every other day'*. The area all along the watercourses from the Mississippi to the Potomac was described in the early 19th century as a 'graveyard', and it was suspected by one authority that *'no changes and no cultivation will ever bring it into a state of salubrity'*. One account from the 1830s describes an exchange between the captain of a boat on the Ohio River and the mother of two young children. The children had crawled out into the warm sun – shivering and with chattering teeth – to watch the boat go past. Their mother, uncertain as to the cause of their fever, was told by the captain of the passing boat:

> *'If you've never seen that kind of sickness I reckon you must be a Yankee. That's the ague. I'm feared you will see plenty of it if you stay long in these parts. They call it here the swamp devil and it will take the roses out of the cheeks of these plump little ones of yours mighty quick. Cure it? No, Madam. No cure for it: have to wear it out … '*

THE 'WHITE MAN'S GRAVE'

Sailors used to sing a shanty containing the warning lines:

> *'Beware, beware the Bight of Benin,*
> *For there's one that comes out for ten that goes in.'*

In the past, Europeans travelling in the continent of Africa were frequently struck down by violent fevers. Some may have had immunity to the northern European form of malaria, but the more deadly *falciparum* form was often lethal. The coast and rivers of West Africa proved particularly deadly, and the area around the Bight (bay) of Benin became known as the 'White Man's Grave'. Almost half of the British soldiers stationed in Sierra Leone between 1817 and 1836 died, mostly from malaria. In India, too, malaria repeatedly struck with a vengeance, accounting possibly for some 1.3 million deaths a year by the 1890s.

UNRAVELLING THE MYSTERY

In the late 19th century, faced with the enormous global toll of malaria, scientists started to unravel the cause of the disease. Was it really spread from the vapours of the swamps and marshes? Alphonse Laveran (1845-1922), a French army surgeon in Algeria, recognized, under the microscope, malaria parasites in the blood of a patient in 1880. Patrick Manson (1844-1922), a Scottish doctor, became known as 'Mosquito Manson' after he discovered the role of the mosquito in lymphatic filariasis (elephantiasis) in 1877 (see pages 108-11). But it was his protégé, a British army doctor called Ronald Ross (1857-1932), who goes down in history as the first scientist to make the connection between mosquitoes and malaria.

While stationed at Secunderabad in India, Ross, inspired by Manson's ideas of a mosquito connection, dissected and examined the stomachs of thousands of mosquitoes in a cramped, hot, humid laboratory until he eventually found 'pigmented cysts' – evidence of the malaria parasite – protruding from the stomach wall of a dappled-wing mosquito that had fed on a patient with malaria. In 1897 Ross reported his remarkable discovery, and in the following year, in Calcutta, was able to elucidate the entire malaria-mosquito cycle in avian malaria.

Italian scientists were hot on Ross's heels, and by 1898 Giovanni Battista Grassi (1854-1925) and other malariologists in Italy had shown experimentally that malaria was transmitted to humans by *Anopheles* mosquitoes. Ross was awarded the Nobel Prize in 1902, but the Italians, justifiably, felt that their vital contributions had been overlooked.

MOSQUITO BRIGADES

Once it was understood that mosquitoes carried the parasite, it was thought that if one could get rid of the mosquitoes, one could get rid of the disease. Ross later recalled his hopes:

> *'In a few more months, perhaps in a year, or in two years, the death-dealing pests would begin to come under control, would begin to diminish entirely in favourable spots; and with them,*

'This day relenting God
Hath placed within my hand
A wondrous thing; and God
Be praised. At His command,

Seeking His secret deeds
With tears and toiling breath,
I find thy cunning seeds,
O million-murdering Death.

I know this little thing
A myriad men will save.
O Death, where is thy sting?
Thy victory, O grave?'

RONALD ROSS CELEBRATING HIS EUREKA MOMENT ON 20 AUGUST 1897, KNOWN AFTERWARDS AS 'MOSQUITO DAY'

slowly, the ubiquitous malady would fly from the face of civilization – not here or there only, but almost throughout the British empire – nay, further, in America, China, and Europe.'

Fired with optimism, 'mosquito brigades' drained swamps and other breeding sites of the mosquito and sprayed them with Paris green (a larvicide of copper acetate and arsenic trioxide) and pyrethrum (from chrysanthemum). People in malarial areas were advised to use bed nets, screens and head nets. Mosquito brigades went into action in India, Malaysia and elsewhere, and even attempted (though failed) to eliminate the indigenous *Anopheles* mosquito from the marshes of Kent in southeast England.

A successful campaign against both the malarial mosquito and the yellow-fever mosquito allowed the Panama Canal to be completed by 1914 (see page 150). Following a major malaria outbreak in 1938–40 in northeast Brazil, Fred Soper (1893–1977), a member of the Rockefeller Foundation and one of the leading forces behind vector control, successfully led a campaign to rid the area of the *A. gambiae* mosquito. But in many parts of the tropics and sub-tropics the mosquito outwitted any attempt at control. The ecology of malaria and its vectors proved far more complex than anticipated.

QUININE – ATTACKING THE PARASITE

Some scientists, including the German bacteriologist Robert Koch (1843–1910), advocated a different tack. Rather than trying to eliminate the mosquito, it would

EARLY REMEDIES

Early remedies for the treatment of malaria included wearing a large fish tooth as an amulet, or eating spiders whole in butter. Purging and bleeding were thought to rectify imbalances in the body's 'humours' and to get rid of 'bad blood'. However, some other early cures have proved highly effective.

In the early 17th century Jesuit missionaries in South America noticed that the indigenous people used the bark of the cinchona tree to control fevers. The Jesuits took the bark – known by a number of names, including Peruvian bark, Jesuit's bark and *quinquina* – back to Rome. It was introduced into England in the 1650s, where the Puritan leader Oliver Cromwell called it 'the devil's bark' because of its association with the Catholic Church. He refused to use it despite suffering badly from malaria, which he probably contracted in the English Fens. Robert Talbor (1642–81), an English quack, made his fame and fortune using a 'secret remedy' based on the bark to cure European royals and nobility. In 1820 the alkaloid quinine was extracted from the bark and is still used as a treatment today.

In the past few decades there has been the remarkable rediscovery of an ancient Chinese herbal cure. This is sweet wormwood, *Artemisia annua*, known in Chinese as *qinghaosu*, which has been used for chills and fevers for over 2000 years. The compound artemisinin is derived from the plant, and combinations of artemisinin derivatives and other anti-malarials are now being used to prevent and treat malaria.

be better, they claimed, to attack the parasite in the human body using the drug quinine. Quinine had been the mainstay of malaria prevention and treatment since the early 19th century (see Early Remedies, left), and was widely used in the tropics. In British India this bitter tasting medicine was added to Indian tonic water – the basis of the still popular gin and tonic. During the US Civil War, every Union soldier in malarial regions was given a daily dose of quinine sulphate dissolved in whiskey.

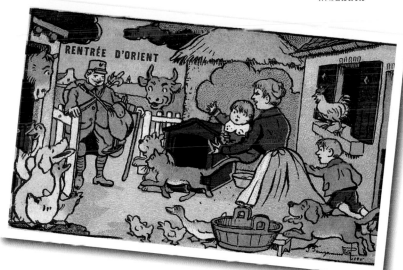

RENTRÉE D'ORIENT

Many campaigns in the early 20th century combined both anti-mosquito and anti-parasite approaches. From the 1920s some malariologists began to think of malaria as a social disease, to be reduced only by improving social and economic conditions in poverty-stricken areas. They based their arguments on the fact that malaria had declined in parts of the temperate north prior to any knowledge of its transmission by mosquitoes. The eventual eradication of malaria from the USA and much of Europe by the mid-20th century confirmed that ecological transformations brought about by socio-economic development play a key role.

In the 1930s and 1940s a number of new synthetic drugs were introduced. The most effective of these was chloroquine, which was synthesized in the 1930s in Germany but not developed until after the Second World War – too late to help the huge numbers of servicemen and civilians affected by malaria during the conflict. Malaria outbreaks caused serious problems for Allied troops fighting in the Middle East, North Africa and, especially, the Pacific – where the daily use of one of the first synthetic drugs, mepacrine (atebrine), which turned the skin yellow and was rumoured to cause impotency, did have some effect in keeping troops fit for active service. In many theatres of operations in both the First and Second World Wars, malaria often proved a greater threat than enemy action.

The benefits of using quinine and a mosquito net are illustrated by this cartoon of a homecoming soldier – one of the lucky ones who did not succumb to malaria. Only the female mosquito bites and sucks the blood of humans. She does so to develop her eggs. Males prefer to sip plant juices. Some people are bitten more often than others: one theory suggests that female mosquitoes use their antennae to seek their blood meal and some people 'smell' more attractive than others. The search is on to find which chemical components of body odour have a repellent effect on mosquitoes.

DDT AND THE PROMISE OF ERADICATION
Discovered in 1874 and synthesized in 1939, the insecticide DDT was heralded by some as a 'miracle', and by the late 1940s it was thought to have enormous potential in the campaign against malaria. In 1950 at a malaria conference held in Kampala, Uganda, a debate ensued about the possibilities of embarking on a global programme to eradicate malaria. By the end of the heated discussion, one of the delegates 'poured oil on troubled waters' and folding his hands said quietly, *'Let us spray'*.

'There is no golden Yale key to open all the doors to all the problems in malaria – it is more like a labyrinth of many doors to many problems, and each key is only the opening of one door to one problem.'

N.H. SWELLENGREBEL (1885–1970), DUTCH MALARIOLOGIST, IN 1938

'The sulfonamides, penicillin, radioactive isotopes, DDT ... foreshadow a new move forward, a new renaissance, a new period in human development when the imagination is endowed with wings ... '

ROCKEFELLER FOUNDATION, 1948

Malaria-control programmes using DDT began to be implemented in a number of countries, and in the mid-1950s the World Health Organization (WHO) endorsed a programme for the Global Eradication of Malaria. Optimistic that global eradication was possible but also aware that mosquitoes were building up some resistance to DDT, the aim was to move forward quickly.

There were some initial and quite spectacular successes, but by the late 1960s the eradication programme had foundered. The reasons for this are complicated. The costs and technical obstacles were far greater than anticipated. As early as 1951 it had been observed that mosquitoes could build up a resistance to DDT, and at the same time some species developed the uncanny ability to alter their resting behaviour to avoid the irritation caused by DDT sprayed onto the walls of huts and houses. The parasite also evolved a resistance to drugs such as chloroquine. The failure of DDT and anti-malarial drugs to fulfil the promise of eradication led to one of the greatest medical disappointments of the second half of the 20th century.

THE COMPLEXITIES AND TRAGEDY OF MALARIA

The late 20th century was the low point in the drive to control malaria. In many developing countries malaria resurged to unprecedented levels. In sub-Saharan Africa today it is estimated that every 30 seconds a child dies of malaria. The recent

Killing waterborne mosquito larvae with insecticides, such as here in Puerto Rico, is an established method of controlling the spread of malaria.

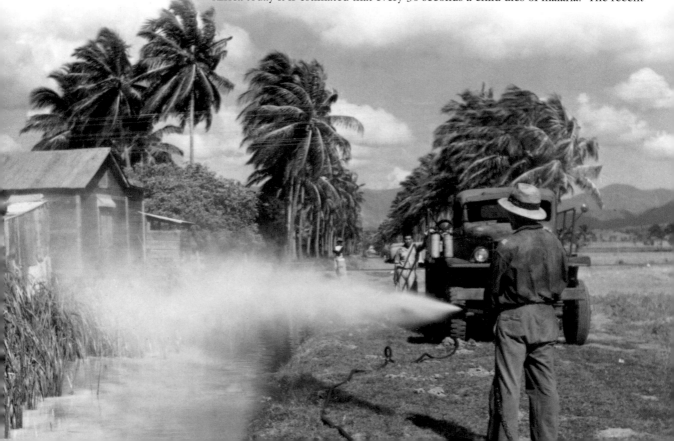

epidemic of HIV/AIDS (see pages 192–201) in the region has made the problem worse, and it is thought that the combination with HIV infection can increase the risk of severe effects of malaria, especially in pregnant women.

Why has the control of malaria proved so difficult? The answer lies, in part, in the puzzling and complex interactions of the mosquito, its parasite and human biology. This has been compounded by problems of resistance to drugs and insecticides, as well as pressure from the environmental lobby since the 1960s to ban DDT, necessitating the use of expensive alternatives. In Africa, political and economic turmoil, war and the pressures of globalization have caused health concerns to be pushed to the side. In some places, rapid and intensive agricultural development has opened up forests, creating additional breeding sites for the mosquito vector and leading to epidemics of so-called man-made malaria. Neglect by international health agencies of tropical diseases that were no longer seen as a direct threat to the developed world has also been cited as a factor in its resurgence.

ROLL BACK MALARIA?

Today malaria is attracting more attention as a serious global problem. Scientists continue to search for answers to the many questions arising from this complex disease, while international agencies are taking a broader view of the links between poverty and ill health. Progress, since the launch of the UN's Millennium Development Goals in 2000, has been promising, but in sub-Saharan Africa up to 40 per cent of the population still subsists on incomes of less than $1 a day.

There are currently various vaccines in development or undergoing trials, though so far none has reached the point of commercial production, and some doubt that a safe and affordable vaccine will be available in the foreseeable future. Various combinations of new and old drugs are more promising, both as prophylactics and treatments, especially the artemisinin-based combination therapies (ACTs), which treat the disease and prevent its transmission. Cost, however, remains an obstacle for many countries, and the appearance on the market of various ineffective counterfeit drugs is both a cruel and potentially dangerous development.

Much scientific knowledge has recently been assembled about the mosquito, its parasite and its effects on the human body. The unveiling of the complete genome sequence of *P. falciparum* was announced in 2002, and that of *A. gambiae*, the world's most dangerous mosquito vector, in 2003. Scientists are mapping malaria risk to develop a more accurate picture of the geographical distribution and burden posed by the malaria parasite and its vectors. Major international initiatives have been launched to tackle malaria with long-term goals and funding, including the Global Fund to Combat AIDS, TB and Malaria. The Bill and Melinda Gates Foundation has committed substantial funds to support this WHO programme.

In the meantime, the revival and wider use of simpler and more economic solutions, particularly insecticide-treated bed nets, are proving highly effective in preventing mosquito bites and malaria transmission. The old adage '*Don't go to bed with a malarial mosquito*' remains as relevant today as it was in the past.

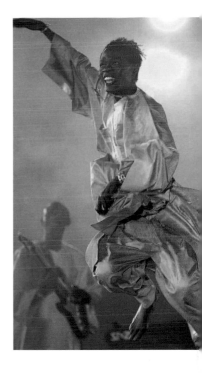

Senegalese singer Baaba
Maal, performing at the WHO
Africa Live Roll Back Malaria
concert. The event in the
Senegalese capital reached
a billion people worldwide.
Malaria is Africa's number
one killer of children.

AFRICAN TRYPANOSOMIASIS

– commonly known as sleeping sickness – is a devastating disease caused by a parasitic protozoan of the genus *Trypanosoma*. It is endemic in the so-called Tsetse Belt, a vast area spanning much of West, Central and East Africa between the Sahara and the Kalahari Desert. The Tsetse Belt is home to the tsetse fly, whose vicious bite injects the trypanosome parasite into both humans and cattle. For centuries the human form of the disease was called 'sleeping sickness' because of its striking symptoms of lethargy and sleepiness, leading eventually to coma and death. Today, both humans and animals continue to be plagued by African trypanosomiasis. Some 60 million people in 36 sub-Saharan countries are at risk, and the impact of the tsetse fly on livestock farming generates a cycle of sickness, poverty, hunger and death.

In the late 14th century news of the death of Mari Jata, the ruler of the great West African empire of Mali, reached the Arab historian Ibn Khaldun:

'Sultan Jata had been smitten by the sleeping sickness, a disease that frequently afflicts the inhabitants of that climate … Those afflicted are virtually never awake or alert. This sickness harms the patient and continues until he perishes … The illness persisted in Jata's humour for a duration of two years after which he died in the year 775 AH.'

When Europeans began to explore and trade along the coast of West Africa over the next few centuries, they too discovered a disease amongst the Africans that led to extreme sleepiness and lethargy. They called it the 'sleepy distemper' or, in French, *la maladie du sommeil*. The peculiarities of the disease and its striking symptoms led to all sorts of speculations as to its cause. Some associated it with drinking too much palm wine, others with smoking hemp or eating rotten food. At the time of the slave trade, a number of physicians examining the disease

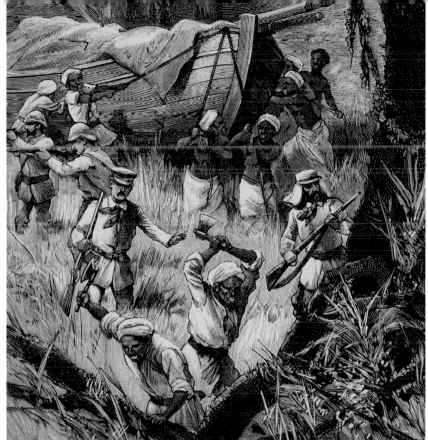

Sir Henry Morton Stanley (1841–1904) and porters crossing Africa. It has been suggested that the movement of people and animals during expeditions by European adventurers to the interior may have aided the spread of trypanosomiasis across the African continent during the late 19th and early 20th centuries.

suggested that the psychological trauma of being uprooted and taken away from their families triggered a mental 'disposition' amongst the slaves that gave rise to the 'African lethargy'.

STALLION SICKNESS, NAGANA AND THE FLY DISEASE

While many of the early European explorers sent back reports of the 'new' and deadly human diseases they encountered in the African rainforests and grasslands, some also described sickness amongst the animals. David Livingstone (1813–73), the Scottish missionary doctor and explorer of the African interior, was struck by the frequent deaths of horses and oxen on his travels in the 1850s, noting that the bite of the tsetse fly was *'certain death to the ox, horse and dog'*.

1901–2 The trypanosome parasite is incriminated for the first time in human cases of sleeping sickness.

1903 The British Sleeping Sickness Commission reports on finding Trypanosoma in the cerebrospinal fluid of patients with sleeping sickness. The tsetse fly (Glossina palpalis) is identified as the vector of the disease.

1905 The arsenical compound atoxyl is introduced as a treatment for sleeping sickness.

1906–7 The German bacteriologist Robert Koch (1843–1910) travels to German East Africa to conduct therapeutic research on trypanosomiasis using atoxyl, which proves to have serious side effects, including blindness.

1908 The Sleeping Sickness Bureau is set up in London.

1912 Another tsetse fly species, Glossina morsitans, linked to the parasite Trypanosomiasis brucei rhodesiense, is identified in Northern Rhodesia (now Zambia).

1917–31 The French physician Eugène Jamot (1879–1937) begins a campaign to eradicate trypanosomiasis from French Equatorial Africa.

(continued ...)

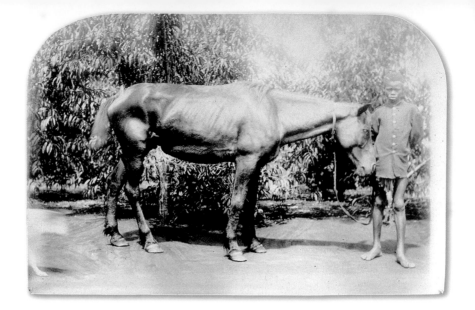

A horse suffering from 'stallion sickness' in the 1890s, brought on by trypanosomiasis. The disease causes wasting and death to other livestock such as cattle.

The effect on the horses was especially troublesome, as it meant that throughout equatorial Africa it was difficult to use them for transport. Livingstone treated horses suffering from 'stallion sickness' with arsenic. He and his luggage bearers were incessantly bothered by humming, buzzing and biting insects, like the tsetse fly, and were warned by the locals to travel during the night when the flies were less active. Livingstone, however, was certain that it was only the animals, and not the people, who suffered as a result of the tsetse bites.

In the era of European colonization that followed, farmers began to report on a fatal disease that was decimating their cattle. The disease was known in Zululand (now northern KwaZulu-Natal in South Africa) as nagana, meaning 'the wasting disease'. The effect on livestock production was dramatic. By the late 19th century both European farmers raising cattle for profit and African pastoralists dependent on the meat and milk of their cattle for subsistence were facing disaster.

Game hunters were also struggling, as their horses died from a wasting sickness. The local Zulus thought that cattle with nagana were being poisoned by food contaminated by game animals. The game hunters, meanwhile, began to suspect, like Livingstone, that their horses were being made ill by the ever-present tsetse fly. They called it the 'fly disease'. It took over half a century, but in the end

timeline

1920s *Major epidemics of sleeping sickness in Africa.*

1960s *Following some effective control pro-grammes, the disease re-emerges with serious epidemics,* including a million victims in the Congo basin.

1990s–present *Severe epidemics of sleeping sickness in Uganda, Sudan, Angola and the Democratic Republic of the* Congo, especially in wartorn areas and amongst refugees.

2000 *The Pan-African Tsetse and Trypanosomiasis Eradication Campaign is launched to tackle the huge impact* of African trypanosomiasis on human and animal popula-tions, to tackle the vector and ultimately to create tsetse fly-free zones.

Early 21st century *Geographical information systems are used to identify grazing areas at most risk and to predict tsetse fly environments, allowing more precise* monitoring. Control efforts lead to some decrease in the annual number of new cases reported.

2005 *The genome of trypanosomiasis is decoded, giving a boost to efforts to find effective treatments.*

scientists worked out the connection between the sleeping sickness of humans, the nagana suffered by cattle, and the stallion sickness of horses.

THE FIRST CLUES AND THE MISSED CONNECTIONS

Between the 1840s and 1880s, an unusual 'new' parasite was observed in fish, frogs, rats, camels and horses. In Paris in 1843 David Gruby (1810–98) saw the parasite in the blood of a frog, and called it *le tire bouchon* – French for 'corkscrew' – after the way it swam through its host, curling and spinning. The scientific name for the genus, adopted shortly thereafter, was *Trypanosoma*, from the Greek words *trupanon*, meaning 'borer' (as in trepanation, the ancient operation of drilling holes into the skull), and *soma*, 'body'.

In Algeria in 1891, Gustave Nepveu (1841–1903) saw and described '*a flagellated parasite*' in a patient with malaria. It was undoubtedly a trypanosome, but the significance of his observation was missed at the time.

The next breakthrough came in 1894 – but at this point the focus was on the animal, not the human form of the disease. David Bruce (1855–1931), a British army surgeon, and his wife Mary (1849–1931) were dispatched to Ubombo (South Africa) by the governor of Zululand, Sir Walter Hely-Hutchinson (1849–1913), to investigate an epidemic of nagana in cattle which were, so to speak, dying like flies. It took the couple several weeks to reach their destination.

It was in the makeshift laboratory that he set up on the verandah of their hut that Bruce, assisted by his wife, observed trypanosomes in blood slides taken from the sick cattle, describing the micro-organism as '*a curious little beast … a creature with a blunt rear end and a long slim lashing whip*'. Bruce then sent dogs and oxen into the 'fly belt' – when they returned and were examined, they too were infected with trypanosomes. His next step was to collect hundreds of tsetse flies from the 'fly belt' and bring them back to Ubombo. The flies were put in a cage made of muslin and left to feed on horses – which, after a month, sickened and died. There was compelling evidence that the tsetse fly might be responsible for the disease in cattle and horses, and that some wild game animals might be the reservoir for the parasite.

In 1899 the parasite found by Bruce in the nagana cattle was named *Trypanosoma brucei*, but still no connection was made with sleeping sickness in humans.

THE FINAL LINKS

Over the next decade, the pieces of the puzzle fell – somewhat haltingly – into place. In 1901 trypanosomes were found in a patient suffering from sleeping sickness in Gambia (see The Cases of Mr Kelly and Mrs S., page 99). At the same time, a major epidemic of sleeping sickness was sweeping through the new British protectorate of Uganda. The urgency of the situation was highlighted by Dr Albert Howard Cook (1870–1951) and his brother Dr John Howard Cook (1871–1946),

GLOSSINA PALPALIS, Rob. Desv.

A tsetse fly. There are a number of species transmitting the trypanosome parasite to humans and cattle. *Glossina palpalis* (above) is the principal vector in West and Central Africa and mainly inhabits humid forests bordering lakes and rivers. *Glossina morsitans* is found in dry savannah and scrub in East Africa. Inset: trypanosomes – the parasites responsible for trypanosomiasis – seen under a microscope.

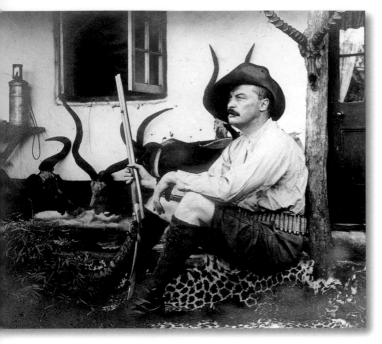

David Bruce, photographed outside his lodge in Ubombo, Zululand (now northern KwaZulu-Natal, South Africa), in the 1890s. Bruce was instrumental in making the link between the protozoan parasite that causes sleeping sickness and its tsetse fly vectors.

who were based at the Mengo Missionary Hospital in Uganda. Three researchers – Count Aldo Castellani (1878–1971), George Low (1872–1952) and Cuthbert Christy (1863–1932) – were sent out to Entebbe, Uganda, in 1902 by the British Foreign Office and the Royal Society of London to solve the puzzle of the human form of the disease. All three were looking for a bacterial cause of sleeping sickness – and so missed the real culprit, the parasitic protozoan.

Exasperated by their lack of results, David Bruce went to Entebbe 'to take control' of the investigation. In 1903 it was confirmed that the trypanosome parasites which caused the wasting disease in cattle were also responsible for human sleeping sickness. The question as to who found what, and who found it first, caused bitter controversy.

The next step was to find how the parasites were transmitted. In 1903 the tsetse fly, *Glossina palpalis*, was identified in Uganda as a vector, and in 1912 another species of tsetse fly in Northern Rhodesia (now Zambia), *Glossina morsitans*, was also found to be a vector. Moreover, it was realized that there were two sub-species of *Trypanosoma brucei*: *T. brucei gambiense* (which causes a chronic form of the disease that eventually leads to coma and death and is endemic in West and Central Africa) and *T. brucei rhodesiense* (which gives rise to an acute form found in East Africa and, if left untreated, kills in a few weeks). Bruce's contribution to their discovery is remembered in the names of both, and Bruce himself was given a knighthood.

The tsetse fly and the trypanosome parasite had finally been established as the links between the sleeping sickness of humans, the nagana of cattle and the stallion sickness or fly disease of horses. It was also discovered that game animals such as waterbuck, hartebeest and antelope could act as reservoirs for the trypanosomes but remain healthy. The trypanosome, adapted to mammalian and non-mammalian hosts, had found its perfect partner in the tsetse fly and, by doing little harm to some of its animal hosts, had evolved to allow the cycle to keep perpetuating.

Sleeping sickness – the 'colonial disease'

Devastating epidemics of sleeping sickness erupted in the British, Belgian, French, Portuguese and German colonies of Africa in the late 19th and early 20th centuries. Between 1896 and 1906, in the British protectorate of Uganda 250,000 Africans died of sleeping sickness and, in the Congo basin, half a million were killed by the disease. Epidemics from the 1920s through to the 1950s continued to claim many more thousands of lives in Africa. Sleeping sickness – which, if

THE CASES OF MR KELLY AND MRS S.

In May 1901, Mr Kelly, the 42-year-old master of the government steamer on the River Gambia in West Africa, began to feel vaguely unwell, with a slight fever. He consulted Dr Robert Michael Forde (1861–1948), the colonial surgeon, who suspected malaria and admitted him to hospital. Malaria was, however, quickly ruled out – Kelly didn't respond to quinine, and there were no malarial parasites in his blood. Dr Forde did, however, notice in some of the blood slides some strange 'wriggly worms', which he had never seen before. These parasites seemed to be more noticeable in the slides taken when Kelly's temperature rose. Forde thought there must be a connection between the 'worms' and the illness. But what?

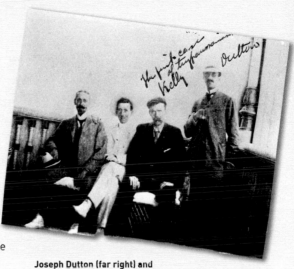

Joseph Dutton (far right) and Robert Forde (left) seen here with Mr Kelly (second from right) and an unknown fourth man.

In December of that year, Dr Joseph Everett Dutton (1874–1905), a young parasitologist from the newly founded Liverpool School of Tropical Medicine, visited the Gambia to conduct a malaria survey. When asked by Forde to look at Kelly's perplexing blood slides, Dutton immediately recognized the 'worms' as trypanosomes – which until then had only been associated with the nagana disease of cattle. Dutton sent a telegram to the Liverpool School: TRYPANOSOMA EUROPEAN, PECULIAR SYMPTOMS. DUTTON.

Kelly's condition showed no sign of improvement, and in 1902 he was sent home to England. His case was presented to the British Medical Association meeting in Liverpool. For some time Kelly continued to get more and more feverish – displaying the characteristic 'moon face' of sleeping sickness, an oedema caused by the leaking of small blood vessels. Eventually Kelly's heart gave up, and on 1 January 1903 he died.

In the meantime, Patrick Manson (1844–1922) in London was investigating a case of sleeping sickness in a Mrs S., a missionary's wife from the Congo. She had first consulted him in 1902 with a fever. The following year Mrs S. became very sick, and her illness was beginning to affect her central nervous system – one of the classic signs of the last stages of sleeping sickness. Mrs S. died in November 1903.

Mr Kelly and Mrs S. were the first two human cases of sleeping sickness to attract the attention of experts in tropical medicine in the early 20th century. The search was now on to find the cause and means of transmission of sleeping sickness in humans and nagana in cattle ...

left untreated, is invariably fatal – attracted huge attention from the colonial authorities. The horrors of the disease appalled the public back in Europe, persuading the colonial powers to send scientists out to Africa to elucidate its cause and to find a solution.

Once the cause of the disease was understood, intensive campaigns were launched in an attempt to control it. Many different methods were employed by the various colonial governments, including forced resettlement away from tsetse-infested areas, systematic surveillance and isolation of patients in lazarettos (quarantine stations), treatments using atoxyl, an arsenic derivative (which could have serious side effects, including blindness), bush clearance, and various attempts to break the cycle of transmission, such as the use of fly traps. Some of these measures conflicted with age-old traditional practices and were often deeply unpopular with the indigenous populations.

Historians looking back over the last 100 years or so have emphasized the inextricable links between sleeping sickness and the ecological disturbances and upheavals brought on by colonization. The opening up of new areas and population centres, the extension of trade routes into the Tsetse Belt, the modification of the environment, the movement of people to work in tsetse-infested areas, and the destruction of local practices that had for centuries enabled many small scattered groups to co-exist with the tsetse fly and the trypanosomes have all been cited as possible factors facilitating the spread of the disease. Concern for animal and human trypanosomiasis in the first half of the 20th century, it has been argued, was as much to do with its threat to the colonizers and the preservation of their health and economic activities as it was to do with the impact on the indigenous populations.

'I used to visit a beautifully equipped research institute outside Nairobi, in Kenya, which specialized mainly in trypanosomiasis, but I was surprised to find, on my first visit, that it was cattle trypanosomiasis that mattered most to them, since it was a major cause of meat shortages and mass under-nutrition.'

JOHN PLAYFAIR, *LIVING WITH GERMS* (2004)

SLEEPING SICKNESS BITES BACK

By the 1960s some progress in the battle against sleeping sickness had been made, and in the 1970s human cases of the disease had dropped to encouragingly low levels. But since then – following widespread political instability, civil wars, large-scale displacements of populations, economic decline, the breakdown of health services and the dismantling of disease-control programmes in many countries – the disease has resurfaced. There have been devastating epidemics in Uganda, the Democratic Republic of the Congo, Sudan, the Central African Republic and Angola, killing millions and disabling many. In some areas, the disease has appeared for the first time.

Today, trypanosomiasis ranks among the top ten diseases of Africa. It is one of several diseases affecting the poorer areas of the world that have been called the 'neglected diseases', because they have been largely overlooked by modern medicine (see Neglected Diseases, page 106). Given the economic and public-health impact of sleeping sickness, the funding for research into this important disease has fallen badly behind in recent decades.

FLY TRAPS, TRYPANO-TOLERANT COWS AND THE FUTURE

There have been a few glimmers of hope for African trypanosomiasis. The genome sequence of the trypanosome was decoded in July 2005 - offering the possibility of finding new ways of treating and preventing the disease. The latest fly traps impregnated with insecticides are proving successful. On the island of Zanzibar the tsetse fly has been eliminated by releasing sterile males into the wild fly population. Scientists have found one breed of African cattle, the n'dama, which, though not as high-yielding as the traditional zebu, is less susceptible to the disease. Researchers are aiming to breed 'trypano-tolerant' cattle, and there are now a number of trypanocidal drugs for both humans and cattle. One of these, eflornithine, is effective in the later stages of human sleeping sickness - hence its nickname, the 'resurrection drug'.

But there is still no vaccine, and some of the older drugs, based on arsenic derivatives, have nasty side effects. Eflornithine is only effective for *T. brucei gambiense* and is difficult to administer, requiring intravenous infusions four times a day (for one to two weeks). The tsetse fly bites during the day, so bed nets are no use. Many puzzles about the epidemiology and immunology of the disease persist, and there is still a long way to go before it can be effectively controlled.

There are currently 60 million people at risk, with about half a million new cases and possibly as many as 60,000 deaths every year. Three million cattle die each year and over 6 million square miles (15.5 million sq km) of land is precluded from stock production because of the presence of tsetse flies, adding to the misery, hunger and despair of many. Elimination of this disease - which has had, and continues to have, such an adverse effect on the world's poorest continent - must surely become a global health priority.

Screening for sleeping sickness in an African village in 2000. A mobile team sets up and takes a blood sample from each villager, which is then tested for the disease. Early detection of cases before the parasites start to destroy the central nervous system is essential for effective treatment.

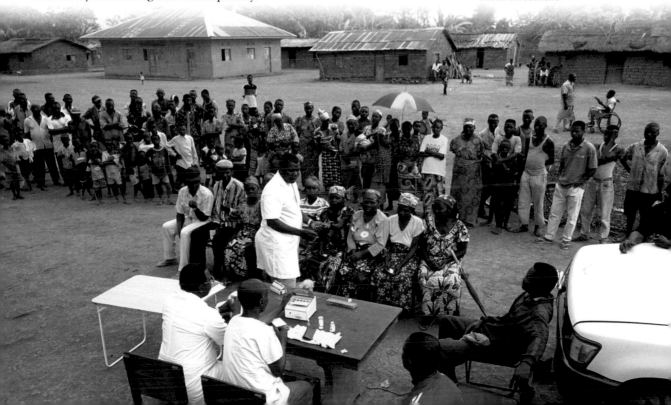

CHAGAS' DISEASE – also called American

trypanosomiasis – is a chronic parasitic infection. It may involve a range of symptoms, including irregularities in the heartbeat and digestive disturbances. The disease is confined to the western hemisphere, and is endemic in many regions of South and Central America and Mexico. Its causative agent, the protozoan *Trypanosoma cruzi*, is transmitted by the triatomine bug – an insect often known as the kissing or assassin bug. The parasite, the vector and the disease were discovered by the Brazilian scientist Carlos Chagas (1879–1934) in the first decade of the 20th century. Today, many millions of people are infected, and Chagas' disease is not only the most debilitating infectious disease in South and Central America, but also the leading cause of heart disease in young adults.

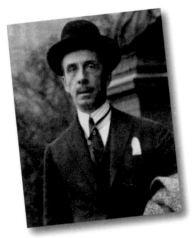

Carlos Chagas. The scientist had already established the main features of the disease before it was given his name.

Spanish and Portuguese missionaries and travellers in South America in the 16th, 17th and 18th centuries have left a number of accounts of the triatomine bug. These writers noted that by day the bug is *'afraid of the light'* and hides away in the thatched roofs and mud walls of huts. But at night, *'guided by the smell of people asleep'*, it drops down on to the face or head of those below. With a bite as *'delicate and sweet'* as a kiss, it gorges itself on the blood of its sleeping victim. As it withdraws, it *'leaves an intolerable pain and an itch that can hardly be borne'*. By the time it has had its blood meal, the bug resembles *'a fat grape ... as big as the tip of the little finger'*. One writer goes on to describe how *'as soon as it has digested, it defecates and this taint makes an indelible spot on the white linen ... and when crushed gives out a strong stench of bedbugs'*.

We now know that the parasitic protozoan that causes Chagas' disease is transmitted via the bug's faeces, when they are rubbed inadvertently into a person's eyes, mucous membranes or abrasions, or when he or she scratches the wound of the bite. The parasite then works its way into the bloodstream and ends up in the tissues of its unsuspecting victim, where it multiplies by binary fission. Infection results in clinical symptoms in a short acute phase followed by

timeline

2000+ years ago Archaeological and DNA evidence from mummies in northern Chile and southern Peru suggest that the disease has been around for millennia – possibly dating back to 9000 years ago.

16th–18th centuries AD Portuguese and Spanish explorers in South America describe the habits of the 'kissing bug'.

1835 *Charles Darwin (1809–82) describes being bitten by a huge triatomine bug in South America.*

1909 *Carlos Chagas (1879–1934) identifies the parasite responsible for Chagas' disease, the role of the triatomine bug as a vector and the first case of a 'new' human trypanosomiasis.*

1935 *Cecilio Romaña (1901–97), a physician from Argentina, describes the swelling at the site where the parasite enters the body – often near the eyelid. This is now known as Romaña's sign.*

1950s *Control programmes aimed at getting rid of the triatomine bug begin.*

1950s and 1960s *It becomes clear that the disease is widespread in South and Central America, although it has many different clinical outcomes.*

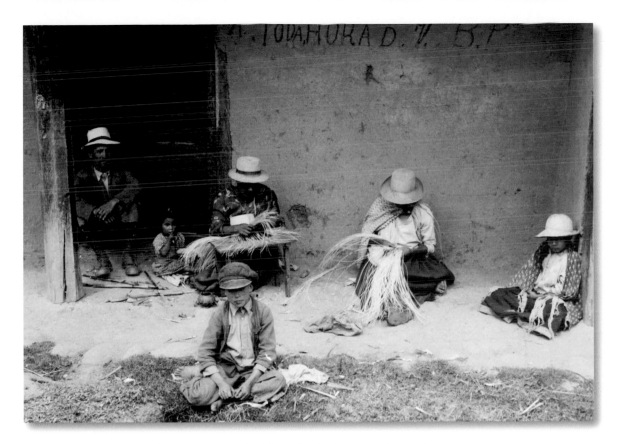

long-term chronic ill health. To complete the life cycle, the bugs can also suck up the parasite from the blood of an infected person or other vertebrate hosts when they feed. The parasite multiplies and develops in the bug's mid-gut and then moves down into its hind-gut, ready to 'assassinate' another sufferer. Gut infection in the insect persists for its whole life – which can be as long as two years.

A house in Ecuador in the early 20th century. Such dwellings were the ideal habitat for the vector of Chagas' disease – an assassin bug which hides away in crevices in walls and roofs.

THE DISCOVERIES OF CARLOS CHAGAS

Carlos Chagas (1879–1934) was a young Brazilian doctor appointed in 1902 to work at a new medical research institute in Rio de Janeiro (then the capital of the country), under the directorship of Oswaldo Cruz (1872–1917). From here, Chagas was sent in 1907 to Minas Gerais, in the interior of Brazil, to investigate and

1980s *Over 20 million people are thought to be infected with Chagas' disease in Latin America.*

1990s *The Southern Cone Initiative is established, followed by the*

Andean Countries Initiative (ACI) and the Central America Countries Initiative (CACI). Such programmes aim to rid the countries of Latin America of the triatomine bug via the application of insecticides.

2000–present *Some countries are declared possibly free of Chagas' transmission, including Brazil, Chile and Uruguay, and overall there is a reduction in the number of cases in Latin America*

from over 20 million in the 1980s to perhaps less than 8 million in 2006.

2005 *The genome sequence of the parasite causing Chagas' disease (along with those leading to African*

trypanosomiasis and leishmaniasis, known collectively as the 'trityps'), is announced. Researchers hope that this may lead to new methods of prevention and treatment.

2007 *Following some successes in eliminating the disease in certain regions, the World Health Organization establishes a new Global Network for Chagas' Elimination, with the aim of*

eradicating the disease entirely by the year 2010.

control a severe epidemic of malaria. While there, he became intrigued by frequent complaints of an insect which, he was informed, *'inhabits human dwellings, attacking man at night, after the lights are out, and hiding during the day in cracks of the walls'*. The locals, he said, called it *barbeiro* (the 'barber' bug) because of it tendency to bite people's faces. Chagas visited many infested homes, curious to find out more about this bug.

Between December 1908 and April 1909, Chagas identified the parasite and the role of the triatomine bug in its transmission. He first observed the parasites in the contents of the bug's hind-gut. The parasites seemed to be similar to – and yet subtly different from – the trypanosomes that had recently been implicated as a cause of African trypanosomiasis or sleeping sickness (see pages 94–101). Some of

DID DARWIN HAVE CHAGAS' DISEASE?

In 1835, while travelling around South America, the young naturalist Charles Darwin (1809–82) wrote a fascinating account of the triatomine bug, which he called the 'Benchuca':

> *'We slept in the village of Luxan, which is a small place surrounded by gardens, and formed the most southern cultivated district in the province of Mendoza [Argentina]; it is five leagues south of the capital. At night I experienced an attack (for it deserves no lesser name) of the Benchuca, a species of* Reduvius*, the great black bug of the Pampas. It is most disgusting to feel soft wingless insects, about an inch long, crawling over one's body. Before sucking they are quite thin, but afterwards they* become round and bloated with blood, and in this state are easily crushed. One which I caught at Iquique (for they are found in Chile and Peru) was very empty. When placed on a table, and though surrounded by people, if a finger was presented, the bold insect would immediately protrude its sucker, make a charge, and, if allowed, draw blood. No pain was caused by the wound. It is curious to watch its body during the act of sucking, as in less than ten minutes it changed from being as flat as a wafer to a globular form. This one feast for which the Benchuca was indebted to one of the officers, kept it fat during four whole months; but after the first fortnight, it was quite ready to have another suck.'*

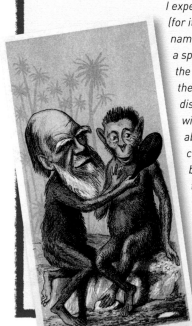

Charles Darwin, seen in a contemporary cartoon which lampooned his views on natural selection.

When Darwin returned to England he began to suffer from a bizarre range of symptoms, including flatulence, heart palpitations, insomnia and hysterical crying, which throughout the rest of his life often incapacitated him. There has been much speculation about the cause of Darwin's illness, including the suggestion that he suffered from Chagas' disease after being bitten by the bug. Retrospective diagnosis is, however, very hard to make, and it is possible we may never know with what illness, or combination of illnesses, Darwin was afflicted.

the bugs were sent back to the Oswaldo Cruz Institute, and their parasites were found to cause disease in monkeys. Chagas then noticed that it was a new species of trypanosome, which he named *Trypanosoma cruzi*, in honour of his mentor, Oswaldo Cruz. Shortly thereafter, returning to Minas Gerais, he discovered the

'While they suck blood, they do it with such care and sweetness, that it cannot be felt; but when they withdraw full, they leave an unbearable pain and itching …'

A DESCRIPTION OF THE 'KISSING BUG', BY JOSEPH GUMILLA (1686–1750)

same parasite in the blood of a sick young girl called Berenice. In April 1909 he announced the discovery of a new human trypanosomiasis. Finally, Chagas found that there were host reservoirs of the disease in animals other than humans. The disease itself was named 'Brazilian trypanosomiasis' but became more generally known as Chagas' disease (or Chagas disease) in honour of his work.

The discovery of all these aspects of the disease's cycle was an amazing achievement. One part of the puzzle that Chagas did not get right was the mode of transmission. Chagas thought that it was the bite of the triatomine bug that injected the disease into the human bloodstream. Emile Brumpt (1877–1951), a Parisian working in Brazil, showed in 1912 that the disease was transmitted not by the bite, but through infected faeces.

WHAT IS CHAGAS' DISEASE?

One of the difficulties faced by Chagas and his contemporaries was how to embrace a multitude of diverse and seemingly unrelated symptoms under the heading of 'Chagas' disease'. In the early decades of the 20th century, scientists investigating Chagas' disease in the bug-infested houses of South America came across people with all sorts of clinical problems, both acute and chronic. Chagas believed that *T. cruzi* infection caused neurological, cardiac and endocrine (mainly thyroid) problems. He thought that endemic goitre, which was common in regions where he found *T. cruzi* infection, was caused by this parasite. From the mid-1910s and through the 1920s, several scientists contested Chagas' claims about the endocrine and neurological forms of the disease. But his ideas about the role of *T. cruzi* in causing cardiac problems in young people were largely confirmed and extended, as was his hypothesis about digestive problems, such as difficulties in swallowing, known as *mal de engasgo*.

By the 1950s and 1960s, it became clear that the disease was indeed widespread and that it manifests itself in diverse and puzzling ways. In general, people experience an initial acute phase of fever and swollen lymph nodes, which may in a few cases prove fatal, especially in

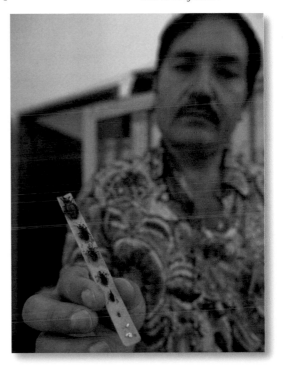

The triatomine bugs responsible for transmitting Chagas' disease via their faeces. The name *vinchuca* is used for the bug in Andean countries. It is derived from the Quechua language of the Incas and means 'that which falls to the ground'.

NEGLECTED DISEASES

Chagas' disease is one of a number of diseases now described as 'neglected diseases'. Such diseases are 'neglected' because they have failed to attract sufficient attention in terms of funding and research, and because their huge impact on the globe, especially amongst the poorer and most vulnerable populations of the tropics and sub-tropics, is often overlooked. It is estimated that 1 billion people – one-sixth of the world's population – are currently affected by one or more of these 'neglected diseases'. Various new initiatives have been launched to address the global problem of these diseases, which hopefully means that they will be neglected no longer.

children. Some of the infected patients, however, may notice a lesion where the bug has bitten and defecated. This sore at the point of infection is known as a 'chagoma'. The most recognized marker of the acute phase of Chagas' disease is called Romaña's sign, which is a swelling of the eyelids on the side of the face near the site of the bite or where the bug's faeces have been deposited or accidentally rubbed into the eye. However, in the majority of cases, it is only after perhaps ten to 12 years that the parasite's cruel attack on its human host becomes visible, when the chronic problems manifest themselves. By then the parasites have invaded some organs of the body, causing damage and swelling of the heart, damage to the intestines and oesophagus, and premature death, mainly by heart failure. The long period of latency makes early diagnosis and treatment difficult.

How to beat the bugs?

Most attempts to control Chagas' disease have been directed against the triatomine bug. In the 1940s the insecticide DDT proved ineffective, but other organochlorine insecticides, such as BHC and dieldrin, seemed to be much more potent. In 1948 two Brazilian researchers, Emmanuel Dias (1908-62) and José Pellegrino (1922-77), who had at that time concluded their experiments proving the efficacy of BHC, expressed to the Brazilian Ministry of Health in Rio de Janeiro their optimism that Chagas' disease would be soon eliminated. The first campaign against the triatomine bug was launched in 1950.

Their optimism has so far proved ill founded, although several programmes have been initiated in recent years with some success. A new programme launched by the World Health Organization (WHO) in 2007 aims to eradicate Chagas' disease by 2010. There are many complex and mysterious aspects of the disease, however, and these create major obstacles to control. Although transmission is primarily via the bug, the infection can also be passed on through blood transfusions or organ transplants from infected donors, by mothers to their unborn or breast-fed children, or by eating meat contaminated with the faeces of the bug. Some cases infected by blood or organ transplants have been identified

'They are as big as the tip of the little finger, longer, brownish and in the shape of beetles. They live in the ceiling of the houses and get out at night guided by the smell of people asleep, and getting down on the beds, bite cruelly, making a big wheal and sucking up to half a thimble full of blood.'

BERNABE COBO (1572–1657) DESCRIBES THE TRIATOMINE BUG AT WORK IN PERU

in non-endemic countries in Europe, and in Canada and the USA. Humans, as a source of parasites for the blood-sucking bugs, may remain infectious for years, and there is also a vast reservoir of the parasite in wild and domestic animals. In parts of South America the bug infests not only houses but also lives in palm trees. Breaking the chain of infection in some of the poorest areas of the world has been fraught with difficulties.

Today, there are glimmers of hope. In the 1980s over 20 million people were thought to be infected in Latin America. Since then, there have been enormous efforts in the region to control the infection, such that some current estimates suggest that less than 8 million people remain infected. Although there are two drugs that can be used in the early chronic phase, control primarily relies on killing the bugs in people's dwellings with insecticides, and substituting plastered walls and metal roofs for adobe-walled, thatch-roofed dwellings, so making them less appealing to the bugs.

A century after Chagas' discovery, Chagas' disease, like its Old World counterpart, African trypanosomiasis, is now dubbed one of the 'neglected' diseases of the 21st century (see Neglected Diseases, left). With a commitment by the WHO and other agencies to give more funding and attention to diseases of the poverty-stricken regions of the world, we can only hope that the target of eliminating Chagas' disease by the year 2010 will be achieved.

A public health campaign in Bolivia in 1997 graphically illustrates both the mode of parasite infection, via faeces, and the role of humans as a blood meal provider for the triatomine bug.

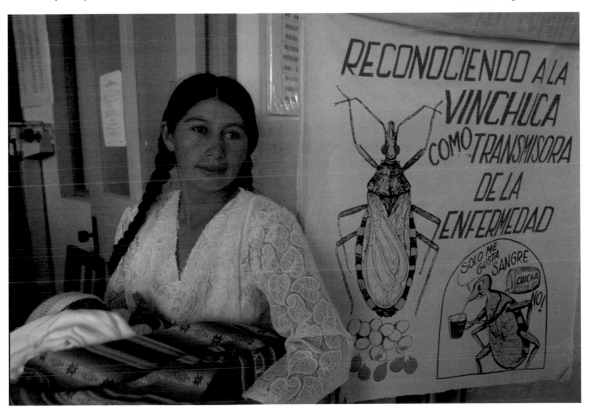

LYMPHATIC FILARIASIS

– or elephantiasis – belongs to a group of tropical diseases caused by thread-like parasitic roundworms (filariae) and their larvae (microfilariae) and transmitted to humans by mosquito bites. Lymphatic filariasis is caused by three types of worms, the most common of which is *Wuchereria bancrofti*. In its advanced stages the disease may cause damage to the kidneys and lymphatic system, as well as gross deformities (such as massive swelling of the limbs, breasts and genitals). With the discovery of the life cycle of the filarial worm and its transmission by mosquitoes in the later 19th century, scientists were optimistic that the vector and its disease could be eradicated. Today, however, millions continue to suffer from lymphatic filariasis.

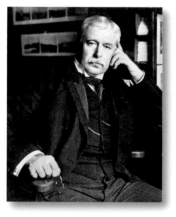

Sir Patrick Manson, the Scottish physician who first discovered that mosquitoes were vectors of lymphatic filariasis.

Lymphatic filariasis was probably known in parts of the ancient world, especially in the Nile Delta. Greek and Roman writers mention *elephantiasis arabum*, and the Persian physician Avicenna (980–1037) described the differences between leprosy and elephantiasis. The clearest early descriptions date from the 16th century, when European explorers in the tropics and sub-tropics witnessed numerous cases of the bizarre 'elephant leg' (the elephantine association derives both from the swelling of legs and genitalia and the rough texture of the skin). Around 1515 Tomé Pires, a Portuguese envoy in India, wrote:

> *'Many people in Malabar, Nayars as well as Brahmans and their wives – in fact about a quarter or a fifth of the total population, including the people of the lowest castes - have very large legs, swollen to a great size; and they die of this, and it is an ugly thing to see … '*

In the same era, Ralph Fitch, an Englishman in India, also noted:

> *'This bad water causeth many of the people to be like lepers, and many of them have their legs swollen as big as a man in the waste, & many of them are scant able to go.'*

timeline

c.2000 BC The swollen limbs of a statue of the Egyptian pharaoh Mentuhotep II suggest elephantiasis.

c.1100 BC Death of Natsef-Amun, a priest during the time of Ramses XI. A recent autopsy on his mummified body has revealed the presence of filarial worms.

AD 16th century Europeans travelling in Africa and Asia begin to bring back descriptions of elephantiasis.

1863 Larval stages (micro-filariae) are seen by the French surgeon Jean-Nicolas Demarquay (1814–75). Three years later they are also seen, independently, by Otto Henry Wucherer (1820–73) in Brazil. Wucherer's name is now remembered in the scientific term for one of the most common of the filarial worms, Wuchereria bancrofti.

1871 Timothy Lewis (1841–86), a British medical officer in India, discovers the presence of microfilariae in blood and urine. His announce-ment in 1872 of the vast number of worms circulating in the blood causes a great deal of scientific interest.

1877 Lewis names the adult male worm Filaria sanguinis hominis. He also recognizes a link with elephantiasis.

The English parasitologist Thomas Spencer Cobbold (1826–86) gives the name Filaria bancrofti (now Wuchereria bancrofti) to the female adult worm sent to him from Australia by Joseph Bancroft (1836–94), who had found it in the abscess of a patient.

Although the disease was chiefly prevalent amongst the local populations, Europeans could also contract it. In the West Indies it was not unknown for plantation owners to suffer from what was known as 'Barbados leg'.

SOMETHING IN THE WATER?

Prior to the later 19th century all sorts of ideas were postulated to explain what caused the disease (see, for example, The curse of St Thomas, below). Several writers noted the close association with 'bad water', even incriminating water in coconuts. Others implicated 'bad airs' or 'consumption of rotting fish'. Some blamed snake venom. One commentator mentioned *'the Knats which never ceas'd tormenting us'* in regions of elephantiasis, but it was not until the endeavours of Patrick Manson in 1877 that the pieces of the epidemiological puzzle began to fall into place.

Patrick Manson (1844–1922) was born in Aberdeenshire, Scotland. While a medical officer in the Imperial Maritime Customs Service in Amoy (now Xiamen) on the southeast coast of China, Manson operated on many elephantiasis patients. One of his patients was a street vendor *'who spread a cloth over his gross deformity and used it as a table to sell his goods'*. He was successfully treated, but, as Manson's son-in-law later recalled, *'instead of showing gratitude to his benefactor he tried to sue him for compensation for loss of his livelihood'*.

It was in Amoy in 1877 that Manson made his remarkable discovery: the mosquito was the 'nurse' of the filarial embryo (see Mosquito Manson, page 111). This was the first disease shown to be transmitted by an insect vector.

THE CURSE OF ST THOMAS

When the Dutch explorer Jan Huygen van Linschoten (1563–1611) visited the Portuguese colony of Goa on the west coast of India between 1588 and 1592, he reported on the belief that those suffering from elephantiasis were the descendants of the murderers of St Thomas the Apostle, who was said to have travelled to India:

' ... and they say that the progeny of those that slew him, are accursed by God, which is that they are all borne with one of their legges and one foote from the knee downewardes as thick as an Elephantes legge ... there are whole villages and kyndreds of them that are borne in the said land of St Thomas ...'

For some time afterwards, elephantiasis in the region became known as the 'curse of St Thomas'.

1877 *Patrick Manson (1844–1922) – later known as 'the Father of Tropical Medicine' – establishes that the filarial parasites are somehow transmitted by blood-sucking mosquitoes – the most significant* early discovery in tropical medicine.

1900 *George Carmichael Low (1872–1952) – following up a suggestion by Thomas Lane Bancroft (1860–1933), son of Joseph Bancroft – shows that it is the bite of the* mosquito that transmits the disease.

1944 *Discovery of diethylcarbamazine citrate (DEC), the first drug effective against filariasis. It is still used, in combination with more recently developed* drugs, such as albendazole and ivermectin.

1997 *The World Health Assembly passes a resolution to launch a Global Programme to Eliminate Lymphatic Filariasis (GPELF).*

2000 *The Global Alliance to Eliminate Lymphatic Filariasis (GAELF) is set up as a joint partnership between the public and private sectors. GlaxoSmithKline and Merck & Co., Inc. pledge to provide free all* the albendazole and ivermectin drugs necessary to eliminate the disease – the largest drug donations in history.

2005 *Annual mass drug administrations reach half of the estimated global* population at risk. However, many endemic areas (mostly in Africa) still remain to be covered. Over 120 million people are still infected, with more than 40 million incapacitated or disfigured by the disease.

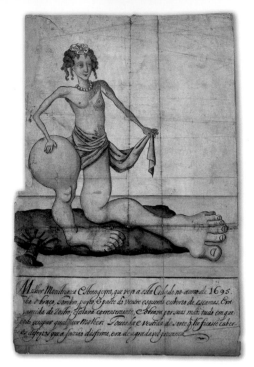

A watercolour from 1695 shows a woman with the rough skin and grossly swollen limbs which characterize lymphatic filariasis. The extreme swelling of the skin and subcutaneous tissue is caused by chronic lymphatic obstruction with filarial worms.

Manson had followed up ideas already put forward by others, especially those who had seen under the microscope 'thread-like worms' (larval microfilariae) in the blood and urine of patients. While being the first to discover the full life cycle of the worm that causes lymphatic filariasis, Manson nevertheless thought that the mosquito sucked up microfilariae from a patient in its blood meal, then when it died a few days later in stagnant water it released the parasite into the water. The next victim, Manson assumed, acquired the disease by drinking the contaminated water.

The final pieces of the puzzle were, however, put in place some 20 years later by the Australian parasitologist Thomas Lane Bancroft (1860–1933) and the Scottish physician George Carmichael Low (1872–1952), who were able to prove that the infective filarial larvae were transmitted not by ingestion but through the bite of the mosquito. By the 1900s the full life cycle of lymphatic filariasis had for the most part been established, though it was shown some time later that there are three different filarial worms capable of causing lymphatic filariasis, with different biological patterns and geographical distributions, and transmitted by different species of mosquitoes.

The most common filarial worm is *Wuchereria bancrofti*. Once in the human system its larvae make their way to the lymphatic vessels where they develop into adult worms and then mate. The adult females release millions of immature microfilariae (tiny larvae), which circulate in the blood, often for several years, and can be taken up by female mosquitoes when they suck blood from the infected human. After repeated infections, the worms lodged in the person's lymph nodes and vessels eventually cause extreme swelling – elephantiasis – of the limbs, breast or scrotum, as well as internal damage to the kidneys and lymphatic system. The disease is usually first contracted in childhood, but its devastating symptoms do not appear until some years later.

A WAY FORWARD?

Manson paved the way for others to unravel the life cycles of many other vector-borne diseases, such as malaria (see pages 84–93) and yellow fever (see pages 146–51). Manson himself hoped that his discovery would lead to the elimination of lymphatic filariasis. Sadly this has not yet come about, although there has in recent years been a push

'This unfortunate, sightless boy was affected in both legs with elephantiasis that he had sustained for a number of years. His ankles were thicker than the thighs; the feet were monstrous … covered with thick, yellowish crusts disposed in scales separated at intervals by deep ulcerated furrows from which oozed fetid, aqueous pus.'

FROM 'DESCRIPTION DE L'ÉGYPTE' COMPILED BY FRENCH SCIENTISTS ACCOMPANYING NAPOLÉON IN 1798

MOSQUITO MANSON

The filarial worm is transmitted to humans by the bite of various species of mosquito – *Culex*, *Aedes* and *Anopheles* – harbouring infected larvae.

In 1877 Patrick Manson (1844–1922), a Scottish physician working in Amoy, China, found microfilariae (larval worms) in the blood of dogs and humans, and had a hunch that perhaps some bloodsucking insect was responsible for transmitting the parasites. He ruled out fleas, lice, bugs and leeches, because they were all distributed far more widely than elephantiasis, but his suspicions fell on a species of mosquito common in Amoy. Manson had found microfilariae in the blood of his gardener Hinlo, and to test his hypothesis he kept Hinlo in a 'mosquito house', into which Manson released mosquitoes to feed on his blood. The mosquitoes were then recaptured in a wine glass and paralyzed with tobacco smoke. When Manson subsequently dissected them, he found larval stages of the filarial worm. The experiment was the first to demonstrate conclusively the insect-borne transmission of any disease.

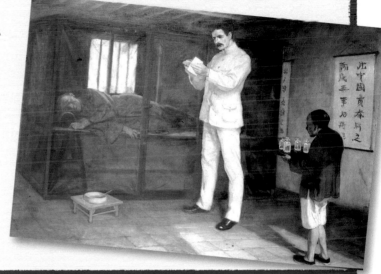

Patrick Manson experimenting with microfilariae on a human subject in China. This picture was painted *c.*1912 by E. Board.

by the World Health Organization and other agencies to interrupt the cycle of transmission and to alleviate the suffering and disabilities caused by the disease.

Unfortunately, efforts to control the mosquito vector using insecticides have not proved successful, but there are a number of microfilaricidal drugs that can kill the parasite in its larval stage and so block further transmission. The microfilaricidal drugs do not, however, kill the adult worm, so that annual treatment is necessary for at least six to eight years – the average lifespan of the adult worm in the human body. Medical care of sufferers also involves dealing with secondary bacterial and fungal infections of the limbs and genitals, which, with treatment and improved hygiene, can dramatically improve the condition.

Lymphatic filariasis, which affects millions of people in 83 countries, remains one of the leading causes of long-term disability in Africa, Asia, Latin America and many islands of the Pacific. For those who suffer from this disfiguring condition – which often affects prospects of marriage for young adults and prevents many sufferers from leading a normal life – there remains much to hope for.

SCHISTOSOMIASIS – also known as bilharzia

— is a nasty disease caused by a parasitic worm belonging to the genus *Schistosoma*, which spends its complex life cycle in both humans and aquatic snails. It is a disease that has been prevalent in China and the Nile Delta of Egypt since ancient times, and today in some villages in the tropics and sub-tropics up to 90 per cent of children may be infected with schistosome worms. The disease is found in areas where people are in close contact with the freshwater habitats of the snail vector. Schistosomiasis can be horribly debilitating, and while it has a low fatality rate it can, in severe cases, lead to chronic bladder, gastrointestinal or liver disease. Although there are effective drugs and an intensive control programme to eliminate the snail, schistosomiasis continues to infect over 200 million people worldwide.

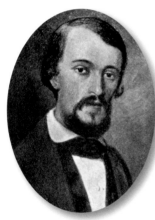

Theodor Bilharz was the first to observe the parasitic worms that cause the disease later to be known as schistosomiasis.

In 1851 a young German doctor called Theodor Bilharz (1825–1862) was working in the Kasr-El-Aini Hospital in Cairo as an assistant to Wilhelm Griesinger (1817–68), the personal physician of the khedive of Egypt. In Egypt at this time many people were afflicted with a strange disease characterized by 'bloody urine'. Bilharz was fascinated by the newly emerging field of helminthology – the study of worms – and while conducting an autopsy on a young man he saw in his portal vein (the great vein that carries blood from the stomach, intestines and spleen to the liver) a number of long white worms. As he peered down the microscope at one 'splendid' worm, he noticed that it had a flat body and a spiral tail. In a letter to his German professor, Carl von Siebold (1804–85), he described his exciting findings, and asked *What then is this animal?*

The first worm Bilharz observed was a male. On examining another specimen he saw, living and moving 'back and forth' within a groove of the male, a slender female worm complete with internal organs and eggs - *'similar to a sword in a scabbard'*. When Bilharz discovered eggs in the bladder wall of a patient, he and his fellow German scientists were quick to recognize that this parasitic worm, or blood fluke, was the likely cause of the 'bloody urine' infection that had plagued humans in the Nile Delta since the dawn of civilization.

timeline

c.1200–1000 BC Egyptian mummies dating from this period contain calcified worm eggs, suggesting schistosomiasis is an ancient disease.

AD 1808 The first clinical description of schistosomiasis is made by a French army surgeon, A.J. Renoult, who described its effect on Napoleon's army in Egypt in 1798.

1847 The Japanese physician Daijiro Fujii travels to Katayama Mountain, near Hiroshima, and describes the symptoms of 'Katayama disease'. According to

local legend, this was caused by the shipwreck of a cargo of lacquer, which poisoned the rice paddies. Fujii's description of the disease, now known to be the first written scientific account of Schistosoma

japonicum, does not come to light until 1909.

1851 Theodor Bilharz (1825–62), a German doctor, discovers the schistosome worm in Cairo, Egypt, during an autopsy. The following

year, with Wilhelm Griesinger (1817–68), Bilharz makes the connection with the 'bloody' urinary disease.

1881 British tropical disease expert Patrick Manson (1844–1922) speculates that a snail may be the intermediate host for lung fluke infection.

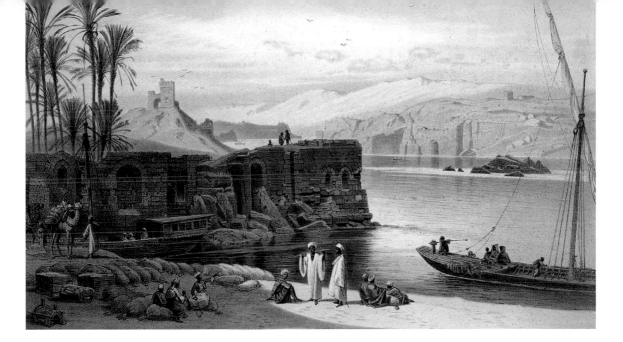

Opening up a can of worms — and finding the answers at a snail's pace

Bilharz's discovery left many questions unanswered. How did the worm enter the human body? Was it through drinking water? Was there an intermediate host before it entered the human? Some 50 years after Bilharz's discovery, the Scottish physician Patrick Manson (1844–1922) examined eggs that were different in shape from those Bilharz had observed in the bladder – the eggs Manson studied were in the faeces. Were there two forms of the disease – one of the urinary tract, the other the bowel – or did the eggs pass out of the body by either route?

Eventually, by 1915, British and Japanese scientists working independently had agreed on the central key to the puzzle – the worm spends part of its life cycle in freshwater snails. And its larvae (or cercariae), emerging from the snail into the water, can penetrate through the unbroken skin of anyone entering snail-infested rivers and lakes. Once in the human body, larvae enter the bloodstream and are carried to the blood vessels of the lungs. From there they migrate to the liver, where they mature and then move to the veins of the abdominal cavity or the bladder. The scientists also established that there were in fact three forms of the

The Nile Delta is one of many places worldwide where schistosomiasis has long been a scourge. In Egypt, the disease has been prevalent from at least the time of the ancient pharaohs.

1903 *Manson suggests there may be two forms of bilharzia with different shaped eggs – one, identified by Bilharz, affecting the bladder (S. haematobium), the other the bowel.*

1904 *Two Japanese physicians, Fujiro Katsurada (1867–1946) and Akira Fujinami (1870–1934), find eggs and adult worms in patients with Katayama disease, naming it S. japonicum.*

1907 *Louis Sambon (1866–1931), at the London School of Tropical Medicine, names the 'bowel' species S. mansoni.*

1908 *Arthur Looss (1861–1923), the German authority*

on parasitology in Egypt, refuses to believe there is more than one species of schistosome, so beginning a series of fierce quarrels with the British parasitologists.

1909–13 *Japanese scientists set up experiments with cattle to prove that the infection occurs through the skin.*

1910 *The British professor of bacteriology at the Cairo Medical School, Marc Armand Ruffer (1859–1917), discovers calcified eggs of S. haematobium in the kidneys of two mummies*

dating from the 20th dynasty (c.1250–1000 BC).

(continued ...)

113

disease, with different pathologies, different passages through the human body, different snail hosts and different geographical distributions.

OLD AND NEW NAMES AND A HOST OF DIFFERENT SPECIES

The disease became known in 1859 as 'bilharzia' or 'bilharziasis' in honour of its discoverer. Since the 1950s it has more commonly been called schistosomiasis – after its causal agent, the flatworm belonging to the genus *Schistosoma*. The name *Schistosoma* comes from the Greek *skhizein*, 'to split', and *soma*, 'body', referring to the way the female is enclosed in the deep cleft of the male during copulation.

Three main types of the disease were initially identified and named. *Schistosoma haematobium* was the disease first seen by Bilharz in Egypt. The worms live in the veins of the bladder and give rise to the blood (Greek *haema*) in the urine. *Schistosoma mansoni* was named after Patrick Manson, who speculated that a different species inhabits the gut. *Schistosoma japonicum*, also affecting the gut, was first identified in 1904 in Japan and, although now eradicated there, it remains a serious problem in parts of the western Pacific area.

Several new species have been discovered more recently: *S. mekongi* (in the Mekong basin of Laos and Cambodia); *S. malayensis* (in the Malaysian peninsula); and *S. intercalatum* (in the rainforest belt of Central Africa). Other species infect mammals and birds, and there are strains of the different species that are quite particular about which of any number of species of snail host they inhabit.

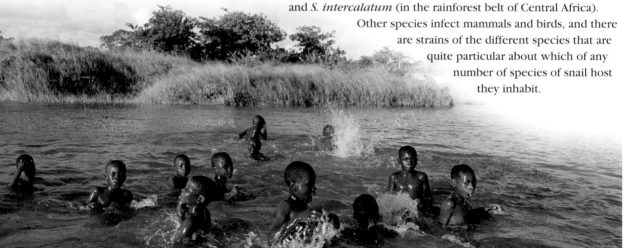

Boys swimming in a seasonal pool in Tanzania. Like many of the country's rivers and pools, it may be infected with schistosomiasis. The resulting clinical symptoms – which can include anaemia, diarrhoea and fatigue – can sap the energy of the infected, and, in serious cases, lead to chronic debilitating and life-threatening complications.

timeline

1914 British scientists Robert Leiper (1881– 1969) and Edward Atkinson (1882– 1929) go to Shanghai in China and Fujinami in Japan. They obtain snails from Katayama to explore the possibility of a snail host.

The whole life cycle of the infection in humans and its intermediate host, the snail, is published (in Japanese and in German)

Arthur Looss remains adamant

by Japanese scientists, describing for the first time the fork-tailed schistosome cercariae (larvae) emerging after a few weeks from snails.

1915 Robert Leiper leads a British Royal Army Medical Corps mission to Egypt

that humans are directly infected by the worm larvae and that there is no intermediate snail host.

and unravels the life cycle of schistosomiasis with the snail as intermediate host. He shows that there are two species of worm attracted to two different species of snail. His work gives little

acknowledgement to the earlier Japanese discoveries.

1930s–60s Various campaigns using a combination of molluscicides (to kill the snails), drugs (to treat

the disease) and improvements in sanitation (to break the cycle) are conducted with varying levels of success.

1944–5 Over 1000 American troops become infected with

The clinical manifestations and severity of symptoms are extensive, ranging from minor irritation at the point where the cerceriae penetrate the skin (often known as 'swimmer's itch') to debilitating and chronic ill health (with local names such as 'big belly' and 'Katayama disease') or, occasionally, life-threatening heart disease, kidney failure and bladder cancer. Much depends on the quirky behaviour of the various worms and their offspring inside and outside the human body.

MUMMIES AND EGGS

In 1910 Marc Armand Ruffer (1859–1917), a pioneer of palaeopathology, came across a remarkable discovery: in the kidneys of two Egyptian mummies he found the calcified eggs of a schistosome worm. The mummies were about 3000 years old – from the 20th dynasty of the New Kingdom (c. 1200–1000 BC). At Manchester University Museum in England, an International Ancient Egyptian Tissue Bank has been set up, with the prime aim of looking at mummies to trace the history and evolution of diseases over the past 5000 years. Using the latest non-invasive technology, scientists are revealing a wealth of information – including confirmation that schistosomiasis was undoubtedly prevalent in ancient Egypt at the time of the pharaohs.

Swimmer's Itch
The larvae of certain schistosome worms, parasitic in birds and other animals, may penetrate the human skin and cause dermatitis, sometimes known as 'swimmer's itch'. These schistosome larvae do not mature into adults. Such infections are found among bathers in lakes in many parts of the world, including the USA and UK.

Eggs of the schistosome worm have also been found in a corpse buried in the province of Hunan in China more than 2000 years ago. Schistosomiasis presumably became a significant human infection in river valleys, such as the Nile in Egypt and the Yellow (Huang He) River in China, when people began to settle, farm and irrigate their land. Snails like to lie on the surface of freshwater plants or hide in reed beds along the banks of rivers and lakes. How, when and why the schistosome worm first appeared on the scene is a puzzling question, but it seems likely that when humans began to use snail-infested waters for domestic and agricultural purposes, the cycle of disease began.

The finding of eggs in mummies and corpses is not simply a reminder of the antiquity of this disease – it is also a key to one of the many peculiarities of schistosomiasis. Unlike many other worm infections, it is not the adult or larval worms that cause the disease – but the eggs. The female worm lays hundreds of eggs each day, and can keep reproducing for several years. About half the eggs

schistosomiasis after landing at Leyte in the Philippines during the Second World War. An extensive campaign is initiated using posters and cartoons to teach soldiers how to prevent infection.

1960s The Aswan High Dam in Egypt and the Volta project in Ghana create vast artificial lakes that prove ideal breeding grounds for the freshwater snail – the intermediate vector in the

life cycle of schistosomiasis.

1970s Three new drugs come on the market for schistosomiasis. One – praziquantel – is hailed as a 'wonder drug'.

2000 The Schistosomiasis Control Initiative (SCI) is launched. In 2002 it receives substantial grants from the Bill and Melinda Gates Foundation to enable it to proceed with implementing and

evaluating control programmes.

2001 Partners for Parasite Control programme (PPC) is launched to tackle worm diseases, with the aim of treating ('de-worming') at least 75 per cent

of all school-aged children at risk by the year 2010.

2007 About 200 million people are infected with schistosomiasis in Africa, Asia, South America and the Caribbean, 80 per cent of them living

in sub-Saharan Africa. The annual mortality is estimated to be in excess of 250,000.

pass out in the urine or faeces, and then hatch in fresh water, after which the larvae enter and live in freshwater snails, thus perpetuating the cycle. The rest of the eggs lodge in the tissues of the liver, bladder or intestine, depending on the species, resulting in the formation of obstructive nodules called glandulomas.

The toll of schistosomiasis

Schistosomiasis has, over the past centuries, taken a huge toll on populations living in areas where the disease is endemic – costing lives, stunting the growth of children, impeding development and seriously affecting productivity through its debilitating effects on the human body.

The effect on communities living and working in the Nile Delta in Egypt has probably been one of the most dramatic examples of the insidious and destructive nature of schistosomiasis. As irrigation schemes were changed or expanded to improve productivity of crops, so people wading and working in the snail-infested waters became more and more at risk from the disease, and, in turn, by urinating or defecating in or near the water, they perpetuated the cycle – from humans to snails and back to humans.

Can the disease be eradicated?

There have been a number of campaigns to control the disease, including that mounted by the Rockefeller Foundation against schistosomiasis and hookworm in Egypt in the 1930s. The Second World War brought schistosomiasis to international attention when Allied soldiers were affected during operations in China, the Philippines and other Pacific islands. Programmes in the Philippines, Japan, China, Venezuela, Puerto Rico and Israel during or shortly after the Second World War were set up to 'defeat' the snail. At a time when the disease was believed to affect up to 150 million people, campaigns were primarily directed against the snail, using molluscicides (initially copper sulphate, and later a range of chemicals including niclosamide). These campaigns also involved mass treatment of infected populations using tartar emetic and other highly toxic drugs. The provision of latrines and improved sanitation was also vital in breaking the cycle, but the effectiveness of efforts to link control with health education and improvements in social and economic conditions have been variable. There have been outstanding successes in some parts of the world, but in others the disease has become, if anything, even more widespread today than it was in the past.

In the 1960s the Aswan High Dam scheme in Egypt, built to provide hydroelectricity and irrigation, created vast artificial lakes, such as Lake Nasser (seen here). These make ideal breeding sites for the snails which are the intermediate host in the life cycle of the parasitic worms causing schistosomiasis.

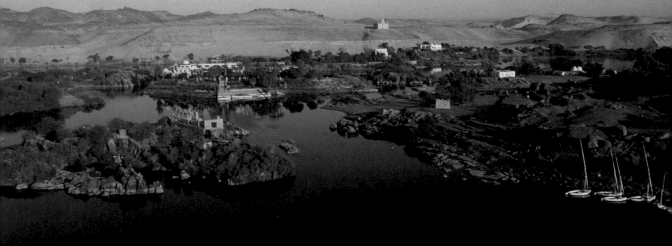

WORMS OF ALL SHAPES AND SIZES

Worms – or helminths' – come in all shapes and sizes: roundworms, hookworms, pinworms, flatworms, whipworms, threadworms and tapeworms. Parasitic worms can be microscopic or can reach several metres in length. Humans are host to at least 300 types of parasitic worms, and many have been around for thousands of years. Worms have been found in dessicated or fossilized human faeces from earliest times.

Some 4 billion people in the world today carry intestinal worms, while perhaps 400 million have worms in their liver, lungs, blood or tissues. The thought of worms penetrating and wriggling through the skin, invading tissues, living, mating and laying eggs in our bodies, exiting through urine or stools, being coughed up or crawling out of legs is enough to make anyone squeamish.

Over the centuries, people have sought ways to kill or get rid of worms. Various concoctions such as turpentine or wormwood have been used to poison the worms. Castor oil, liquorice and other plant extracts have been given to people as purgatives. The Guinea worm (*Dracunculus medinensis*) has traditionally been extracted by winding it round a stick.

There are effective drugs for some helminth infections. The best way is to break the cycle of contact between worms and humans – ideally by improvements in hygiene and public health. Even simple solutions – such as wearing shoes, having access to safe water, washing hands, or cooking food properly – can have huge benefits. One of the most remarkable programmes has been the near elimination of the Guinea worm, which causes a disease called dracunculiasis, through a concerted campaign to filter drinking water.

One of the many formidable campaigns to eradicate schistosomiasis was launched in 1949 by China. At the start of the campaign, some 10 million Chinese were heavily infected with worms. The Chinese used many different approaches to target the disease and employed millions of farmers, barefoot doctors and others in the 'People's War against the Snail'. It is even said that peasants walked through irrigation ditches plucking snails one by one - using chopsticks. Today schistosomiasis has been eliminated from many, though not all, parts of China. In other areas of the world, the construction of dams, reservoirs and irrigation canals for hydroelectric power and agriculture has allowed the snail population to explode massively. In some villages, many of the children have subsequently become burdened with worms.

The first drugs to be developed for schistosomiasis were highly toxic and nearly as bad as the disease itself. Since the 1970s three new drugs have come on the market. One - praziquantel - is safe and effective against all schistosome species, but it does not prevent re-infection, and the cost and logistical difficulties of treating people with the drug in the poorest parts of the world are huge. The World Health Organization in the last decade has set up a worldwide Schistosomiasis Research Project with the aim of developing new methods of preventing, diagnosing and treating the disease. Global eradication in the near future is, however, unlikely, and today schistosomiasis remains, after malaria, the second most serious parasitic disease in the world, infecting over 200 million people, especially school-age children and young adults, in 70 countries of the developing world.

HOOKWORM is a parasitic infection caused by a bloodsucking

roundworm. It is a disease that has affected humans since ancient times. Its chief symptom is severe anaemia, which leaves the sufferer physically weak, lethargic and incapacitated. One of the first major campaigns to control an infectious disease was that launched by the Rockefeller Sanitary Commission in the early 20th century in an attempt to eradicate hookworm from the southern states of the USA. This was succeeded by a number of international anti-hookworm programmes. Today, however, there are still as many as 800 million to 1 billion people infected with hookworm in the developing nations of the tropics and sub-tropics.

The lethargy resulting from the anaemia caused by hookworm led the Chinese in the third century BC to call it the *'able-to-eat-but-lazy-to-work yellow disease'*. In the early 20th century a journalist in the southern states of the USA dubbed it *'the germ of laziness'*. In Egypt in the 19th century it became known as 'tropical chlorosis', reflecting the pallor and greenish yellow skin of those afflicted (rather like the anaemic Victorian girls in England who were diagnosed with 'chlorosis' or 'green sickness'). It has also been called 'angel wings' or 'pot belly' because it can lead to misshapen shoulder blades and a distended abdomen. Other names, such as 'ground itch' or 'dew poison' in the southern USA, and 'water itch' or 'coolie itch' in India, have been used to describe the initial dermatological symptoms, when the larval hookworms penetrate the skin of the feet. Its scientific name, ancylostomiasis (from Greek *ankulos*, 'hooked', and *stoma*, 'mouth'), was coined in the mid-19th century.

The 11th-century Persian physician Avicenna (980–1037), seen opposite expounding pharmacy to his pupils, discovered hookworm in some of his patients and even linked the infestation with their disease.

AN ANCIENT INFECTION

The many colloquial names (there are over 150) reflect the breadth of symptoms, characteristics and outcomes of this nasty disease. Although only a small proportion of those infected eventually die from the disease, it can lead to severe iron-deficiency anaemia, protein malnutrition and chronic ill health, which, in turn, can have serious consequences for daily life and intellectual and physical

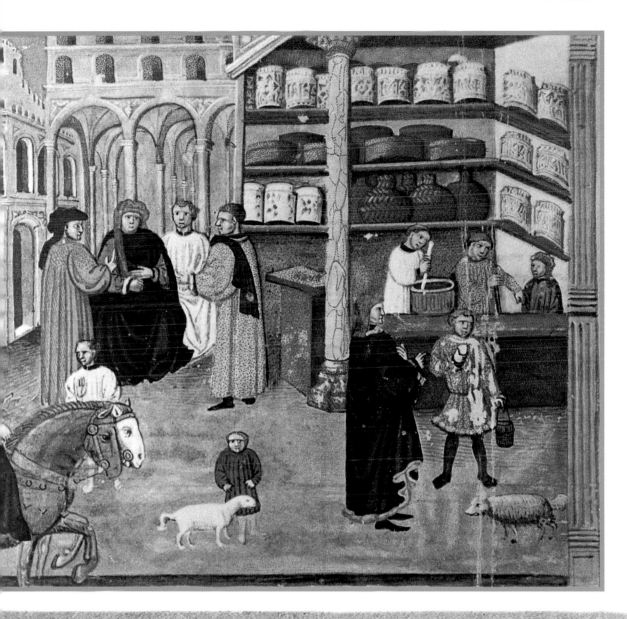

1902 *Charles Stiles (1867–1941) identifies a second species of hookworm, which he names Necator americanus ('American killer'). This species is soon found in other places, such as Africa, India and Australia.*

1903–14 *Anti-hookworm campaigns take place in Costa Rica and in Puerto Rico, where the disease is rampant among workers in the sugar-cane fields.*

1909–10 *The Rockefeller Sanitary Commission for the Eradication of Hookworm Disease is set up, initially focused on the southern states of the USA but later extended to other parts of the 'Hookworm Belt'.*

1913 *The Rockefeller Foundation, based in New York City, is created, with its central mission 'to promote the well-being of mankind throughout the world'.*

1914–1920s *Rockefeller anti-hookworm programmes are set up in many parts of the world, but the disease proves very hard to eliminate.*

1960s *By this time hookworm is largely* neglected by the global medical community.

2000 *The Human Hookworm Vaccine Initiative (HHVI) is set up to develop a safe, efficacious and cost-effective vaccine.*

2001 *The World Health Organization (WHO) advocates the anti-helminthic treatment ('de-worming') of 75–100 per cent of all at-risk school-aged children by the year 2010.*

development. If left untreated, those with a heavy worm load – maybe with some hundreds or thousands of worms drinking blood from their gut – are barely able to carry out even the most simple everyday activities. Its threat to pregnant women is especially serious, with an increased risk of death and complications for both mother and infant.

Eggs and larvae, possibly of hookworms, have been found in human coprolites (fossilized faeces) from Brazil dating from 430 to 340 BC, while the remains of adult worms have been discovered in the intestines of an ancient Peruvian mummy dating from about AD 900. There are also a number of early written records of a hookworm-like anaemia, including hieroglyphic entries in the Egyptian Ebers Papyrus (c.1550 BC) and descriptions in the Hippocratic Corpus (fifth century BC) – all suggesting that humans in many parts of the world have long been plagued by this debilitating scourge.

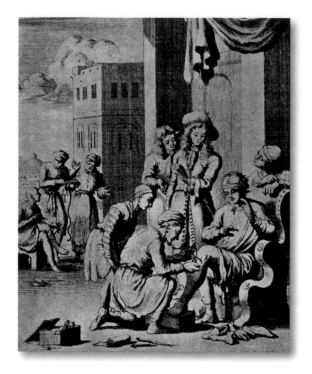

A historical illustration showing a surgeon extracting a guinea worm from a man's leg. In the background, after a successful operation, another surgeon is holding a long worm. Guinea worms are one of the many other worm diseases of the ancient and modern world.

A YEAR IN THE LIFE OF A HOOKWORM

Like many worm infections, the life cycle of the hookworm - inside and outside the human - is extraordinary. The adult worm, which is about 1 centimetre (0.4 in) long, lives in the small intestine, where it attaches itself to the lining and feeds on blood. One species of human hookworm, *Ancylostoma duodenale*, locks itself on with its sharp teeth, while the other species, *Necator americanus*, uses cutting blades. The female lays her eggs - up to several thousand a day - in the host's intestine, from where they are passed out in the faeces.

In areas of the world where human faeces are left untreated in backyards or spread onto the fields to be used as fertilizer, the eggs hatch in the warm, moist soil and grow through three larval stages. The third stage, known as 'wriggling larvae', can then penetrate through the skin of anyone living or working barefoot in contaminated areas.

'[If a person were freed of hookworm, he would have] more money in his pocket with which to buy better food, better clothes, better houses and better schools. With better schools there will come enlightenment. Intelligence will displace ignorance, and with intelligence there will come a true social revolution.'

AN OFFICER OF THE ROCKEFELLER COMMISSION IN MEXICO, 1925

In the next phase, the larvae that have burrowed through the skin, most usually through the feet, make their way via the bloodstream to the lungs. But rather than settle here, they continue to migrate through the respiratory tract to the back of the mouth, where they are swallowed. And so the larvae return to the gut, where they become adults, mate, lay eggs and live for up to a year or more on human blood. Somehow, throughout its life, the adult parasite has a way of keeping its host alive and the blood flowing.

The main stages of this intricate life cycle were unravelled by a number of scientists from the mid-19th to the early 20th century. These researchers painstakingly looked at the intestines of cadavers and endless stool samples, examined the worms under the microscope, measured 'worm burdens', and watched as larvae placed on skin burrowed and disappeared, leaving only their 'abandoned cuticles' on the surface. One of the most remarkable investigations was the 'accidental' experiment of Arthur Looss in the late 19th century (see Wormy Tales, below).

'THE GERM OF LAZINESS'

In 1909 the Reverend Frederick T. Gates (1853–1929) and Dr Wallace Buttrick (1888–1926), both Baptist pastors, were on a trip

WORMY TALES The first key scientist to report on the discovery of a hookworm in a human was the Italian physician Angelo Dubini (1813–1902), when in 1838, during an autopsy, he saw the worms in the bowel of a peasant. In 1854 Wilhelm Griesinger (1817–68), a German physician working in Egypt, suggested there was a connection between the worm and the disease known as 'tropical chlorosis'. Further evidence came during an epidemic of anaemia and diarrhoea among Italian workmen digging the St Gotthard Rail Tunnel in the Alps in the 1880s. Hundreds of miners were examined and found to be infected with hookworm; one postmortem examination in Turin found 1500 worms in a single miner. The link between worm infestation and anaemia was established. Scientists also noted that the men had to defecate in the 9-mile (15-km) tunnel, and often wore worn-out shoes. But just how did the worm get into the human body?

When the German scientist Arthur Looss (1861–1923) was working in Cairo, Egypt, in the late 19th century, he accidentally spilled a culture containing hookworm larvae on his hand. His hand began to turn red and burn – and two

Coloured scanning electron micrograph of the head of the hookworm, *Ancylostoma duodenale*.

months later, examining his stools, he found the eggs of the hookworm. After several experiments – including one in which he put larvae on the leg of a boy who was to have it amputated – Looss was able to confirm in 1901 that the hookworm larvae entered the body through the skin.

Looss is not the only scientist to have discovered the pathway of worms – albeit, in his case, accidentally. The Italian scientist Giovanni Battista Grassi (1854–1925) infected himself with the eggs of *Ascaris lumbricoides* (the large roundworm) and subsequently found eggs in his faeces. In the mid-19th century Friedrich Küchenmeister (1821–90), in much criticized experiments, fed pig meat containing some worm larvae to two criminals who were condemned to death, and subsequently recovered adult tapeworms – one of them 1.5 metres (5 ft) long – from their intestines after they had been executed.

'[Hookworm,] silent and insidious ... in my view outranks all other worm infections of man combined ... in its production, frequently unrealized, of human misery, debility, and inefficiency in the tropics.'

NORMAN STOLL, ROCKEFELLER SCIENTIST, 1962

Hookworm was rife among poor people in the southern US states during the early 20th century. Up to 40 per cent of the population may have been suffering from the disease.

to the southern states of the USA. They were travelling in luxury in the private railroad car of the oil magnate John D. Rockefeller Senior (1839–1937) to investigate the prevalence and consequences of hookworm. As they looked out of the windows they saw scenes of unimaginable poverty and despair – pallid, listless children with pot bellies and matchstick-thin legs, dull-eyed and stunted in growth. Such sights were to have a profound impact on the understanding of the so-called 'germ of laziness' and led to one of the first major philanthropic public-health initiatives.

At that time the 'Hookworm Belt' extended across many parts of the globe, between latitudes 30° S and 36° N, with extensive foci in Latin America and the southern states of the USA. Hookworm was also a common condition amongst miners and construction workers in underground tunnels in temperate countries. Gates and Buttrick were able to persuade Rockefeller to fund a commission to mount a major anti-hookworm campaign in 11 southern states of the USA. The commission was headed by Wickliffe Rose (1862–1931), and the chief scientist was Charles Wardell Stiles (1867–1941), nicknamed the 'Privy Councillor' (because of his insistence on hygiene and clean privies).

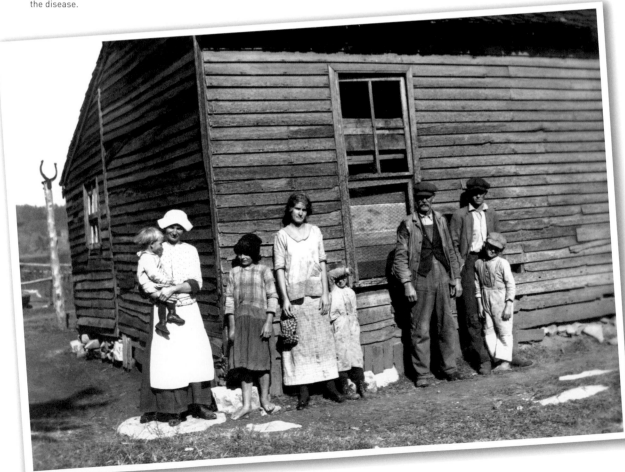

The prime emphasis of the campaign was health education, aimed at over 1 million people. Some 25,000 public meetings were held, more than 2 million handbills were distributed, stool samples were collected, and people were taught the importance of wearing shoes, how to build sanitary privies and about the significance of hookworm as a major factor in ill health and low productivity. The campaign also dispensed thousands of treatments – although the first drug used to kill the worms, thymol, could have toxic side effects.

In the days before wireless and TV, this campaign was a massive public-health enterprise. It had some immediate successes in reducing the burden of hookworm, but it proved hard to eliminate the infection entirely. There was also some public resistance to the programme – it was rumoured that the shoes being 'peddled' were made in Rockefeller-owned factories. In the first two decades of the 20th century, many other anti-hookworm programmes were set up around the world. But in spite of intensive efforts, the results were often negligible, and by the mid-1920s disillusionment had set in.

Although not without critics, Rockefeller's enduring legacy was to pave the way for the development of other major international public-health programmes. His commission also acted as a model for the League of Nations Health Organization, set up after the First World War, and its successor, the World Health Organization, established in 1948.

HOOKWORM AND HUMAN HEALTH

Hookworm has receded or disappeared from some parts of the world over the last century, but has remained a continuous though often neglected problem in many parts of the tropics and sub-tropics. The USA is now virtually free of the disease, as are Europe and Japan. In part, these successes can be attributed to specific anti-hookworm campaigns, but perhaps more broadly to improved living conditions, better sanitation, greater public-health awareness, and the availability of safe and effective anti-helminthic ('de-worming') drugs, and of iron supplements to counteract the anaemia. Endeavours to find an effective vaccine are currently under way, which could transform future control programmes and reduce dramatically the human suffering caused by hookworm.

In the meanwhile, tackling the remaining endemic foci of hookworm and breaking its cycle are still enormous tasks in the impoverished rural areas of sub-Saharan Africa, Southeast Asia, China and Latin America, where the disease remains entrenched.

THE TURN OF THE WORM

In 2006 scientists at Nottingham University in Great Britain infected themselves with hookworm larvae – deliberately. They had discovered that hookworms produce chemicals that can calm the human immune system, possibly reducing symptoms of allergic diseases such as hay fever and asthma. But before testing out the worms on patients they needed to find out just how safe worm infestation is. So they volunteered themselves. The worm's potential as a form of biotherapy is currently being tested.

Hookworms are being investigated for other medical uses. The worms produce molecules that clasp perfectly with clotting factors in human blood, and biotechnology companies are now putting them through trials to assess their potential value as blood thinners for surgery.

ONCHOCERCIASIS – which is often known as 'river blindness' – is a chronic parasitic disease

caused by a filarial worm, *Onchocerca volvulus*, and transmitted from person to person by the bite of an infected female blackfly of the genus *Simulium*. The small, fiercely biting blackfly breeds in fast-flowing rivers in the tropics and sub-tropics, and for centuries the disease has plagued people living in the vicinity of such rivers. As well as being a leading cause of blindness, especially in Africa, onchocerciasis has had serious economic consequences. There is, however, some hope for the millions still at risk following a successful Onchocerciasis Control Programme in West Africa initiated in the 1970s, aimed at eliminating the blackfly and treating the disease.

For people living in many parts of the tropics and sub-tropics, the river valleys have always been the most productive areas, offering fertile soils, fish and fresh water. But they are also the favoured breeding grounds of the blackfly. In the past, to farm and survive in such areas often became economically impossible. Settlements were frequently abandoned as those tormented by swarming flies, skin lesions, unbearable itching and progressive blindness moved away from the rivers to healthier but less fertile lands. In the drier uplands the pressure on the land led to erosion and poor harvests – and so set up a vicious circle that has been described by one scholar as *'a cyclical pattern of advance and retreat'*, with farmers *'caught between malnutrition and land shortages on the one hand and the perils of onchocerciasis on the other'*.

'Nearness to rivers can eat your eyes.'

AFRICAN PROVERB

It took many decades for scientists to unravel the life cycle of the disease, and to recognize its role in mass blindness and the abandonment of riverside settlements.

CRAW-CRAW, WORMS AND BLACKFLIES

In 1875 Irish naval surgeon John O'Neill (1848–1913), who was working in Addah Fort Hospital in the Gold Coast (now Ghana), examined and described minute filarial larvae measuring about 0.25 mm (1/100th of an inch) long. Under the microscope, O'Neill had seen these microfilariae wriggling, twisting, curling and coiling in skin snips cut off with a scalpel from patients suffering from 'craw-

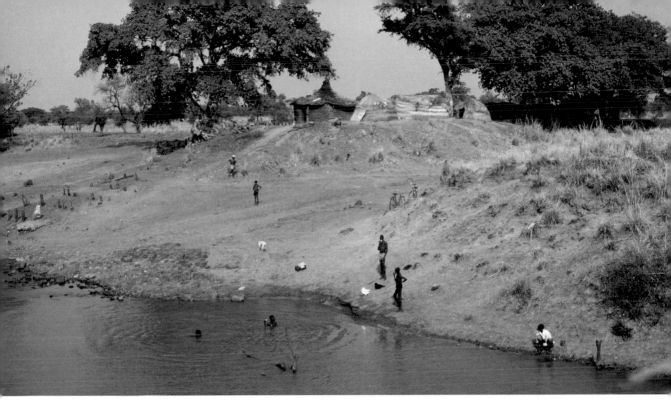

craw'. Craw-craw (or *kru kru*) was the local name for a condition that gives rise to intense itching that can be so maddening that sufferers use knives and stones to scratch themselves. Some are even driven to suicide. We now know that craw-craw is in fact one of the characteristics of the early stages of onchocerciasis. O'Neill noted that sulphur, used to treat scabies, was ineffective against craw-craw and was intrigued by the question as to how the worms, seen under the microscope, entered the human body.

Around this time various scientists – including the Scottish physician Patrick Manson (1844–1922), known as the 'father of tropical medicine' – were beginning to suspect that parasitic infections might be transmitted to humans by insect vectors. A number of culprits were suggested for craw-craw, including bedbugs, ticks, mosquitoes and the Congo floor maggot. It was not until the 1920s, following the studies of the Guatemalan investigator Rodolfo Robles (1878–1939) in the Americas and the Scottish parasitologist Donald Breadalbane Blacklock

Villagers in Burkina Faso in West Africa bathe in a river which has been made safer following a World Health Organization project to control onchocerciasis. This photograph was taken in c.1980.

1932 *Jean Hissette (1888–1965), working in the Belgian Congo (now the Democratic Republic of the Congo), suggests that the eyes of* sufferers of river blindness might be infected by the microfilariae. In the ensuing years it is realized that onchocercal blindness in Africa is widespread. **1930s–1960s** *Various schemes get under way in endemic areas to reduce the number of blackflies, initially by clearing vegetation in* streams where the blackfly breed, and from the late 1940s using chemical larvicides, including DDT. **1974** *The Onchocerciasis Control Programme in West Africa begins, followed by the African Programme for Onchocerciasis* Control and the Onchocerciasis Elimination Programme for the Americas.

1988 *Introduction of ivermectin, a microfilaricide,* donated free by Merck and Co. to all those who need it for as long as necessary. It is described as 'one of the milestones of tropical disease treatment'.

(1879–1955) in Sierra Leone, that the blackfly (also known as the 'coffee fly' or the 'buffalo gnat') was finally incriminated in the transmission of the disease.

What these studies revealed was that the infectious agent, the filarial worm *Onchocerca volvulus*, is transmitted through the bite of infected female blackflies of the genus *Simulium*. In the human host the adult worms live in nodules in the skin, producing over 1000 eggs per day. The larval worms (microfilariae) migrate from the nodules, mainly to the skin and eyes. When a female blackfly next takes her blood meal from an infected host she ingests any living microfilariae, which after a period of further development are ready to be passed on through her bite to the next person in the chain. Once infected, people can continue to infect flies as long as the adult worms produce microfilariae, often for ten to 15 years. The clinical manifestations of onchocerciasis - agonizing itching, visual impairment and eventual blindness - are due to an inflammatory response to dead or dying microfilariae. In a heavily infected person, 100,000 or more microfilariae die daily.

Photomicrograph of a nodule of the type which typically occurs over bony protuberances caused by the presence of the filarial worm *Onchocerca volvulus*.

At first, researchers focused their attention on the skin lesions and pigment changes, especially prominent on the lower limbs (known as 'leopard skin'). Loss of skin elasticity and other complications, including 'hanging groin', were also striking features, but the fact that the microfilariae reach the eyes and cause blindness was not fully appreciated until the 1930s. Indeed it was only in the 1940s that the association between widespread depopulation of river valleys, mass 'river blindness', onchocerciasis and the blackfly vector finally became clear.

HOPE FOR THE FUTURE

In 1974 the serious impact of onchocerciasis, especially in Central and West Africa, led the World Health Organization (WHO) to initiate a major campaign to eliminate the disease. At the start of the programme more than a

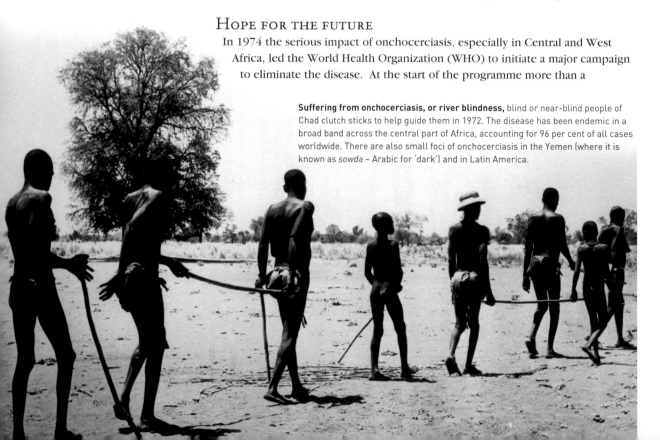

Suffering from onchocerciasis, or river blindness, blind or near-blind people of Chad clutch sticks to help guide them in 1972. The disease has been endemic in a broad band across the central part of Africa, accounting for 96 per cent of all cases worldwide. There are also small foci of onchocerciasis in the Yemen (where it is known as *sowda* – Arabic for 'dark') and in Latin America.

million people in West Africa were suffering from onchocerciasis. Of these, 100,000 had chronic eye problems, and 35,000 were blind. In some West African communities, 50 per cent of men over the age of 40 had been blinded by the disease.

The Onchocerciasis Control Programme (OCP) involved reducing the local blackfly population using aerial spraying of larvicides over the rivers, and removing people from villages in high-risk areas. Since 1988 it has also involved treating infected people with the safe and highly effective microfilaricidal drug ivermectin. By killing the microfilariae, ivermectin both reduces clinical symptoms and lowers the chances of further transmission of the disease.

Personal protection – avoiding being bitten – is also a high priority. Unlike many vector-borne diseases, the blackfly bites during the day, and it takes several bites for a person to become infected. In particularly badly infested areas, some people are bitten up to 20,000 times a year. The greater the number of infective bites, the higher the likelihood of blindness. Interrupting and reducing transmission is therefore of paramount importance.

BLINDNESS – AN ANCIENT PROBLEM

There are many conditions and diseases that can lead to blindness. Ninety per cent of the world's blind people live in developing countries; 1.5 million children in the world are blind, and another 500,000 go blind every year, many dying soon after. Among the most common causes is trachoma, a serious and potentially blinding bacterial eye disease which affects about 150 million people.

Eye problems – probably caused by infections spread by flies and eye gnats – were especially common in ancient Egypt. It is possible that the popularity of kohl in ancient Egypt – worn like an eyeliner by both men and women – derives partly from the fact that it contains the black mineral galena. Galena would have helped to reflect the glare of the sun, and its lead content may have repelled the flies that caused eye infections and blindness.

It is estimated that in the last three decades the OCP has prevented blindness in some 600,000 people, including many children. It has also made vast areas of fertile land suitable for resettlement and farming, with the potential to feed 17 million people. Today the number of infected people within the original area of operations is practically zero, and vector-control efforts have almost ceased – although continual vigilance is needed to prevent the disease from returning.

Further programmes have been initiated to try to eliminate onchocerciasis from other remaining endemic areas in Africa, and also in the Americas. Research is under way to develop safe and effective drugs to sterilize or kill the adult worm, which can live and continue to reproduce in the body for up to 15 years. Such drugs are urgently needed to supplement ivermectin.

In the past, it was common in Africa to see groups of blind villagers holding hands in a chain, led by those who still had their sight. Today, outside the headquarters of the WHO in Geneva, Switzerland, stands a statue of a child leading his blind father. It commemorates the successful OCP campaign against river blindness conducted in West Africa since 1974. It is a poignant reminder of the suffering inflicted by onchocerciasis, but at the same time a symbol of hope that it can be eliminated from other parts of the world where it is still endemic.

SMALLPOX was for centuries one of the most dreaded, lethal and common of all infectious diseases.

It is probably an ancient disease, but it became increasingly virulent in many parts of the world during the early modern period. The pocked and scarred faces of those who survived this horrific viral infection marked them out for life. No cure has ever been developed, but inoculation against smallpox began to be widely practised in Europe and North America in the 18th century, until at the end of the century it was superseded by vaccination. By 1979 a worldwide vaccination campaign led by the World Health Organization (WHO) achieved the ultimate goal of completely eradicating smallpox – the only major disease so far eliminated by human intervention.

In the late 18th century Edward Jenner (1749-1823), a country doctor in the English village of Berkeley in Gloucestershire, became aware of a local story that cowhands and dairymaids who had contracted cowpox from infected cows' udders might be protected from the much more serious smallpox. As Jenner and other country folk observed, *'what renders the Cow-Pox virus so extremely singular … is that the person who has been affected is for ever after secure from the infection of the Small-pox'.*

Jenner spent some years wondering whether there was a way that this link could be put to beneficial use for humankind. In May 1796 he decided to act on his hunch. He chose the son of his gardener – a healthy eight-year-old boy called James Phipps – and a young dairymaid, Sarah Nelmes, for his experiment. The dairymaid had contracted cowpox from a cow called Blossom. Jenner took a scraping of material from a cowpox pustule on her hand and then scratched it into the skin of young James Phipps. The next stage was to be the tricky one. Six weeks later, he inoculated the boy with smallpox virus taken from a pustule of a smallpox patient. It didn't 'take'. The boy did, indeed, appear to be protected against smallpox. He then went on to vaccinate his own son with cowpox and

timeline

c.1157 BC *Burial of Pharaoh Ramses V. Lesions found by archaeologists on his mummified face suggest he may have suffered from smallpox.*

1112 BC *A Chinese manuscript refers to a dreaded disease that may be smallpox.*

AD 570 *Bishop Marius of Avenches uses the term 'variola' to describe an*

epidemic that affects both Italy and France.

735–7 *The 'Great Smallpox Epidemic' in Japan – the first of a series – claims countless lives.*

c.900 *Smallpox is first clearly described by the Persian physician Rhazes (c.865–925).*

1500s *Smallpox reaches the New World with devastating consequences.*

1717 *Lady Mary Wortley Montagu (1689–1762) has her six-year-old son inoculated against smallpox in Constantinople. The method subsequently becomes popular on both sides of the Atlantic.*

1796 *Edward Jenner (1749–1823) tries out his cowpox vaccine on young James Phipps.*

1798 *Jenner publishes a pamphlet on his experiments in vaccination.*

1800s onwards *Smallpox vaccination (the first-ever human vaccination) is undertaken in many parts of the world.*

1872 *Endemic smallpox eliminated in*

128

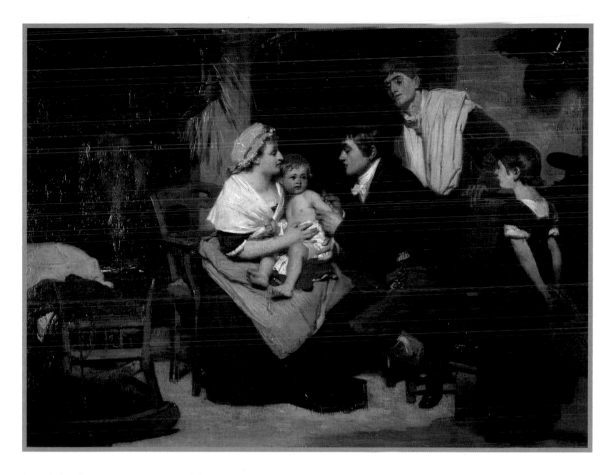

found that he, too, was protected from smallpox. Jenner was convinced that he had found a way of preventing this terrible scourge.

Jenner's story and the discovery of vaccination has been told and retold many times, as befits a milestone in the history of medicine. In honour of Jenner's discovery, Louis Pasteur (1822–95) gave wider currency to the term 'vaccination', a word derived from Latin *vacca*, meaning 'cow'.

The eradication of smallpox was made possible through the use of a modern version of the vaccine first developed by the pioneering physician Edward Jenner, seen here vaccinating a small boy.

Ireland, followed by Sweden (1895), Norway (1898) and Denmark (1901).

1907 Ireland is free of smallpox.

1934 The UK is free of smallpox.

1942 Canada is free of smallpox.

1949 The USA is free of smallpox.

1953 Portugal is the last European country to eliminate smallpox.

1966 With smallpox remaining serious in parts of Africa, South America and Asia, the World Health Assembly agrees to embark on a ten-year Smallpox Eradication Programme.

1972 Smallpox is eliminated in South America.

1975 (October) The world's last case of Variola major smallpox occurs in Bangladesh. The victim is a three-year old girl; she survives.

The disease is eliminated from Southeast Asia, leaving only the Horn of Africa to be cleared.

1977 (October) The last naturally occurring case of smallpox in the world occurs in Somalia, where a hospital cook contracts Variola minor smallpox. He also recovers.

1979 The World Health Organization (WHO) announces the global eradication of smallpox. In 1980 it is officially removed from the list of world diseases.

The speckled monster

The origin of smallpox remains an enigma. It is likely that it is a disease of great antiquity, possibly spreading from person to person around the time of the first agricultural settlements in the river valleys of Egypt, the Middle East, India and China. Smallpox has no animal reservoir, although it may in the dim and distant past have evolved from an animal virus such as cowpox, horsepox or (the most likely candidate) 'camelpox'. But once established as a solely human disease, smallpox can be spread only when there is a sufficient number of infectious people in the population in close proximity to a reservoir of people who have no immunity. To what extent smallpox was present in ancient Egypt or responsible for some of the great epidemics and 'plagues' of the Greek world and the Roman empire is a topic of lively scholarly debate.

We arrive at a more scientific historical basis of the disease in the tenth century, when the Persian physician ar-Razi (c.865–925), known in the West as Rhazes, wrote an account in which he differentiated measles from smallpox. At this time it seems that smallpox was a common childhood disease, and not as severe as measles. Certainly, over the next few centuries, smallpox did not carry the same fear as bubonic plague – indeed, it was not until some 200 years after the Black Death of the mid-14th century that smallpox emerged as one of the major killers of the early modern world.

In Europe by the 16th century, smallpox had become the dreaded 'speckled monster', attacking princes and peasants alike, and accounting for some 10 to 15 per cent of all deaths. It established itself as an endemic disease in cities and as a frightening periodic epidemic in towns and villages. At least 80 per cent of its victims were under the age of ten, and it could kill between 25 and 40 per cent of its victims. Survivors were left scarred and sometimes blind for life.

Smallpox and the New World

The most devastating impact of smallpox at this time was in the New World. Shortly after the arrival of Columbus in 1492, smallpox crossed the Atlantic from Europe and Africa. It spread rapidly and quite likely contributed to the collapse of the Aztec empire in Mexico and the Inca empire in Peru. The Native Americans had never before experienced smallpox and, as a 'virgin' population, they were exceptionally vulnerable. Estimates vary, but it is possible that 90 per cent of the indigenous population of the New World (amounting to between 50 and 100 million people) may have been wiped out by a combination

WHY THE 'SMALL' POX?

The term 'smallpox' came into general usage in the 16th century, replacing the word 'variola' (from the Latin *varius*, 'spotted'). 'Pox' (the plural of 'pock', a pustule, from the Old English word 'pocc') was used widely in Medieval times to describe a number of 'pestilences', including plague, variola and other diseases with pustular eruptions on the skin. There are two main types of smallpox – *Variola major* and the milder *Variola minor* – and prior to the 16th century the milder form may have been the more prevalent of the two. The disease was possibly called 'small' pox to differentiate it from the 'great pox', or syphilis, which struck across Europe with alarming consequences from the late 15th century. Perhaps the pockmarks of smallpox, though many, seemed 'small' in comparison with the repulsive pustules that spread over the entire body of the earliest victims of syphilis. It is also possible that at the time smallpox seemed the lesser of the two evils.

of factors, including 'new' diseases (especially smallpox and measles) and superior European military technologies (guns, steel swords and cavalry).

Accounts tell of masses of corpses piled up along the roadsides, of the stench of death pervading the villages, of dogs and vultures devouring the dead. The Mayans called smallpox *nokakil* – the great fire. One chronicler of the destruction of the civilization of the Aztecs wrote:

> *'More than half the population died ... in heaps, like bedbugs. Many others died of starvation, because, as they were all taken sick at once, they could not care for each other, nor was there anyone to give them bread or anything else. In many places it happened that everyone in a house died, and, as it was impossible to bury the great number of dead, they pulled down the houses over them in order to check the stench that rose from the dead bodies, so that their homes became their tombs.'*

Another observer wrote that *'a man could not set his foot down unless on the corpse of an Indian'*.

However, few of the Spanish conquistadors appear to have caught smallpox in the Americas. It may have been introduced, initially, by Europeans, but many of them may have already experienced smallpox and acquired immunity, protecting them from further attacks. The psychological impact on the indigenous populations was as devastating as the physical harm, as the hideous infection sapped their will to resist. Tribes and communities broke up and scattered, spreading smallpox far and wide, and the mighty empires of the Aztecs and the Incas crumbled amidst fear, anguish and panic.

Wave after wave of smallpox continued to devastate the indigenous inhabitants of the New World, carried across the Atlantic by traders, soldiers, sailors, slaves and settlers. The disease also hit the newly founded colonial settlements along the eastern seaboard of North America. Boston experienced eight epidemics during the 18th century, and in some of these epidemics more than half the population were infected.

'The streets, the squares, the houses ... were covered with dead bodies; we could not stop without treading on them, and the stench was intolerable ... all the causeways were full, from one end to the other, of men, women and children, so weak and sickly, squalid and dirty, and pestilential that it was a misery to behold them.'

THE SPANISH CONQUISTADOR BERNAL DÍAZ DEL CASTILLO OBSERVES THE EFFECTS OF SMALLPOX IN THE NEW WORLD, 1521

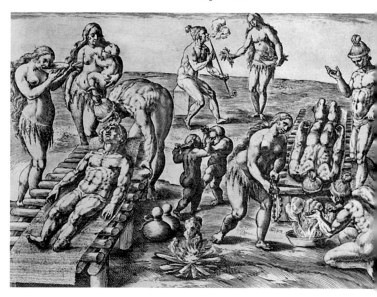

South American Indians were devastated by diseases such as smallpox, for which they had no immunity. This engraving from *c.*1591 shows tribespeople attempting cures using traditional healing methods.

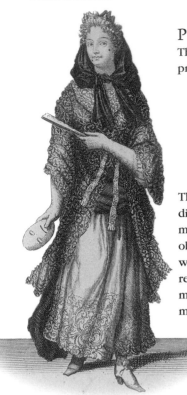

A London courtesan from about 1688 with her beauty spot, mask and fan. Such 'beauty aids' were used to hide scars from smallpox or venereal disease.

POCKMARKS, PUS AND INOCULATION

The great historian Lord Macaulay (1800–59), writing about England in the previous century, made this sombre observation:

'*The smallpox was always present, filling the churchyards with corpses, tormenting with constant fears all who it had not yet stricken, leaving on those whose lives it spared the hideous traces of its power, turning the babe into a changeling at which the mother shuddered, and making the eyes and cheeks of the betrothed maiden the objects of horror to the lover.*'

The permanent pockmarks suffered by survivors often caused considerable distress, and fashionable ladies, robbed of their smooth skins, did all they could to mask their scars with paints, potions and beauty spots. At the same time, it was observed that those who carried the telltale signs of once having had smallpox were not likely to catch the dreaded disease again. Adverts for servants often requested that they had already had 'the smallpox in the natural way', and in many parts of the world, parents were anxious that their children should only marry someone who had previously had the disease.

These observations regarding what we would now call acquired immunity inspired a method of preventing the disease. This was known as 'variolation' (after variola, the scientific name of the disease) or 'inoculation'. Might it be possible to take some of the infectious agent and transmit it to someone who had not yet caught the disease, in the hope that they might get a milder – rather than the full-blown and potentially fatal – form and thus become immune?

The technique of inoculation probably originated in India and then spread to other countries. In the tenth century the Chinese removed scabs from the drying pustules of a smallpox patient, pounded them into a powder, and then blew a few grains into the nose of people who had not had the illness – up the right nostril for a boy and the left one for a girl. In other parts of Asia and the Arab world, pus from the 'pocks' of an infected person was inoculated into a scratch in the skin of healthy people.

In the early 18th century Lady Mary Wortley Montagu (1689–1762), wife of the British ambassador to the Ottoman court, learned of this practice from the locals during her residence in Constantinople (now Istanbul). Her own stunning beauty had been destroyed by an attack of smallpox when she was 26 years old, leaving her badly scarred and without

'I went and made a visit to Mrs Graham … her eldest son was now sick there of the smallpox, but in a likely way to recovery, and other of her children ran about and among the infected, which she said she let them do on purpose that they might whilst still young pass that fatal disease she fancied they were to undergo one time or other, and that this would be for the best … '

JOHN EVELYN (1620–1706), DIARY, 1685

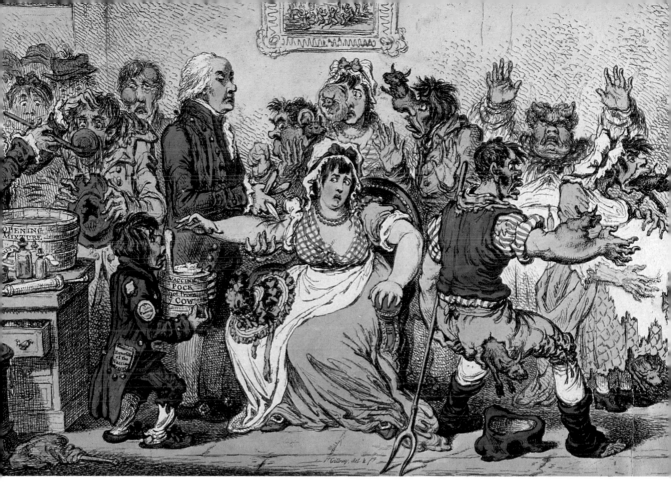

eyelashes. In a letter to a friend she described the 'smallpox parties' in which peasant women would routinely perform inoculation:

> *'Apropos of distempers, I am going to tell you a thing that will make you wish yourself here. The smallpox, so fatal and so general amongst us, is here rendered entirely harmless by the invention of engrafting, which is the term they give it. There is a set of old women who make parties for this purpose … an old woman comes with a nutshell full of the matter of the best sort of smallpox, and asks what veins you please to have open'd. She immediately rips open that which you offer her with a large needle (which gives you no more pain than a common scratch) and puts into the vein as much of the venom as can lie on the head of her needle …'*

In 1717 Lady Mary decided to have her six-year-old son inoculated, and in 1721, back in England, her three-year-old daughter was inoculated by the eminent surgeon Charles Maitland (1677–1748). This aroused much publicity. Princess Caroline (1683–1737), wife of the future King George II, was also keen to have her two daughters inoculated. But first she took the precaution of having six condemned felons in Newgate Prison inoculated on the promise of reprieve. She also had 12 charity schoolchildren inoculated and, once reassured that the attacks were mild, went ahead with the two little princesses. Catherine the Great of

This cartoon from 1802 depicts Edward Jenner at the Smallpox and Inoculation Hospital at St Pancras, London, vaccinating the local population with cowpox. According to the original caption, the treatment had *'Wonderful Effects!'* In some quarters, there was initial concern about vaccination and the introduction of an animal disease into humans.

133

'Medicine has never before produced any single improvement of such utility. You have erased from the calendar of human affliction one of its greatest ... future nations will know by history only that the loathsome smallpox has existed and by you has been extirpated.'

THOMAS JEFFERSON, LETTER TO EDWARD JENNER, 14 MAY 1806,
SOME 170 YEARS BEFORE SMALLPOX WAS FINALLY 'EXTIRPATED'

Russia (1729-96) had her family inoculated by Thomas Dimsdale (1712-1800), an English surgeon who was awarded £10,000 and a Russian barony for his services. With these royal marks of approval, the technique attracted huge attention in Europe.

Meanwhile, in Boston, Massachusetts, Reverend Cotton Mather (1663-1728) had learned of the same practice from one of his African slaves. He inoculated his own son, but the idea of interfering in this way with Divine Providence led to outrage amongst many Bostonians. Nevertheless, during a severe epidemic of smallpox in Boston in 1721, Mather persuaded the medical practitioner Zabdiel Boylston (1680-1766) to inoculate those not yet infected. Although some of those inoculated died, the numbers were few by comparison with those who died of smallpox 'in the natural way'.

Inoculation gradually became popular on both sides of the Atlantic, especially in the latter half of the 18th century when the technique was made safer, cheaper and easier by a number of practitioners, including Robert Sutton (1708-88) and his son Daniel (1735-1819) of England, and James Kirkpatrick (1676-1743) of South Carolina. Nevertheless, there were still many who questioned the efficacy and safety of inoculation. One of its main problems, apart from a 1-3 per cent risk of death, was that during the mild attack of smallpox people were actually infectious, and needed to be isolated. Thus inoculation was only a partial solution, and at the end of the 18th century smallpox was still exacting a huge toll across the world.

For example, smallpox devastated the Aboriginal population in Australia after the disease arrived there in 1789, possibly from Indonesia, just a year after the first European settlement in New South Wales. Eyewitnesses described the horrors of finding corpses washed up on the shore. About half of those who had contact with the British settlement of Port Arthur (Sydney) died, and it was probably one of the greatest demographic and psychological shocks in the history of Australia.

VACCINATION IS ADOPTED ACROSS THE GLOBE
When Edward Jenner sent his first report of his cowpox vaccination experiments on young James

DID JENNER INVENT VACCINATION?

Some 20 years before Jenner's 1796 experiment on James Phipps, a farmer in Dorset, Benjamin Jesty (1736–1816), had come up with the same theory about the protective nature of cowpox. He had rubbed matter from cowpox pustules into scratches on the arms of his wife and two children using a darning needle.

However, he did not subsequently expose them to the smallpox virus. It may be that Jesty was the first person to use this technique, but it was certainly Jenner who put vaccination into everyday medical practice.

Phipps to the Royal Society of London in 1797, it met with a cold reception. Although Jenner had already been elected a Fellow of the Royal Society for his work on cuckoos, the Society rejected his paper on the grounds that Jenner *'ought not to risk his reputation by presenting to the learned body anything which appeared so much at variance with established knowledge, and withal so incredible'.*

The following year, with more cases and evidence to support his theory, Jenner privately published a pamphlet entitled *An Inquiry into the Causes and Effects of the Variolae Vaccinae, a Disease, Discovered in some of the Western Counties of England, particularly Gloucestershire, and Known by the Name of The Cow Pox.* Although there were some critics (especially those who feared the consequences of transferring an animal disease to humans), the speed with which vaccination was subsequently adopted around the world was extraordinary. By 1801 more than 100,000 people had been vaccinated in England, and by 1811 over 1.7 million in France: the emperor Napoleon managed to have half his army vaccinated. Between 1804 and 1814, 2 million were vaccinated in Russia, and in the USA the practice was taken up with great enthusiasm by Dr Benjamin Waterhouse (1754–1846) of Boston. By the 1820s vaccination against smallpox had spread to much of the world. Its benefits for humankind were quickly recognized, and Jenner was richly honoured and rewarded.

A fold-out colour plate from 1803, published in Spain, illustrating the scars left by smallpox vaccination.

One of the most remarkable aspects of the story is the way in which the vaccines were transported around the world. Dried vaccine on quills and lancets, dried scabs, or cotton threads impregnated with matter from pustules, were just some of the methods used. For long sea voyages the 'serial method' was adopted, in which children were successively vaccinated, one after the other, using ripe pustular matter, until the destination was reached. Between 1803 and 1806 Don Francisco Xavier Balmis (1753–1819) used this arm-to-arm technique to take the vaccine from Spain across the Atlantic to Spanish America, on to the Philippines and China, and then back to Spain, vaccinating en route possibly 450,000 people. From one small village in Gloucestershire, the vaccine circumnavigated the globe.

The great advantage of vaccination over inoculation was that the former not only left the recipient non-infectious and immune, but also involved a far milder and less dangerous reaction. (It was realized some time later, however, that vaccination did not give lifelong protection, and people needed to be re-vaccinated after several years.) In some countries, mass vaccination centres were set up. There were objectors to the practice – on ethical and religious grounds – and a number of anti-vaccinationists fought hard to suppress it.

Especially unpopular was the policy in some countries of making vaccination compulsory, at least for infants. There was also the possibility of transferring other infections, such as syphilis, via the vaccine, and the risk of complications, such as post-vaccinial encephalitis. But on the whole vaccination proved highly successful, especially with the refinements and improvements made to the vaccine in the later 19th century.

It is difficult to document the success of smallpox vaccination in terms of number of lives saved, but it is likely that millions of people in the 19th and early 20th centuries were spared the horrors of the disease – not only death and disfigurement, but also blindness. In the late 18th century, about one-third of cases of blindness in Europe were probably from smallpox.

An early photograph shows a nurse tending a smallpox sufferer at an isolation hospital – possibly at Ilford, Essex, a small town outside London. Smallpox is an acute infectious disease caused by an *Orthopoxvirus* and transmitted by airborne droplets or the pus from pustules of an infected person. It produces a distinctive pustular rash. The scabs which form fall off after three or four weeks, leaving permanent pitted pockmarks.

THE ERADICATION OF SMALLPOX

The widespread practice of vaccination against smallpox was undoubtedly a major factor in the decline of mortality rates in the Western world over the past 200 years. In the early 20th century, although the incidence of smallpox was significantly less in the industrialized world than it had been a century earlier, smallpox remained endemic in almost every country, with periodic outbreaks of *Variola minor* (a milder form of the disease) in parts of Europe and North America. By the 1950s smallpox was no longer endemic in Britain and the United States, and by 1967 it had been eliminated from both Europe and North America, as well as China, Japan and Australia.

However, smallpox persisted in parts of Africa, Asia and South America. In the 1960s, 10 to 15 million people in some 43 countries across the world contracted the disease each year, with about 2 million deaths. In a trailblazing decision, the 19th World Health Assembly meeting at Geneva in 1966 agreed (albeit by just two votes) to embark on what they called an Intensified Ten-Year Smallpox Eradication Programme. At the time there were many doubts as to its feasibility, and even the director-general of the World Health Organization (WHO) was not optimistic that it would succeed. The programme was nevertheless launched the following year, with the backing of a small multinational team led by Donald Henderson (b.1928) of WHO.

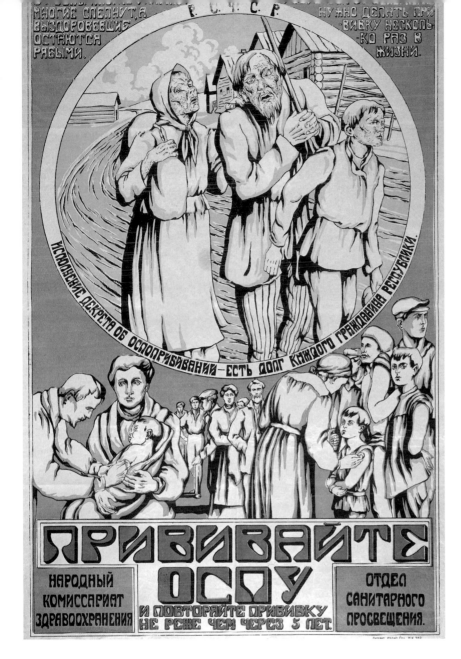

Pockmarked and blinded peasants who have suffered from smallpox are contrasted with children and adult citizens who are vaccinated against the disease in this Russian poster dating from the 1920s.

A successful programme of mass vaccination – made easier with the development of a freeze-dried vaccine that remained stable in tropical climates – led to the eradication of smallpox from South America by 1972. In parts of Africa and Asia, however, the task remained formidable. Health workers faced technical, logistical and cultural barriers. They crossed jungles, deserts and mountain ranges, worked in countries scarred by civil war and transcended political boundaries (this was one field in which the USA and the Soviet Union fully co-operated). 'Surveillance' and 'containment' were the operative words. Wherever they went their aim was to search for active cases of smallpox and trace and vaccinate contacts, as well as vaccinating the local population, so imposing a 'ring' around each outbreak.

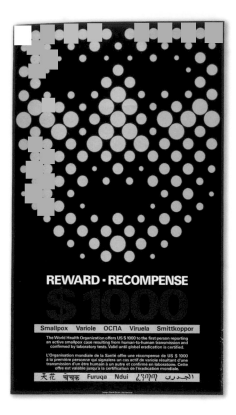

This poster from about 1977, with red and yellow circles (smallpox pustules) in the form of an open-mouthed face, offered a reward to *'the first person reporting an active case of smallpox resulting from human-to-human transmission and confirmed by laboratory tests'*. This reward – the last and highest ever offered – was never claimed, and the eradication of smallpox was certified just two years later.

Messages about the campaign were spread via newspapers, radio and posters, and rewards were offered to those who reported active cases of smallpox. Technological developments also played their part: new jet injector guns could vaccinate a thousand people in an hour, while the special bifurcated needles, needing only a tiny amount of vaccine, enabled thousands of people to be vaccinated by local health workers.

In October 1975 the last case of *Variola major* smallpox on the Indian subcontinent made headline news. The victim was a three-year-old girl in Bangladesh, and she survived. The last naturally occurring case in the world was a hospital cook in Somalia who contracted *Variola minor* in October 1977. He also recovered. In 1979 the WHO felt confident enough to announce that smallpox had been completely eradicated from the world. Jenner's goal, *'the annihilation of the Small Pox – the most dreadful scourge of the human species',* had finally been realized.

In some ways, smallpox was easier to deal with than some other infectious diseases. Vaccination had been available and proved effective since the early 19th century. Smallpox had no reservoir outside the human population – so there were no complex life cycles to crack, no dormant animal reservoirs of the virus to contend with, no insect vectors to transmit the disease. Within the human body, the smallpox virus has an incubation period of 12 to 14 days; it spreads only during the time of the rash, making it possible to trace contacts, isolate them prior to the infectious stage and thereby break the chain of transmission. In addition, smallpox has no long-term latency – once a person is over the attack, he or she is no longer infectious and there are no 'silent' carriers. Finally, the disease makes such distinctive marks on the skin that it was easily recognized, diagnosed and contained. The vaccination procedure also left its distinctive scar, so it was relatively easy to observe who had or had not been vaccinated. Despite all these advantages, Donald Henderson of the WHO recalled that the great campaign he co-ordinated *'only just succeeded'*.

THE VIRUS LIVES ON

Following the global eradication of smallpox, there was one further case of smallpox – in Birmingham, England, in 1978. A photographer was working above a smallpox research laboratory, and somehow the virus escaped – possibly through the ventilation system – and infected her. The young woman died. Her mother also came down with the disease, but she survived. The laboratory director committed suicide while in quarantine. There has been no known case of smallpox since.

Whether stocks of the smallpox virus and the vaccine should be kept in laboratories has remained a contentious issue. In 1995 governments began to destroy the stores of smallpox virus and the vaccine, and it was finally agreed that only two heavily guarded labs – one in Atlanta, Georgia, and one in Koltsovo, Siberia, in the Russian Federation – would keep the virus frozen in liquid nitrogen.

SOME FAMOUS VICTIMS OF SMALLPOX

King Henry VIII's fourth wife, Anne of Cleves, survived the disease, but was left scarred. Henry divorced her soon after their marriage had taken place, repelled by her physical appearance.

In 1562 Queen Elizabeth I of England became seriously ill with smallpox, but recovered. Rumour had it that her refusal to marry arose from an unwillingness to reveal her scars.

Pocahontas, the daughter of a Virginian chief, died in 1616 aged 21 on a visit to England, possibly of smallpox.

Mary II, queen of England, Scotland and Ireland, and wife of William of Orange, died aged 32 in 1694 of 'black' smallpox – one of the very worst forms, with massive haemorrhaging into the skin, lungs and other organs.

Prince William, the only offspring of the future Queen Anne of Great Britain to survive infancy, died of smallpox in 1700, at the age of 11.

Tsar Peter II of Russia died of smallpox in 1730, when aged 14.

Tsar Peter III of Russia suffered an attack of smallpox in 1744. The 1911 edition of *Encyclopaedia Britannica* commented: *'Nature had made him mean, the smallpox had made him hideous, and his degraded habits made him loathsome'*.

Wolfgang Amadeus Mozart contracted smallpox during an epidemic in Vienna in 1767. He became delirious and was lucky to survive. *'Te Deum Laudamus!'* wrote his father. *'Little Wolfgang has got over the smallpox safely!'*

President Abraham Lincoln suffered a mild attack of smallpox in 1863.

The Soviet dictator Joseph Stalin was badly scarred by a youthful bout of smallpox. He would often have photos retouched to hide his pockmarks.

Queen Elizabeth I of England, seen here in her robes of state, was a victim of smallpox. She painted her face with white lead and vinegar to cover up her smallpox scars.

It has been argued that there is a need to keep such stocks in case there is ever a recurrence of smallpox – for example, if terrorists should use the smallpox virus as a biological weapon. The outcome could be disastrous, as many young people today have never been vaccinated, and those who were vaccinated before the 1970s may no longer have the necessary immunity to fight off an attack. Those who oppose the maintenance of existing stores of the virus point out that with available stocks of cowpox, it should be possible for scientists to reintroduce the vaccine quickly. The completion of the genome map of the smallpox virus has also led to questions about the need for maintaining the existing stocks of smallpox.

We can only hope that, following the enormous efforts over the past centuries to eradicate one of the most dreadful diseases of history, there will be no reappearance of this deadly virus – either naturally or through the deliberate use of the pathogen for bio-terrorism.

MEASLES – or rubeola – is a highly infectious viral disease, characterized by fever and

a reddish rash over the body. It has probably been around for some 5000 years in the Old World, establishing itself as a common childhood disease when people first began to live in cities. Although often not serious, measles can prove fatal, especially in populations not previously exposed to it. A measles vaccine was introduced in the 1960s, and this, like the infection itself, confers life-long immunity. Many children in Western countries are now protected from the disease. Measles does, however, remain a major cause of childhood mortality in some parts of the developing world.

In 910 the Persian philosopher and physician ar-Razi (*c.*865–925), known in the West as Rhazes, wrote *A Treatise on the Smallpox and Measles*. His account, which was later translated from Arabic into Latin, is one of the first to draw a distinction between these two highly infectious diseases, both of which cause skin rashes. Rhazes suggested that measles was *'more to be dreaded than smallpox'*. Whether a person suffered from smallpox or measles depended, he believed, on their underlying constitution:

> *'Bodies that are lean, bilious, hot and dry are more disposed to the measles than to the smallpox.'*

'Count your children after the measles has passed.'

ARABIC PROVERB

The earlier history of measles is difficult to document, but it may have evolved from the canine distemper of dogs or the bovine rinderpest of cattle several thousand years ago, when humans first began to domesticate their animals. Once adapted to humans, measles probably spread out from its original urban hearth in Mesopotamia around 3000 BC. Diseases such as measles that spread from person to person are often known as 'crowd diseases' or 'diseases of civilization': they need a certain density of population before they can establish themselves as endemic.

In the case of measles, it is thought that once cities grew to a size of one-quarter of a million inhabitants or thereabouts, the disease became endemic as a common infection of children. In smaller cities and rural areas, measles was more likely to erupt from time to time in epidemic waves, affecting wider age groups of non-immune or susceptible individuals.

timeline

910 *The Persian physician Rhazes (c.865–925) writes an account of measles and smallpox.*

1492 *Europeans reach the Americas, and measles becomes one of the major 'virgin soil' epidemics.*

1758 *Francis Home (1710–1801) of Edinburgh attempts to inoculate subjects against measles.*

1846 *The Danish physician Peter Panum (1820–85) unravels the epidemiology of measles while reporting on an outbreak on the Faeroe Islands.*

1875 *A measles epidemic in Fiji results in a death rate of 25–30 per cent.*

1954 *The American microbiologist J.F. Enders (1897–1985) and his colleague T.C. Peebles isolate the measles virus.*

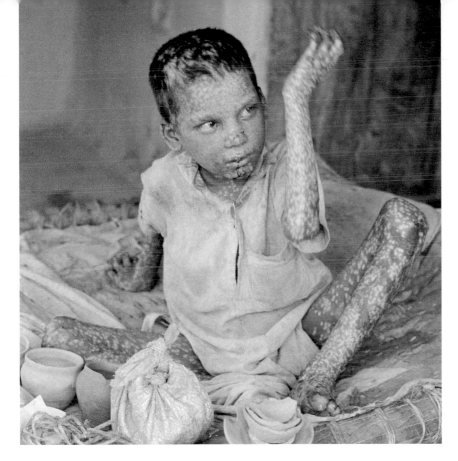

A child with a severe case of measles. The first signs of measles are usually a fever with a cough, coryza (runny nose) and conjunctivitis (red eyes) – symptoms known as 'the 3 Cs'.

MEASLES ADAPTS TO THE OLD WORLD

The Arabic word for measles, as used by Rhazes, was *hasbah*. In the following centuries various names were given to the disease, including rubeola (from the Latin *rubeus*, 'reddish') and *morbilli* (a diminutive of the Latin *morbus*, hence meaning the 'little plague'). The origin of the word 'measles' is uncertain, although some scholars trace it to the Old German word *masa*, 'spot', which became in Middle English *maselen*, 'many little spots'. In 11th-century Japan, the disease was known as the 'red pox' or the 'red rash pox', and in Europe a range of colloquial terms – 'red measles', 'red spots pox', 'red smallpox', 'hard measles', 'nine-day measles' – was used to highlight its characteristic appearance: the reddish rash that spreads rapidly over the body and generally lasts for nine days or so. Thomas Sydenham (1624–89), the London physician sometimes known as the 'English Hippocrates', wrote a classic description of measles epidemics

1962 *J.F. Enders develops an effective vaccine against measles, which is licensed in 1963.*

1963–4 *CDC (Centers for Disease Control) begin a programme for the elimination of measles in the USA.*

1974 *The World Health Organiza-tion (WHO) announces its Expanded Programme of Immunization, covering six common diseases:* *measles, polio, tuberculosis, diphtheria, tetanus and whooping cough.*

2005 *The WHO and UNICEF announce Global Immunization Vision and Strategy (GIVS) to reduce global* *measles deaths by 90 per cent by 2010.*

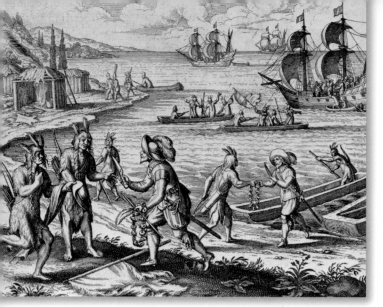

in London in 1670 and 1674. Although the disease accounted for only a small fraction of all childhood deaths, the London Bills of Mortality record deaths from measles in every year from 1629. It was clearly a disease to be feared.

Some outbreaks seemed to be mild, but others could be deadly. In 1808 a particularly severe epidemic hit the city of Glasgow:
The disease has never before been nearly so mortal there, nor had any infection since the time of the plague, not even smallpox itself, engrossed the burial registers so much as measles did in the months of May and June.'

Contact with Europeans, such as through trade in the 1600s as shown here, led indigenous Americans to catch diseases for which they had no immunity. Measles and many other illnesses exacted a huge toll on the population. The Amerindians described the measles epidemics in their picture writing.

Measles continued to take its toll during the 19th century – its variable impact possibly depending as much on the general health, living standards, nutrition and age group of those affected rather than any differences in the virulence of the disease.

MEASLES STRIKES THE NEW WORLD

Measles was totally absent from the Americas prior to the arrival of Europeans. The conquest of the New World has often been described as one of the greatest of all demographic disasters. From a population of anywhere from 50 to 100 million people before the arrival of Columbus in 1492, the indigenous population of the Americas was reduced to perhaps just one-tenth of its original level. Historians have debated the possible reasons for this 'holocaust'. Some have attributed it to the brutality of the conquistadors, others to the ensuing break-up of the social and economic fabric. But most historians now concur that it was mainly 'germs' and not 'guns' that wiped out so many people in the post-Columbian era.

Measles, along with smallpox (see pages 128–39), was one of the major killers of the Native Americans, who had no immunity against such 'new' diseases. All age groups were affected. Young adults were particularly hard hit, and this removed a vital section of the population who might otherwise have provided food and care for their families. The result was helplessness and despair. The Europeans, by contrast, were mostly already immune to measles and smallpox, and thus, as they set about their conquests, found they had the upper hand not just technologically – with horses and firearms and steel swords – but also epidemiologically.

MEASLES ADAPTS TO THE AMERICAS

During the later 17th and 18th centuries, measles became a leading cause of death in the eastern seaboard cities of North America. Mirroring patterns in the Old World, the disease was often mild, but occasionally severe and disruptive. In large metropolitan communities it attained epidemic proportions every second or third year; in smaller communities and areas, outbreaks tended to be more widely spaced and somewhat more severe.

In Fairfield, New Jersey, in 1759 – the 'never to be forgotten year' – a contemporary witness, Ephraim Harris, recounted how:

> 'The Lord sent the destroying angel to pass through this place, and removed many of our friends into eternity in a short space of time; not a house exempt, not a family spared from the calamity. So dreadful was it, that it made every ear tingle, and every heart bleed; in which time I and my family were exercised with that dreadful disorder, the measles. But Blessed be God, our lives are spared.'

Measles in the United States spread westward in the 19th century as new areas were opened up by settlers. One of the most serious outbreaks was during the Civil War of 1861–5 when many thousands of Union and Confederate troops are thought to have died of the disease.

MEASLES TOUCHES ALMOST EVERY OTHER CORNER OF THE GLOBE

Over the course of the 19th and early 20th centuries measles was carried by explorers and travellers to many far-flung places. The Faeroe Islands, Iceland, Alaska, Australia, New Zealand, Hawaii, Samoa, Fiji and other Pacific islands often witnessed dramatic epidemics and, occasionally, sustained huge losses when they encountered measles for the first time. Two of the best documented cases were the 1846 epidemic in the Faeroes and the 1875 epidemic in Fiji.

In 1846 a young Danish doctor, Peter Ludwig Panum (1820–85), was sent to the Faeroe Islands – which lie in the Atlantic between the Shetlands and Iceland – to investigate a violent epidemic of measles that was occurring there. Although this was not the first time measles had hit the islands, the 1846 epidemic affected 6100 inhabitants out of a total population of some 7800. Those who were over 65 years old and had lived through the previous epidemic of 1781, however, did not contract measles. In his report of the epidemic, Panum recognized that measles conferred life-long immunity.

The number of deaths from measles was relatively low during the epidemic in the Faeroes. By contrast, the 1875 epidemic that struck the islands of Fiji killed possibly as many as one-quarter of the Fijian population in little over three months. The disease was introduced by the royal family on their return from a state visit to New South Wales in Australia. The king of Fiji, Ratu Seru Cakobau, had contracted measles

TERROR AND DESPAIR IN FIJI

Describing the devastating Fiji measles epidemic of 1875, the German physician and medical historian August Hirsch (1817–94) wrote:

> 'Later in the epidemic, when it is said to be like plague ... the people, seized with fear, had abandoned their sick ... the people chose swampy sites for their dwellings, and whether they kept close shut up in huts without ventilation, or rushed into the streams and remained in the water during the height of the illness, the consequences were equally fatal. The excessive mortality resulted from terror at the mysterious seizure, and [from] the want of the commonest aids during illness ... Thousands were carried off by want of nourishment and care, as well as by dysentery and congestion of the lungs.'

August Hirsch, *Handbook of Geographical and Historical Pathology* (1883–6)

'Love is like the measles: we all have to go through it.'

JEROME K. JEROME, *IDLE THOUGHTS OF AN IDLE FELLOW* (1886)

in Sydney but was recovering as their ship, HMS *Dido*, reached the Fijian capital, Levuka, on the east coast of Ovalau Island on 12 January 1875. His two sons, however, were very sick and, undoubtedly, infectious.

The *Dido* did not fly the yellow flag to indicate that there was sickness on board, and no quarantine was imposed. Over the next ten days the royal party entertained a great number of chiefs, their families and entourages, who came from distant islands to welcome home the king and his sons. After the festivities, as they returned home, measles spread like wildfire through the islands. Some 40,000 Fijians – out of a population of 150,000 scattered over 700,000 square miles (1.8 million sq km) on 100 inhabited islands – died in this single epidemic. Some attributed the huge mortality to the practice of 'plunging' young children with a high fever into cold water. Others blamed the disaster on poisoning, treachery or bewitchment. Lack of medical care for those infected was also a serious problem. The epidemic has been described as '*one of the great tragic events in Pacific history*'.

By the end of the 19th century measles had reached almost every corner of the globe, becoming one of the most ubiquitous of all infectious diseases. Some of the last pockets of population to be visited by measles were the isolated and remote communities of the sub-Arctic region. In 1900 mainland Alaska had an epidemic of measles with rates of mortality that reached 40 per cent among the isolated Native American populations. Iceland was struck several times – in 1846, 1882 and 1904. The 1904 outbreak arrived in late April in the northwest fjords with a crew of whalers from Norway. It spread rapidly after a confirmation ceremony in a little church on a remote fjord. Children and non-immune adults were packed into the church, and by the end of August local doctors were overwhelmed. Further periodic waves occurred in Iceland through the 20th century, becoming even more frequent after the increase in air travel in the 1950s.

MEASLES – MILD OR MORTAL?

Over the centuries, measles epidemics were invariably described as either 'mild' or 'mortal'. In the developing world today measles carries a high death toll, killing between 5 and 10 per cent (sometimes more) of all those infected. The reasons for the variations in mortality are complex, but it seems clear that for impoverished children living in crowded conditions, suffering from malnutrition and lacking basic medical care, measles can lead to severe consequences. Complications of the disease include pneumonia, diarrhoea, otitis media (infection of the eardrum), damage to the nervous system and encephalitis (inflammation of the brain). The risk of a malnourished child dying from diarrhoea associated with measles is especially high. Measles can also precipitate acute kwashiorkor (a form of malnutrition caused by lack of protein) and exacerbate vitamin-A deficiency, which may in turn lead to blindness.

The reasons for the significant decline in mortality attributed to measles in the USA and Europe from the early 20th century (several decades before immunization was introduced) is still a puzzle, but may relate to improvements in nursing care, standards of living and nutrition.

'MAKE MEASLES A MEMORY'

The last major 'virgin soil' epidemic of measles was in Greenland in 1951, when only five people out of a population of 4262 in the southern part of the island escaped the disease. A decade later, scientists in the United States developed the first effective vaccine for measles. The search for a vaccine had begun in the mid-18th century, when the Scottish physician Francis Home (1710–1801) attempted to inoculate children, either through the skin or into the nose, with cotton swabs soaked in the 'fresh blood of a measly patient' at the height of their fever. Unlike the successful vaccine for smallpox developed by Edward Jenner (1749–1823) (see pages 128–9), Home's procedure did not catch on, and it was not until 1963 that the first live-attenuated measles vaccine was licensed.

By this time measles had already begun to decline as a cause of death in America, Europe, parts of Asia and Oceania. Indeed, by the 1940s – two decades before the introduction of the vaccine – it is estimated that measles mortality was already one-tenth of its level at the turn of the 20th century. With the introduction of the measles vaccine (which is now usually combined with a mumps and rubella vaccine – the MMR vaccine) the downward trend was accelerated in developed countries. In the United States a mass immunization programme – which became known as the 'make measles a memory' campaign – has been successful in practically eliminating measles from that country. With effective childhood immunization programmes in many other industrialized countries, measles cases have dropped by 99 per cent over the past half century.

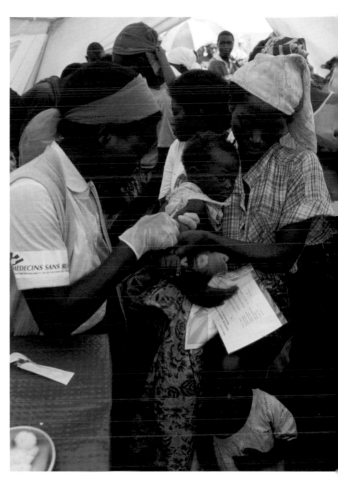

However, in the developing world, measles, although significantly reduced, remains a serious childhood disease, with nearly 1000 victims dying every day. In the pre-vaccination era, there were an estimated 100 million cases and 6 million measles deaths per year globally. By the early 21st century, this had fallen to approximately 35 million cases and 600,000 measles deaths worldwide. From 2000 to 2005, more than 360 million children worldwide received the measles vaccine, and the current figures are 20 million cases each year and 345,000 deaths – a promising reduction, but still an unacceptably high death rate. Over 90 per cent of deaths occur in countries with a per capita GNP (gross national product) lower than $1000, over 75 per cent in children under five years, and over 50 per cent of all measles deaths are in Africa. Despite the existence of a safe, effective and inexpensive vaccine for over 40 years, measles remains the leading vaccine-preventable killer of children worldwide.

Médicins Sans Frontières health workers administering measles vaccinations to Rwandan refugees at Benaco refugee camp, Tanzania, c.1994.

The World Health Organization has launched a number of programmes over the past few decades to try to extend the coverage of measles vaccination for children in poorer countries, with the aim of making measles 'a memory' worldwide. When Rhazes in the tenth century conjectured that measles was 'more to be dreaded' than smallpox, his words would ring true for the 21st century. Smallpox has been eradicated – there is still hope that measles will follow it into oblivion.

YELLOW FEVER – an acute viral disease in which

victims become jaundiced and vomit up black blood – was at one time amongst the most dreaded of all diseases. It was particularly rife during the era of European global exploration, when sailors, soldiers and slaves may have carried the virus and its mosquito vector from Africa to the New World. There has been a vaccine for yellow fever since the 1930s, but there is as yet no cure. Like other mosquito-borne diseases, it continues to evade our efforts to eradicate it.

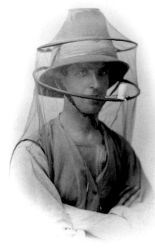

Anti-mosquito clothing, such as this net, was one of the methods people used to avoid contracting insect-borne diseases. However, today vaccination is the single most important measure for preventing yellow fever.

The name yellow fever - reflecting the typical yellow skin and eyes of victims - was first coined by Griffin Hughes in 1750, in his *Natural History of Barbados*. The disease can vary in severity. In some cases it is a mild illness of short duration, but in the worst cases yellow fever attacks the liver, leading to jaundice (from the French *jaune*, 'yellow'), and the kidneys. Between 20 and 50 per cent of those with the severe form of the illness will die.

Although yellow fever has probably been around for centuries, it was not until 1900 that it was finally proved that it was transmitted by the bite of mosquitoes (notably the female *Aedes aegypti*), and not until the 1930s that the causative organism was found to be a virus - one belonging to the same family as the virus causing dengue fever (see pages 152-5).

'YELLOW JACK' AND BLACK VOMIT

In the past yellow fever was so common among sailors that ships carried a special 'Yellow Jack' flag. Infected ships were isolated outside ports and obliged to fly the flag as a warning. Neither sailors nor passengers were allowed to leave the ship for up to 40 days, and anyone trying to escape took the risk of being shot by police or vigilantes. The 'Yellow Jack' became such a distinctive emblem that it was often used as a nickname for the disease itself.

While the word 'yellow' in the English name of the disease reflects the outward appearance of sufferers, the Spanish name for yellow fever, *vomito negro*, reflects

timeline

1647 First recorded epidemic of yellow fever occurs on the Caribbean island of Barbados. It is called the 'Barbados distemper' by Massachusetts governor John Winthrop (c.1587–1649),

who establishes North America's first quarantine regulations to protect his English colony from infection.

1654–5 Many French soldiers die of yellow fever during an attempt to capture the island of St Lucia in the Caribbean.

17th–19th centuries Huge death tolls from yellow fever are experienced time and again in the Americas, the Caribbean and, occasionally, in Europe.

1741 Admiral Edward Vernon (1684–1757) of the British Royal Navy loses half his force to disease, notably yellow fever, while attempting to capture Spanish strongholds off the coast of New Grenada (now Colombia).

1764 Earliest recorded evidence of yellow fever in West Africa.

1802–3 French troops ravaged by yellow fever in Haiti.

1878 Devastating outbreak of yellow fever in the Mississippi and Ohio valleys, infecting over 100,000 people, with some 20,000 deaths.

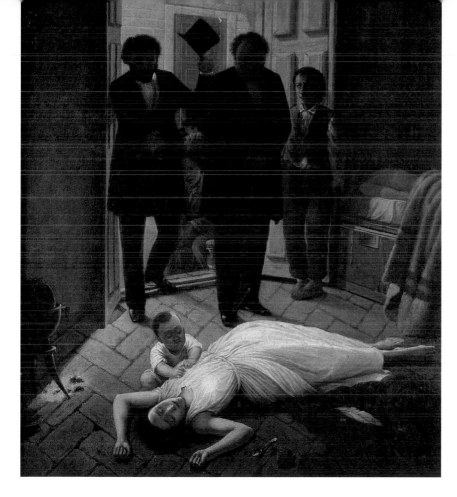

A yellow-fever victim in Buenos Aires, Argentina, 1901. In the Americas, the disease is still endemic in nine South American countries in a band from 15° N and 10° S of the equator, as well as in several Caribbean islands.

its other notorious symptom: 'black vomit'. This is the result of internal bleeding, especially into the stomach and intestinal tract. Copious bleeding may also occur from the eyes, nose, gums and rectum.

In a letter written in 1897 in Memphis, an uncle describes his niece's final hours:

> ' ... to me the most terrible and terrifying feature was the "black vomit" which I never before witnessed. By Tuesday evening it was as black as ink and would be ejected with terrific force. I had my face and hands

1881 *Cuban physician Carlos Finlay (1833–1915) suggests that mosquitoes are the agent for the transmission of yellow fever.*

1897 *British doctor Ronald Ross (1857–1932) discovers the role of mosquitoes in transmitting malaria.*

1900 *British doctors Herbert Durham (1866–1945) and Walter Myers (1872–1901) visit Cuba. They suspect, like Finlay, that mosquitoes might transmit yellow fever, and this may have influenced*

Walter Reed (see next entry) in following up the idea.

1900–2 *US Army doctor Walter Reed (1851–1902) and associates conduct experiments in Havana, Cuba, which finally prove that mosquitoes transmit yellow fever.*

1901–2 *Under the direction of US Army doctor William Gorgas (1854–1920), sanitary squads successfully destroy the breeding grounds of mosquitoes in Havana, freeing the city of yellow fever.*

1903–8 *The Brazilian physician Oswaldo Cruz (1872–1917) uses anti-mosquito strategies to combat yellow fever in Brazil.*

(continued ...)

spattered but had to stand by and hold her. Well it is too terrible to write any more about it …'

YELLOW FEVER AND THE TRANSATLANTIC WORLD

Like many diseases, it is hard to know when or how yellow fever began to infect humans. It is possible that for thousands of years yellow fever was a disease of monkeys in the African (and possibly the South American) rainforests. At some time in the past, as people moved into the jungles, the mosquitoes that transmitted yellow fever started to feed on humans.

'There was one thing nearly everybody … had been agreed upon for nearly two hundred years, and that was this: when folks of a town began to turn yellow and hiccup and vomit black blood, by scores, by hundreds, every day – the only thing to do was to get up and get out of town … '

PAUL DE KRUIF, *MICROBE HUNTERS* (1926)

The first major recorded human epidemics were in the 17th century in the Caribbean and the Americas. Some historians have suggested that yellow fever and its vector crossed the Atlantic from Africa on slave ships, where it had devastating effects on both the European colonists and the indigenous population, neither of whom had ever before been exposed to the disease.

In 1647 yellow fever appeared in Barbados, where some 5000 people died of '*a new distemper*'. In the following year the disease struck both Cuba and the Yucatán Peninsula. From that date on, it regularly visited the ports and cities of the Americas during the summer months - from Quebec in the north to Rio de Janeiro in the south. With its close trading connections with the Caribbean, the city of Philadelphia became one of the hotbeds of the disease, and in 1793 some 4000–5000 people, one-tenth of the city's population, died in a single epidemic. A similar number fled in panic.

Over the following century, not only Philadelphia but also New Orleans, Savannah, Charleston and other US cities were repeatedly struck by yellow fever. In 1853 in New Orleans there were so many dead that there were not enough grave diggers to bury them all. European ports - including Lisbon in Portugal, St Nazaire in France and Swansea in Wales - also suffered visitations of yellow fever.

timeline

1905 *Last major epidemic of yellow fever in the USA.*

1914 *The Panama Canal is opened after a huge effort to eliminate mosquitoes from the region.*

1926 *The first large epidemic amongst native West Africans occurs in the British colony of Gold Coast (now Ghana).*

1927–1930s *Yellow fever re-emerges in Brazil,* and the American public-health physician Fred Soper (1893–1977) identifies the jungle or sylvatic yellow-fever cycle, transmitted by wild mosquitoes with a host in monkeys.

1935–7 *The first effective vaccine for yellow fever is developed by South African-born US physician and bacteriologist Max Theiler (1899–1972) of the Rockefeller Institute, New York.*

1939–52 *Yellow fever cases almost vanish from French West Africa following intensive vaccination campaigns.*

1960–2 *Ethiopia experiences one of the worst yellow-fever epidemics of the 20th century, with thousands of deaths.*

1986–91 *Severe yellow-fever epidemic in Nigeria, with* nearly 20,000 cases and more than 4000 deaths. There is a subsequent upsurge of the disease in parts of tropical and sub-tropical Africa and South America.

MOSQUITOES, FILTH AND GRISLY EXPERIMENTS

In 1900 in Havana, Cuba, Walter Reed (1851–1902) of the US Army and his medical associates – James Carroll, Jesse Lazear and Aristides Agramonte – showed once and for all that yellow fever was transmitted by mosquitoes. Carroll allowed mosquitoes that had fed on four patients with yellow fever to bite him. He became very sick but just about survived. Lazear was bitten by a mosquito in a hospital ward and also contracted the disease. Such was the wildness of his delirium that it took five men to hold him down before he died.

In order to confirm the mosquito theory, Reed built an experimental establishment, which he named 'Camp Lazear' in honour of the dead physician. One group of recruits was put in a mosquito-free but filthy building filled with the vomit- and blood-covered clothing and bedding of yellow-fever victims. Another group was left in isolation in a screened clean building and then bitten by mosquitoes that had previously fed on yellow-fever patients. The mosquito-bitten volunteers caught yellow fever, while the other group remained 'as fit as fiddles' – although gasping for fresh air.

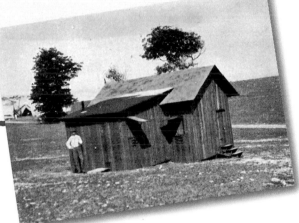

'Camp Lazear', where Walter Reed carried out his experiments to prove that yellow fever was not transmitted by means of infected clothing.

THE BAFFLING 'CAUSE' OF YELLOW FEVER

To the peoples of the New World, yellow fever proved baffling. Some blamed it on filth and foul smells and burned bonfires of aromatic herbs in the streets; others believed it was a contagious disease passed from person to person. One doctor attributed it to *sickly and tasteless* oysters, another to rotting coffee beans. Mysteriously, it seemed that yellow fever was a disease that only, or primarily, afflicted Europeans – especially newcomers to the New World – and was often called the 'strangers' disease'. African slaves seemed to resist the disease, possibly having experienced it mildly in childhood, giving a rather sinister justification to plantation owners for the use of slave labour.

THE ROLE OF THE MOSQUITO

In the early 1880s Carlos Finlay (1833–1915), a Cuban doctor of Anglo-French descent, conducted a number of experiments and surmised that yellow fever was transmitted by mosquitoes. Finlay was right in his conjecture. Others, however, remained convinced that yellow fever was caused by filth, contaminated clothing and bedding, or poisonous airs arising from stagnant water. It was another two decades before Finlay's hunch was finally shown to be correct.

After the Cuban War of Independence (1895–8) and the Spanish-American War (1898), in which the US Army lost more men to disease, including yellow fever, than to enemy action, the American army doctor Major Walter Reed (1851–1902) was sent to the Cuban capital, Havana. Around half a million American troops remained in Cuba after the war, and Reed was appointed head of the US Army Yellow Fever Commission to find the true cause of the disease. Despite a major

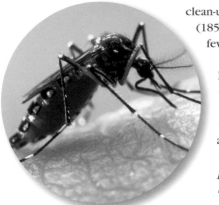

The mosquito responsible for transmitting both yellow fever and dengue fever – *Aedes aegypti* – breeds close to human habitation. The female lays her eggs in all sorts of artificial water containers.

clean-up of the city, conducted by army medical officer William Crawford Gorgas (1854–1920), and an overall fall in mortality from a number of diseases, yellow-fever deaths had, paradoxically, increased.

In 1900, following up earlier leads – especially Carlos Finlay's crucial observations and the subsequent identification of the mosquito's role in malaria (see pages 84–93) – Reed proved beyond doubt that yellow fever is transmitted by the bite of *Aedes aegypti* mosquitoes (see Mosquitoes, Filth and Grisly Experiments, page 149). On 31 December, Reed wrote to his wife: ' … *the prayer that has been mine for twenty years, that I might be permitted in some way or some time to do something to alleviate human suffering has been granted! A thousand Happy New Years …* '

Tragically, Walter Reed died of appendicitis shortly after this great discovery.

With the knowledge that it was a vector-borne disease, strategies were implemented to rid cities of their mosquitoes. *Aedes aegypti* lives in close proximity to human settlements, the female laying her eggs in any source of temporary water. Water receptacles were oiled, houses were screened and dusted with pyrethrum powder, patients isolated and sick rooms mosquito-proofed.

Shortly after Reed's discovery, Gorgas – who had contracted and survived yellow fever in Texas in 1882 and was therefore immune to the disease – carried out a successful campaign of eradication in Havana, which was free of the disease by

POURING OIL ON TROUBLED WATERS

'The Panama Canal was dug with a microscope.'
Ronald Ross
(1857–1932)

Since the 16th century, navigators and merchants had longed to cut a swathe through the 50-mile (80-km) Panama Isthmus in Central America to link the Atlantic and Pacific Oceans. But technical, financial and political constraints, inhospitable conditions and deadly mosquitoes were a serious hindrance to such plans.

In 1851–5 a railroad was built across the Panama region; it is said that for every sleeper laid, one labourer died. Ferdinand de Lesseps (1805–94), the French engineer, had to abandon the first attempt to build a canal across the isthmus in

1889. Tens of thousands of workmen died on the project, notably from yellow fever and malaria.

With the discovery in 1900 of the yellow-fever mosquito vector, *Aedes aegypti*, US Army medical officer William Crawford Gorgas (1854–1920) set about the task of ridding the area of mosquitoes and mosquito-borne diseases during a renewed attempt to build a canal. He tried draining ponds and swamps, pouring oil over open water to kill mosquito eggs and larvae, building sewerage systems and hospitals, putting screens on every door and window and isolating yellow-fever patients in mosquito-proof rooms. Although the death toll for workers was still high, by 1906 Gorgas had successfully eliminated yellow fever from the region, and the Panama Canal was finally opened in 1914 – one of the greatest engineering marvels of the modern world.

1901. With further anti-mosquito programmes, including that which enabled the completion of the Panama Canal in 1914 (see Pouring Oil on Troubled Waters, left), it was hoped that the disease could be eradicated from the world.

YELLOW FEVER PERSISTS ...

In the 1930s yellow fever was found to be a viral disease – the first human disease to be identified as such. In the same decade a vaccine was developed. In the 1940s the introduction of the insecticide DDT provided another weapon in the battle. Epidemics of yellow fever declined in ports on both sides of the Atlantic, and there was optimism that 'urban' yellow fever would be eradicated.

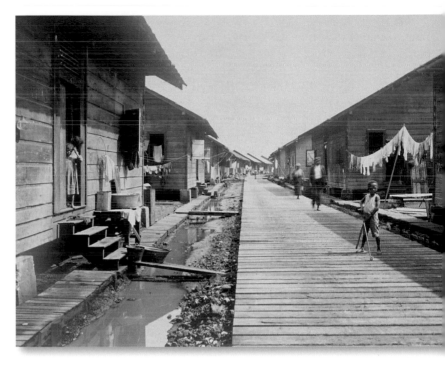

Panama Canal workers' houses, photographed in 1910. Diseases such as yellow fever initially killed many workers, making the construction of the canal a slow and deadly business.

As early as 1926, Paul de Kruif (1890–1971), in his popular book *Microbe Hunters*, was confident enough to write:

> *'There is hardly enough of the poison of yellow fever left in the world to put on the points of six pins; in a few years there may not be a single speck of that virus left on earth – it will be as completely extinct as the dinosaurs.'*

His optimism was, however, premature and in recent decades there has been a resurgence of yellow fever, especially in parts of Africa and South and Central America where mosquitoes persist in large numbers. At present, yellow fever is endemic in 33 countries in Africa, nine in South America, and on several Caribbean islands. There are currently about 200,000 reported cases a year with some 30,000 deaths, though this is likely to be an under-estimate. Curiously, yellow fever has never been reported in Asia, in spite of the abundance of the *A. aegypti* vector.

One of the main reasons for this resurgence in endemic countries is the lapse of immunization programmes in many poorer countries (although routine childhood and mass vaccination campaigns are now under way in various places). Rapid urbanization and a lack of mosquito-eradication programmes are also factors in its recent re-emergence. The outlook has been further complicated by the discovery of jungle vectors (such as mosquitoes of the *Haemogogus* genus in South America) and non-human hosts (including monkeys) in the Amazon and African rainforests – which present an increasing threat as people begin to move into these hitherto sparsely uninhabited regions. Thus the threat of yellow fever – a centuries-old scourge – remains a real problem for the 21st century.

DENGUE FEVER was often known as 'break-bone

fever' and is a viral infection transmitted by the bite of a female mosquito. It can cause a high fever and agonizing pain, followed by debilitating after-effects. In the past dengue evoked less fear and horror than many other diseases, but with the recent emergence of more deadly forms of the disease – notably dengue haemorrhagic fever (DHF) – it has become a serious health threat in many parts of the world.

The origin of the word 'dengue' (pronounced 'deng-gy', the last 'g' being hard) is something of a puzzle. One suggestion is that it derives from the Swahili phrase *ka dinga pepo,* meaning a sudden cramp-like seizure caused by an evil spirit. Alternatively, 'dengue' may be a corruption of 'dandy' – slaves in the West Indies called the disease 'dandy fever' because sufferers were crippled with pain and had a 'dandified' manner of walking. Another explanation is that it comes from the Spanish *denguero,* meaning 'affected' or 'finicky', perhaps referring to the stiffness that afflicted victims. It was the American physician Benjamin Rush (1746-1813), one of the signatories of the Declaration of Independence, who first described the disease, aptly calling this crippling condition 'break-bone fever'.

THE AGONIZING SYMPTOMS OF DENGUE FEVER

Benjamin Rush made his historic description of 'break-bone fever' following an outbreak in Philadelphia in 1780:

> *'The pains which accompanied this fever were exquisitely severe in the head, back and limbs … the pains in the head were sometimes in the back part of it, and at other times they occupied the eyeballs … its more general name among all classes of people was the break-bone fever … '*

Rush treated his patients with *'a gentle vomit of tartar emetic'* to empty the stomach. He also advised *'a liberal supply of opium, oysters, a generous amount of porter and some gentle exercise in the open air'*. To this day there is no cure for dengue or its close relative, yellow fever (see pages 146-51). But while a safe, effective vaccine for yellow fever has existed since the 1930s, there is still no vaccine for dengue, although candidate vaccines are being evaluated.

timeline

1780 *Outbreak of 'bilious remittent fever' in Philadelphia, later recognized as dengue fever and described as 'breakbone fever' by Benjamin Rush (1746-1813) in 1789.*

1826-8 *Serious outbreaks of dengue strike parts of the southern United States and the Caribbean, followed by further outbreaks in 1850-1 and 1878-80.*

1906 *Thomas Bancroft (1860- 1933) in Australia shows that the Aedes aegypti mosquito (then known as Stegomyia fasciata) transmits dengue fever as well as yellow fever. He suggests* that the infectious agent, too small to be seen under a microscope, is neither a parasite nor a bacterium.

1940s *Albert Sabin (1906-93) cultivates the dengue organism in the laboratory and shows it to be a virus.*

1941-5 *Dengue fever is a major problem in the Pacific theatre* during the Second World War.

1945 *The last outbreak of endemic dengue fever in continental USA occurs in Louisiana.*

1950s *Programmes to eradicate dengue and Aedes aegypti, primarily using DDT, begin in South and Central America.*

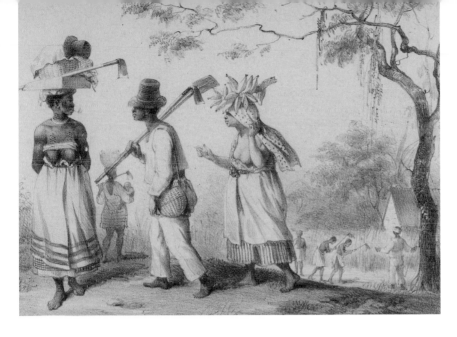

Slaves en route to work in Surinam (formerly Dutch Guiana), c.1839. It is possible that dengue fever was brought to the West Indies and the Americas from Africa by transported slaves infected with the disease.

The classic form of dengue is characterized by the sudden onset of fever, vomiting, a rash, severe frontal headache, intense pain behind the eyes, and searing joint and muscle pains, especially in the lower back. It is not very often fatal, although – as Rush also noted – the disease could leave its victims seriously debilitated and *'uncommonly dejected'* for a long time after recovery.

UNRAVELLING THE CAUSE OF DENGUE

The origins of dengue fever are uncertain. It may have been endemic in Africa and spread to the West Indies and the Americas via the transatlantic slave trade. Its chief vector, the *Aedes aegypti* mosquito, possibly originated in Africa, but as humans started to travel across the globe the mosquito established itself in far-flung places. Simultaneous epidemics occurred in the 1780s in Asia, Africa and North America, and throughout the following century there were many outbreaks of dengue fever, mostly in tropical and sub-tropical regions but occasionally also in temperate areas.

'I attended two young ladies, who shed tears while they vented their complaints of their sickness and weakness. One of them very aptly proposed to me to change the name of the disease, and to call it, in its present stage, instead of the break-bone, the break-heart fever.'
BENJAMIN RUSH (1746–1813)

1953 *Dengue haemorrhagic fever (DHF) is first identified in the Philippines, and is originally called Philippine haemorrhagic fever. It is later designated as a clinical entity* separate from the classical form of dengue fever.

1958 *DHF hits Bangkok, Thailand, and persists for five years, with over 10,000 cases and 694 deaths.*

1960s *Many Southeast Asian countries are afflicted by dengue fever and DHF. The Singapore government institutes measures to reduce its* incidence, including fining or imprisoning residents who allow mosquitoes to breed on their property.

1970s *Dengue fever and DHF erupt in other parts of Asia and the southwest Pacific.*

1981 *Major epidemic of dengue fever and DHF in Cuba, with 344,000 sick and 158 deaths.*

Late 20th–early 21st century *Resurgence of serious epidemics of dengue fever in many parts of the world, including Vietnam in 1987, Brazil in 2002 and Paraguay in 2007.*

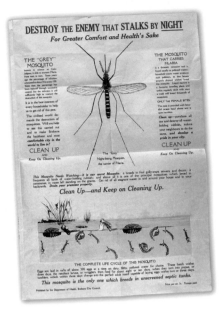

Initially, no one knew how the disease was transmitted. Then in 1906, following the discovery of the role played by mosquitoes in the transmission of diseases such as malaria and yellow fever, the Australian physician Thomas Lane Bancroft (1860–1933), using human volunteers for his experiments, showed that the *Aedes aegypti* mosquito responsible for yellow fever also carried dengue fever. Some decades later, the infective agent was found to be a virus.

SEARCHING FOR A SOLUTION

Following the discovery of the vector, there was considerable optimism. Successful control programmes virtually eliminated mosquito-borne diseases in Cuba and the Panama Canal Zone (see page 150), and there was tremendous hope that they could be tackled in other regions of the world. In the Americas, the Pan American Health Organization mounted a campaign to wipe out *Aedes aegypti* from most Central and South American countries in the 1950s and 1960s.

An Australian public health information poster of 1928 warns of the dangers posed by mosquitoes. Although *Aedes aegypti* has, historically, been the most important vector for dengue, another mosquito, *A. albopictus* (the Asian tiger mosquito), is now responsible for outbreaks of dengue in Asia. In 1985 this mosquito reached the Americas and spread rapidly across the eastern states of the USA, raising fears of the possible re-introduction of dengue fever to the USA.

DDT was widely used in mosquito-control programmes, but by the 1960s, following revelations of its toxic effects on the environment and problems of resistance, it was no longer considered a magic weapon. By the 1970s some of the anti-mosquito programmes were allowed to lapse, and it was increasingly difficult to control dengue fever in countries where it was endemic. With the growth of uncontrolled high-density urbanization in the developing world, often without adequate systems of water supply and sewerage, ideal conditions were created for the proliferation of the mosquito and the transmission of dengue.

Poor medical care and deteriorating public-health infrastructures are further problems in endemic regions, while an increase in global air travel has aided the worldwide dispersal of the dengue virus and a mixing of its various sub-types and strains.

'The presence of albopictus dramatically increases the probability that exotic viruses will be brought into the urban human environments of the Americas … the tiger mosquito will feed on anything, a rat for example, and then turn right around and feed on a human.'

DUANE GUBLER, SPECIALIST IN DENGUE FEVER, UNIVERSITY OF HAWAII

NEW AND DEADLY FORMS OF DENGUE EMERGE

Partly as a result of these factors, in recent decades there has been a dramatic increase in dengue fever, especially in Southeast Asia, the Pacific region (including northern Queensland, Australia), the Caribbean, South America and parts of the Middle East and Africa. An average of 900 cases per annum were recorded in the late 1950s, but by the end of the century this had jumped to over half a million. Even more worrying has been the emergence of more deadly forms of the disease – dengue haemorrhagic fever (DHF) and dengue shock syndrome (DSS).

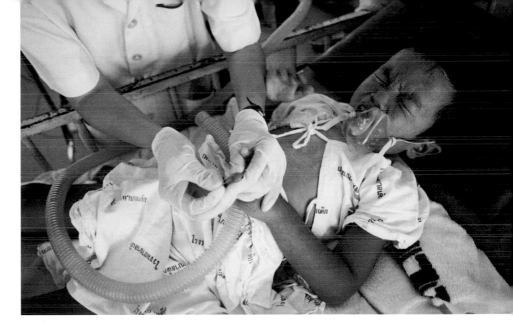

The first epidemic cases of DHF were reported in Manila in the Philippines in 1953. A small child with dengue fever started bleeding uncontrollably, then other children fell victim to this strange new syndrome. By the following year a serious epidemic of DHF was sweeping though the area, thereafter reaching Thailand and other parts of Asia. In 1981 a six month epidemic of dengue and DHF occurred in Havana, Cuba, killing 158 people, including 51 children, and further outbreaks were reported in Latin America. This apparently new clinical syndrome seems to have arisen in Southeast Asia and the Pacific during and after the Second World War, linked to the movement of troops and populations, and associated with ecological disruption. It has rapidly become a significant public-health problem in many towns and cities in the tropics and sub-tropics.

DHF, with its ominous symptoms of pinpoint-sized spots of blood, bleeding under the skin, convulsions and fevers reaching over 104° F (40° C), can lead to multiple haemorrhaging or, in the case of DSS, circulatory shock. It is currently a leading cause of hospitalization and death in Southeast Asia, especially in young children. There is no cure, but fatality rates can be kept down (to 5 per cent) with good medical care and fluid-replacement therapy. DHF and DSS are puzzling and frightening outcomes of dengue fever – one hypothesis is that they are triggered by a complex hyperactive immune response following a previous (and usually mild) infection with a different serotype of dengue fever.

Dengue today

Today some 2.5 billion people – two-fifths of the world's population – in more than 100 countries live in areas where dengue is endemic. Tens of millions of cases of dengue fever have been reported so far in the 21st century, and hundreds of thousands of cases of DHF/DSS occur each year. Dengue is now thought to be the most important viral disease transmitted by mosquitoes.

The best advice at present to avoid contracting the disease is to cover up, avoid mosquito bites, remove any potential 'mosquito-breeding' containers, use insect repellents in areas where dengue fever poses a risk – and to remember that unlike the malarial mosquito, which bites after dusk, *Aedes aegypti* likes to bite by day – especially favouring a few hours after sunrise and a few hours before sunset.

A child with dengue haemorrhagic fever at the Children's Hospital in Bangkok, Thailand. Many children contract dengue fever during the rainy season when there is a lot of standing water. There are no cures but mortality can be kept down with medical care and intravenous fluid replacement.

RABIES is an acute viral infection of the central nervous system, transmitted via the saliva of an

infected animal. Although rabies has not been responsible for devastating epidemics like cholera and plague, it is one of the most frightening of all diseases. The very word 'rabies' – from the Latin word meaning 'to rave' – conjures up images of 'mad' dogs foaming at the mouth and biting people in a frenzied attack, resulting in horrific symptoms and almost certain death for the victim. Although there are now effective vaccines, there are still parts of the world where rabies is a very real danger.

In the 23rd century BC, a legal document, called the Eshnunna Code of Babylon, was drawn up in Mesopotamia. It stipulated the amount of compensation that an owner of a 'mad' dog had to pay in the event that the animal caused the death of a person - 40 shekels of silver in most cases, or 15 shekels if the victim was a slave. Today, in the 21st century AD, there are all sorts of strict and costly regulations to ensure that domestic animals are vaccinated or put into quarantine before entering a rabies-free country. In the intervening 4000 or so years, societies have struggled to understand, contain and prevent rabies. It is a story of insights and dead ends, brilliant scientific discoveries and worldwide fear.

THE BITE OF A MAD DOG

In ancient Mesopotamia, China, India, Greece and Rome, the consequences of the bite of a rabid dog were all too familiar. There was no cure, and the victim had no chance of survival. The cause of the human form of the disease - the bite of a rabid animal - was one of the most clearly recognized and dreaded diseases of the ancient world. But what caused dogs and other rabid animals to go 'mad' in the first place? For Roman and Greek physicians, rabies somehow had to fit into their 'humoral doctrine' of disease, based on the idea that the body was made up of four 'humours' or fluids: black bile, yellow bile, phlegm and blood. When these were in balance, a person remained healthy. But if the humours became unbalanced, disease resulted. All sorts of factors could upset the balance. Animals, it was believed, developed rabies following 'a corruption of the humours', caused possibly by cold, heat, poisoning, stress or by devouring corpses. The next part of the puzzle was how the bite of a rabid animal transmitted the disease to humans.

timeline

23rd century BC
The Babylonian Eshnunna Code contains the first known mention of rabies.

c.420 BC *The Greek philosopher Democritus (c.460–c.370 BC) mentions rabies.*

1st century AD *The Roman philosopher Celsus (25 BC–AD 50) makes the first accurate description of rabies.*

1500s *During the Spanish conquest of the Americas, a bishop describes small animals that bite soldiers' toes as they sleep, resulting in their death. It is possible that* the soldiers were bitten by rabid vampire bats.

1708 *The first well-documented outbreak of dog rabies in Italy.*

1804 *The German scientist Georg Gottfried Zinke (d.1813) publishes a small book on rabies and carries out experiments transmitting rabies from animal to animal.*

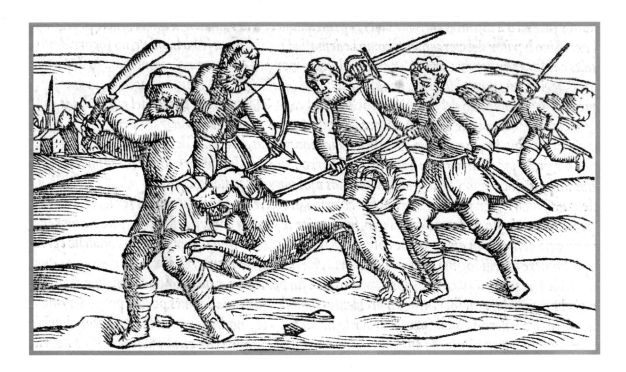

In the first century AD, Aulus Celsus (25 BC–AD 50), the Roman philosopher and writer, used the word 'virus' in connection with dog bites. In Latin *virus* means 'something slimy and poisonous'. Celsus suggested that if anyone was bitten by a rabid dog, 'the virus must be drawn out with a cupping glass'. As it happens, Celsus had the right word for the infection, but it was not until the 1930s that any 'virus' – a tiny micro-organism that can only reproduce inside another living cell – was actually 'seen', using an electron microscope.

For many centuries, the ideas of the ancients about rabies continued to dominate as well as to confuse and perplex. Some (correctly) narrowed the virus down to the 'poisonous' saliva in the bite of the rabid animal. In 1735 an anonymous contributor to the *London Magazine* wrote that rabies was transmitted by means of *'minute particles or animalculae mixt with saliva'* inserted through a wound into the *'nervous juice'*, and that these particles then affected the brain. Others

A woodcut from the Middle Ages showing a group of people using a variety of weapons to slay a rabid dog.

1885 *Louis Pasteur (1822–95) successfully vaccinates Joseph Meister after he has been attacked by a rabid dog.*

1922 *Britain is declared free of rabies.*

1930s *Scientists establish connection between bites of bats and paralytic rabies.*

1996 *A new rabies virus is identified in several species of flying foxes and other bats in Australia, and has been associated with two human deaths from rabies-like illnesses.*

1999 *Rabies in wildlife is eliminated in Switzerland, followed by other European countries.*

2007 *World Rabies Day takes place on 8 September to increase world awareness of rabies and to raise support and funding towards its control and prevention.*

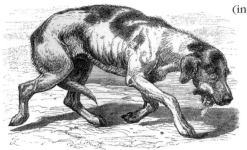

Late-stage rabies, from an 1872 illustration. Over the millennia, all sorts of regulations have been imposed in an attempt to prevent the spread of the disease. In Britain, the Victorians passed laws that required all dogs in public places to be muzzled, and allowed policemen to shoot any unmuzzled dog. Elsewhere, dogs had their teeth filed down to prevent them inflicting deep bites.

(incorrectly) questioned the physical nature of the disease, suggesting that its deadly symptoms were a result of imagination and fear.

TO CURE OR CONTAIN

Physicians searched for ways of curing the terrible scourge – drugs and purges, bloodletting and cauterizing the wound with hot irons, jumping into the sea, electrical shocks, ingesting the liver of mad dogs – but to no avail. In Korea, medicines were made up using cats as the main ingredient – the idea, possibly, being that the cat medicine would neutralize the dog poison. The French physician Joseph-Ignace Guillotin (1738–1814), who is more commonly associated with the decapitation device that bears his name, wanted to set up some experiments whereby condemned criminals would be bitten by 'mad' dogs and used to try out various remedies. The idea was not taken up.

THE TERROR THAT LED TO THE TREATMENT

In July 1885 the story of rabies control was transformed by a remarkable experiment by the French chemist Louis Pasteur (1822–95), one of the founders of modern bacteriology. As a nine-year-old child he had witnessed the mutilation and deaths of several people when a 'mad' wolf had rampaged through his village in the Jura Mountains of eastern France, biting people on their hands and faces. The experience gave him a lifelong fear of rabies, a fear shared by millions. By 1885, Pasteur already had an international scientific reputation. He had discarded the old notion of 'spontaneous generation' (by which it was thought that

SPASMS, RAVING AND THE FEAR OF WATER

The word 'rabies' has its origins in ancient languages. In Sanskrit, the word *rabhas* means 'to do violence'. The Greeks used the word *lyssa*, meaning 'frenzy'. In Latin *rabere* means 'to rave', and the associated adjective *rabidus*, 'furious, raging', gives us the term 'rabid'. In French, rabies is *la rage*. The words aptly describe the symptoms of this terrible disease.

Rabies is caused by the *Lyssavirus* virus, which is present in a rabid animal's saliva. It is communicated either by a bite or by the infected animal licking a break in the victim's skin. From the site of entry it travels along the nerve pathways to the brain. Sometime after the bite or lick (the incubation period can be anything from nine days to more than a year, though usually three to eight weeks) the most horrible symptoms manifest themselves. The infected do, indeed, appear to go 'mad' in all sorts of ways. They foam at the mouth, become vicious and aggressive, suffer seizures, hallucinations and extreme thirst – but when they try to drink they are crippled by severe muscle spasms in the throat; in spite of their desperate need for water, its very sight can lead to terror, followed by delirium and convulsions. In Europe in the Middle Ages, the disease was also known as hydrophobia, meaning 'fear of water'. In the end, the victim falls into a coma and death, when it comes, is often due to respiratory paralysis. There have only been a handful of recorded cases of a person surviving rabies after the onset of symptoms.

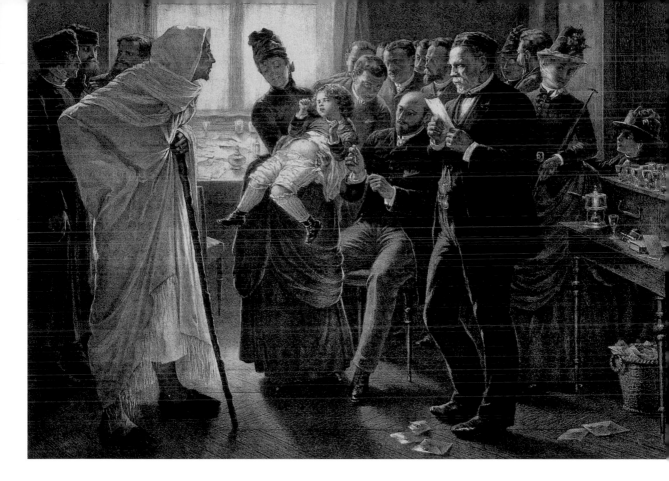

A contemporary lithograph showing a rabies vaccination session at Pasteur's clinic in Paris. Unlike most preventive vaccines, Pasteur's was intended to stop the disease spreading once a victim had been bitten by a rabid animal.

decaying meat, for example, spontaneously generated maggots), and had replaced it with the 'germ theory' of disease (in which he proved that it was infectious agents or germs that caused the decay and not the other way round). He had also found a way of eliminating microbes from milk ('pasteurization'), and had developed vaccines for chicken cholera and anthrax. But there was still one thing that he was determined to discover: a treatment for rabies.

After years of exhaustive work, Pasteur and a team of researchers in Paris eventually developed a vaccine using the dried spinal cord of rabbits, which they found was effective in rabid dogs. But would it work on humans? On 6 July 1885 a badly bitten little boy from Alsace named Joseph Meister (1876–1940) was brought to Pasteur by his distraught mother and Théodore Vone, the owner of the rabid dog. The boy was not expected to live. Pasteur took the chance. He and two doctors vaccinated the boy and, after another 12 injections over a period of ten days, he survived.

In October of the same year, Pasteur successfully vaccinated a second child – Jean-Baptiste Jupille,

'As the death of this child appeared inevitable, I decided, not without deep and severe unease, as one can well imagine, to try out on Joseph Meister the procedure which had consistently worked on dogs.'

LOUIS PASTEUR, DESCRIBING HIS DECISION TO ATTEMPT TO VACCINATE A RABIES VICTIM IN JULY 1885

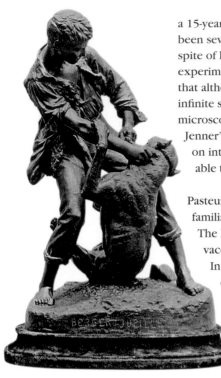

A sculpture representing Jean-Baptiste Jupille struggling with a rabid dog. The 15-year-old shepherd boy was the second person to be successfully treated with the rabies vaccine by pioneering bacteriologist Louis Pasteur in 1885.

a 15-year-old shepherd boy from Pasteur's home district of the Jura, who had been severely bitten as he tried to protect other children from a rabid dog. In spite of his initial successes, there was some scepticism and criticism of Pasteur's experimental vaccine in the medical profession. Even Pasteur had to acknowledge that although he suspected the infective agent of rabies to be 'a microbe of infinite smallness', he could not actually see the microbe in question using the microscopes then available. His discovery of the rabies vaccine, like Edward Jenner's vaccine for smallpox nearly a century earlier (see page 128), was based on intuition and trial and error, and it was many decades before scientists were able to 'see' the virus responsible and understand how it acted.

Pasteur's rabies vaccine was different from most vaccines with which we are familiar today. It was not given in order to prevent the disease but to cure it. The long incubation period of rabies, following the initial bite, meant that vaccination at this stage could stop the dreaded symptoms from developing. In 1886, even after the long train ride to Paris to seek the vaccine, 35 out of 38 Russian peasants mauled by rabid wolves were apparently saved by Pasteur's injections.

In 1888 a new scientific research centre opened in Paris, named the Institut Pasteur in honour of the great man's achievements. Joseph Meister went on to become the concierge of the institute. Tragically, Meister shot himself in 1940 after the Fall of France, devastated that he had been unable to prevent the Nazis from entering the crypt inside the institute where Pasteur's remains were interred.

CANINE RABIES

Pasteur's vaccine, with various later refinements, continued to be used in the control and prevention of rabies for nearly a century. Recently, safer and more effective vaccines for post-exposure rabies have been developed, as well as a preventive vaccine for people who are at high risk. There is also a vaccine for dogs, cats, sheep, cattle and horses. The control of rabies in domestic animals has been highly successful in some parts of the world. Britain, for example, has been free of canine rabies since 1922. Some other nations with strict measures of inspection, vaccination, quarantine of pets and control of stray animals have also successfully exterminated canine rabies. Fox rabies, once widespread across continental Europe, has also declined considerably in recent decades since the introduction of an oral rabies vaccine for foxes (contained in chicken heads and distributed across the countryside).

Western, central and eastern Europe, including the Russian Federation, currently report less than 50 rabies deaths each year. In Latin America, a canine rabies control programme established in 1981 has led to an 84 per cent reduction in human deaths, with only 56 cases reported in the early 21st century. Throughout the world, 50 million dogs are vaccinated each year, though in parts of Africa and Asia the vaccine coverage in the dog population (30–50 per cent) is not high enough to break the transmission cycle of the disease.

The number of humans infected and killed still remains horribly high. Over 10 million people receive the post-exposure vaccine every year, and an estimated 55,000 people worldwide die of the disease. The majority of all human cases occur in Africa and parts of Asia (mainly India), and most human deaths in these continents follow dog bites for which post-exposure vaccination was not or could not be provided.

WILD CARNIVORES AND VAMPIRE BATS

Although 'mad' dogs are usually singled out as the culprits as far as human rabies is concerned, dogs and other domestic animals can themselves be infected by bites from feral or wild animals, such as wolves, foxes, jackals, coyotes, raccoons, skunks and mongooses. Such animals may also directly infect humans: in South America, for example, more people now die from rabies following bites from wildlife than from dogs. Bats, such as the flying fox in Australia and the blood-sucking vampire bat in South and Central America, are also reservoirs for the rabies virus. Since 1985 cases of bat rabies have been reported in Europe (including Great Britain), as well as in the USA and Canada. In North America the most recently documented human rabies deaths have occurred as a result of infection from the silver-haired bat. Alarmingly, a new rabies virus, closely related to but not identical to the classical rabies virus, was identified in 1996 in several species of flying foxes and bats in Australia, and has been associated with two human deaths from rabies-like illnesses.

As with many other diseases with a reservoir in wild carnivores, breaking the cycle of transmission is far from easy. Wild animals are not subject to inspection at international border controls. The main advice is to steer clear of any animal behaving bizarrely, to avoid flying foxes and other bats, and, if in doubt, remember Joseph Meister and seek early treatment.

Dumb Rabies

Not all sick dogs or animals infected by rabies display the typically alarming symptoms of foaming at the mouth and hydrophobia. A form of rabies, known as 'dumb rabies', leaves the animal or human victim listless and progressively immobile. In avoiding rabid animals, it is important to watch out for any bizarre behaviour as both the 'furious' and 'dumb' forms can mean almost certain death if a person is bitten and left unvaccinated.

A photograph taken outside the Pasteur Institute at Kasauli, India, in 1910, shows patients in front of the inoculation rooms. Although the hospital prepared vaccines against a number of diseases, for many years it was known locally as the 'mad dog' hospital, for its treatment of rabies.

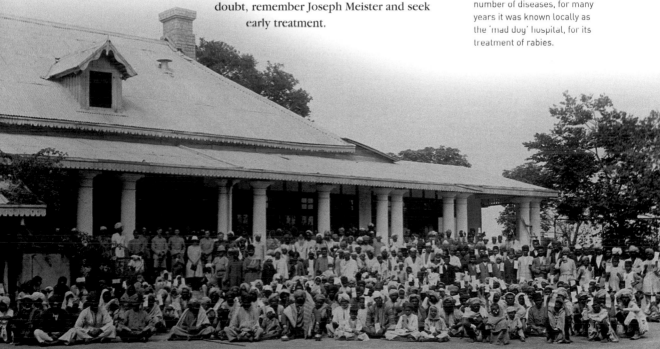

POLIO is a cruel disease that has disabled many people

– especially children – over the last century or so. It is caused by a virus, and is passed from person to person via unwashed hands or contamination of food or water. In most cases the infection provokes only a mild illness, but in some cases the virus may invade the central nervous system, leading to muscle degeneration and paralysis. Its full scientific name is poliomyelitis, so named because of inflammation of the 'grey matter' of the spinal cord (in Greek, *polios* means 'grey' and *myelos* means 'matter'). Polio is probably an ancient disease, but it was not until the end of the 19th century that outbreaks of polio attracted serious attention. The first vaccines were developed in the mid-20th century, and with mass immunization the incidence of polio around the world has fallen dramatically.

In the summer of 1916 in Brooklyn, New York City, a small child lay sick. She was gasping for air, struggling to take each breath. Her desperate parents had no idea what was wrong. Late that night, the local doctor was summoned. He held the child's hand and felt her pulse. She was feverish, delirious and clearly in intense pain. She began to lose all feeling and movement in her little legs. She lay on her bed soaked in sweat – listless and apparently almost lifeless. The doctor arranged to take her to hospital. Her parents were distraught that she was being taken away. She was admitted as an emergency. She had all the signs and symptoms of poliomyelitis or, as it was then known, 'infantile paralysis', and she was one of thousands of cases in the world's first most serious recorded epidemic of polio in 1916–17 in New York.

INFANTILE PARALYSIS

'Infantile paralysis' in 1916 was a diagnosis without hope, without treatment and with no known cause. Many children died, others spent months in hospital. There was little to be done but to wait and watch. By 1917, nearly 9000 cases of infantile paralysis had been recorded in New York City. Some victims were left permanently paralyzed, and around 2400 people, mostly children, had died. Many of the survivors spent the rest of their (often short) lives in 'callipers' or braces.

timeline

1400 BC An Egyptian stele shows a young priest with a shortened, deformed foot typical of polio. The disease may be as old as humankind, but there are very few early descriptions.

AD 1789 A British surgeon-apothecary, Michael Underwood (1736–1820), makes the first known clinical description of polio, calling it 'debility of the lower extremities'.

1831–5 One of the earliest recorded outbreaks of polio occurs on the island of St Helena; small epidemics follow in England and the USA.

1840 Polio is recognized as a clinical entity by the German physician Jacob von Heine (1800–79). He names it 'infantile spinal paralysis'.

1890s–early 1900s Further epidemics in Scandinavia and New England, USA.

1908–9 The Austrian biologist and physician Karl Landsteiner (1868–1943) shows that polio is contagious by injecting a monkey with an emulsion made from the spinal cord of a polio victim; he then successfully transfers the virus from that monkey to another.

1916 At New York City's Rockefeller Institute for Medical Research, Simon Flexner (1863–1946) describes polio germs that he and his colleagues have seen under a microscope as 'innumerable bright dancing points, devoid of definite size and form'.

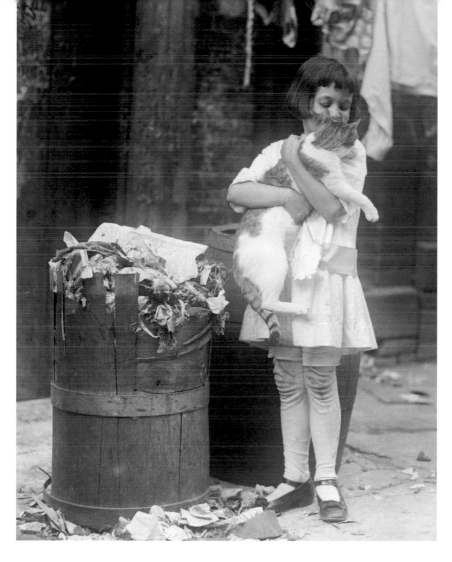

Linking dirt with disease, this picture was intended to demonstrate how illnesses like polio spread: a girl hugs a stray cat picked up whilst feeding on rubbish.

The authorities dealt with the epidemic in ways that were reminiscent of reactions to bubonic plague in earlier centuries. Road blocks were imposed and vehicles with children under 16 years of age were not allowed to come into the city. Some of the wealthier families fled to the countryside, but many others who tried to escape the pestilential city were sent back. In the poorer areas of the city,

1916–17 The world's first most serious recorded epidemic occurs in the USA. In New York City alone over 9000 cases are reported, while nationwide there are more than 27,000 cases and 6000 deaths.

1921 Franklin D. Roosevelt (1882–1945) contracts what was thought to be polio.

1927–8 Philip Drinker (1894–1972) and Louis Shaw (1886–1940) at Harvard School of Public Health, Boston, USA, develop an air-tight chamber that pushes air in and out of an immobilized polio patient's lungs. In 1928, a young girl at Boston Children's Hospital becomes the first to use the 'iron lung'. Commercial production begins a few years later.

1920s–1950s Major epidemics of polio occur regularly in the USA and other industrialized countries.

1933 Elizabeth Kenny (1880–1952) opens her first clinic in Townsville, Australia, for the care of polio victims. Her methods include physical therapy and heat treatment.

1938 Franklin D. Roosevelt sets up the National Foundation for Infantile Paralysis – the first public-health organization in the USA to rely on the general public for funds. Its annual 'March of Dimes' fundraising drives are highly successful, raising an estimated $630 million between 1938 and 1962.

(continued ...)

'polio houses' were quarantined, warning placards were posted and 'crippled' children were forcibly removed to isolation hospitals. Cats and dogs, as possible carriers, were abandoned or killed; public places were shut or avoided; immigrant families were shunned and blamed. The city reeked of disinfectant as officials battled to sanitize and contain the spread of this mysterious summer sickness.

DIRT, DISEASE AND THE DANGER OF THE HOUSEFLY

Across the USA, there were 27,000 cases of polio and over 6000 deaths between 1916 and 1917. Almost all were children under the age of five. Americans were gripped by fear, panic and, above all, hopelessness. It was a terrifying disease, one that struck young children and inflicted appalling suffering. Polio has probably been around for centuries but, for reasons that remain obscure, it seems to have become a serious problem only in the last hundred or so years (see Polio Puzzles, page 166).

In 1916 no one knew how the disease spread. Was it through the air or through water and food? There was no shortage of theories, from both medical and lay people. Some blamed summer fruits, ice creams, candy, maggots in the colon, insects, raw sewage, garbage, dust, poisonous caterpillars, mouldy flour, contaminated milk bottles or even bananas infected by tarantula spiders. Others advised parents to avoid close contact with their children, believing the disease to be transmitted through sneezing, coughing, spitting and kissing.

'In one house I went into the only window was not only shut, but the cracks were stuffed with rags, so that the "disease" could not come in. You can imagine what the dark, dirty room was like; the babies had no clothes on, and were so wet and hot that they looked as if they had been dipped in oil, and the flies were sticking all over them ... '

A LETTER FROM A SOCIAL WORKER DURING THE 1916 NEW YORK EPIDEMIC, REPRINTED IN A NEW YORK NEWSPAPER

In the USA and Europe in the late 19th and early 20th centuries, polio was predominantly a disease of the summer months. Drawing parallels with cholera, typhoid and other 'filth diseases', doctors linked polio with dirty environments and insanitary conditions, especially in hot, smelly summers. Initially, in the wake

timeline

1942 The Sister Kenny Institute is established and directed by Elizabeth Kenny in Minneapolis, Minnesota, USA.

1948–9 John Enders (1897–1985), Thomas Weller (b.1915) and Frederick Robbins (1916–2003) at the Children's Medical Center in Boston, Massachusetts, succeed in growing the polio virus in non-neurological human tissue in the laboratory, paving the way for the development of a vaccine.

1952 In Pittsburgh, Pennsylvania, USA, Jonas Salk (1914–95), supported by the National Foundation for Infantile Paralysis, tests his inactivated vaccine on volunteers, including himself, the laboratory staff, his wife and children.

1954 The Salk vaccine is tested on nearly 1.8 million schoolchildren in the USA.

1955 The Salk vaccine is licensed following the announcement of the success of the Salk trials. In the notorious 'Cutter Incident', however, 200,000 people are injected with 'Salk vaccine' prepared by the Cutter Laboratories in California. The 'vaccine' turns out to contain virulent, non-attenuated polio virus: 70,000 become ill, 200 children are left paralyzed, and ten die. A storm of controversy follows in the USA.

1961–2 Following successful trials in the USSR and elsewhere, the attenuated vaccine developed by the American scientist

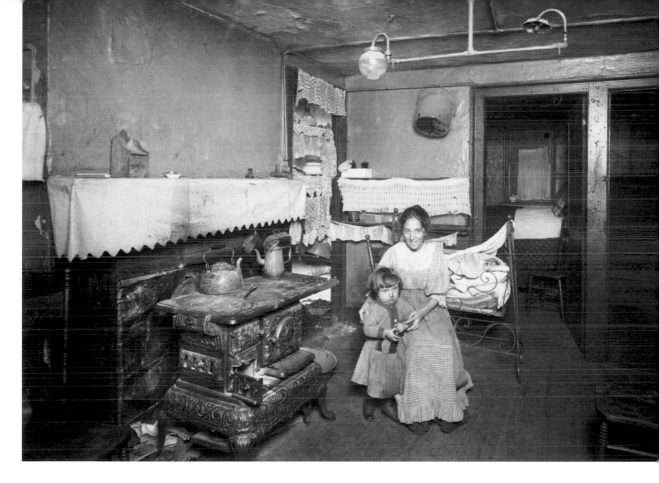

of the New York epidemic, immigrant ghettos and slum areas were targeted as the likely source of the disease. But in the summer of 1916 it became clear that the epidemic, while striking hardest at the young, affected both rich and poor, long-time residents as well as recent immigrants.

The association between dirt and disease was extended to the idea that maybe the ubiquitous housefly carried the germs of polio – from filth to food, from the 'dirty' immigrant quarters to the sparkling 'clean' houses of the leafy suburbs. Discoveries in the field of tropical medicine in the late 19th and early 20th

A poor New York City tenement room from 1911. The source of the outbreak of polio in the city in 1916 was blamed initially on slum dwellings such as this one.

Albert Sabin (1906–93) is widely taken up in the USA and throughout the Pan-American Health Organization countries. The Sabin vaccine largely replaces the Salk vaccine

since it can be administered orally rather than by injection.

1979 The last cases in the USA of paralytic polio caused by endemic transmission of 'wild' polio virus.

All subsequent cases are either imported or vaccine-related.

1988 The Global Polio Eradication Initiative, spear-headed by governments, the World Health Organization

(WHO), Rotary International, the US Centers for Disease Control and UNICEF, launches a campaign to eradicate polio by 2000 – one of the largest public health initiatives ever seen.

1994 The Americas are certified as 'polio free', followed by the western Pacific region in 2000 and the European region in 2002.

2003 The number of polio cases worldwide de-creases from 350,000 in 1988 to under 700 in 2003.

2007 The WHO states that the world now has its best chance ever to eradicate polio, but it still remains endemic in a few hotspots in Nigeria, India, Pakistan and Afghanistan.

centuries had shown that mosquitoes, fleas, flies and lice could transmit diseases like malaria, yellow fever, plague, sleeping sickness and typhus. The housefly was everywhere, buzzing on the piles of horse dung in the streets of New York, swarming in the garbage cans, then alighting on babies or infecting food. Attacking the housefly became a major preoccupation. Garbage bins were sealed, houses were screened, windows shut, fly-swatting contests were held, while posters and pamphlets featured an image of a giant housefly menacing the children of the city.

'We have a gospel to preach. We need to make America "polio conscious" to the end that the inexcusable case of positive neglect will be entirely eliminated.'

FRANKLIN DELANO ROOSEVELT, 1932

We now know that the housefly is capable of carrying over a hundred pathogens. Polio, however, is spread primarily through contaminated water, food or unwashed hands. The polio enterovirus is ingested and passes into the gut. It is shed in the faeces, and can then infect those with poor sanitary facilities or inadequate hygiene. This pathway of transmission is known as the faecal-oral route. A high proportion of the population infected with the virus get a mild fever or show no symptoms but can act as carriers (an observation that was first made in Sweden early in the 20th century). The 1916 campaign in New York, involving quarantine, cleansing and disinfecting, arose out of desperation and uncertainty, but in retrospect some measures were not far off the mark.

A FAMOUS VICTIM

In a minority of people, for reasons still not fully understood, the virus moves from the intestinal tract into the bloodstream and then invades the central nervous system (the brain and spinal cord) where it causes serious damage, leading to muscle weakness, paralysis and sometimes death. In the early decades of the 20th century, finding a way of helping those who survived 'infantile paralysis' was as problematic as understanding its cause. Some doctors recommended

POLIO PUZZLES

A curious feature of polio is why paralysis occurs in only about 1 per cent of all those infected, while 85–90 per cent have no symptoms at all, and the rest only a mild fever. This varying severity may depend on the virulence of the polio strain, genetic factors, or possibly excessive muscular activity while the disease is incubating or during its early onset.

Another puzzle is why, over the course of the first half of the 20th century, polio in the West became associated with increased prosperity and cleanliness. A disease spread by the faecal-oral route that flourishes at a time of improved hygiene is something of an epidemiological paradox. It has been suggested that over the past two millennia infants and children were constantly exposed to the disease in areas of poor sanitation and, while developing a mild fever, they were able to build up life-long immunity. Only when general standards of hygiene and public health improved did the mild form of the disease cease to be a constant part of life so that, when it did strike, children and adolescents had little early exposure, and thus little or no immunity.

heavy massaging and exercising affected limbs, while others suggested putting them into plaster casts or callipers, recommending long periods of immobility to prevent deformities. Various experimental therapies such as lumbar puncture and injections of anti-polio blood serum were tried out in hospitals. Home remedies and preventions included anything from 'earthworm oil' to bathing in ox blood.

Heart-rending images of children crippled by infantile paralysis became all too familiar, but when in the summer of 1921 a prominent member of a wealthy New York family was struck down with polio, it became clear that the disease could affect anyone, no matter how old or how privileged. The victim was Franklin Delano Roosevelt (1882–1945), a rising star in the Democratic Party, and later four-times president of the USA. Roosevelt, then aged 39, had been taking his summer vacation on the island of Campobello, off the coast of New Brunswick and Maine, when, on the night of 10 August 1921, he was suddenly struck by the disease.

Roosevelt survived, but for the rest of his life he battled with his pain and disabilities. In 1924 a visit to Warm Springs, Georgia, inspired him to organize major fund-raising events to transform the spa town into a hydrotherapy and rehabilitation centre for polio sufferers. He also began to put the needs of the disabled on the political agenda.

THE MARCH OF DIMES

As president of the United States from 1933 until his death in 1945, Roosevelt shouldered many burdens, first taking upon himself the task of mitigating the worst effects of the Great Depression, and then leading his country through the Second World War. He also had his own physical disability to cope with, but this was one thing he was determined to hide from the public: as far as we know, there are only two pictures of him in his wheelchair. While hiding his affliction, he remained committed to finding a way of helping his fellow sufferers.

What started out as Roosevelt's personal mission at Warm Springs became in 1938 the National Foundation for Infantile Paralysis, whose aim was to *lead, direct, and unify the fight against every aspect of the killing and crippling infection of poliomyelitis*. Shortly after a radio appeal asking everyone to send their dimes (10 cents) to the president at the White House to fight polio, the sum of over a million dollars was collected. The annual 'March of Dimes' – the catch phrase for the polio crusade – raised $630 million between 1938 and 1962. The Foundation did much to provide long-term care for sufferers, and also funded research and promoted awareness of the disease. Its propaganda film, *The Daily*

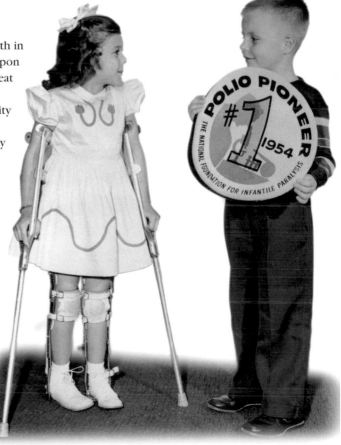

Mary Kosloski, 1955 March of Dimes poster girl and polio sufferer, meets Randy Kerr, the US's first Polio Pioneer to receive the Salk vaccine the previous spring. Together, they represented the two aims of the March of Dimes – polio treatment and cure.

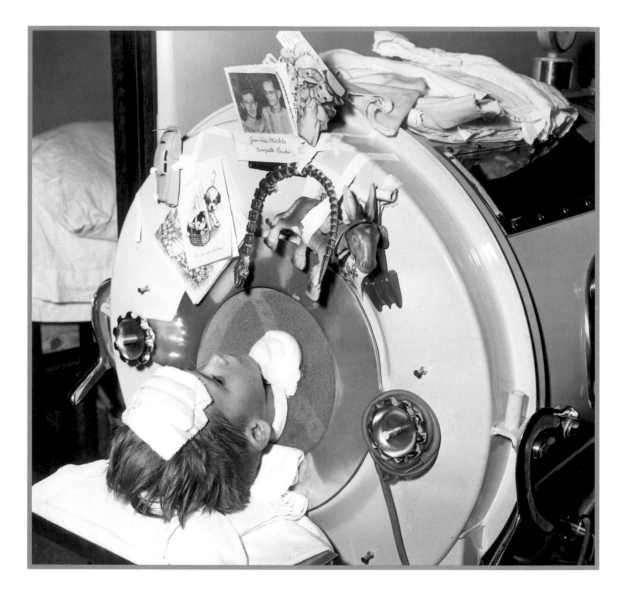

Because polio can paralyze the muscles used to breathe, some polio sufferers became dependent on a mechanical respirator, known as an iron lung, to assist with breathing.

Battle, features a nearly invisible figure leaning on a crutch. This figure, known colloquially as 'The Crippler', stalks the land intoning the sinister but true words: '*And I'm* especially *fond of children*'.

IRON LUNGS

The thermal baths at Warm Springs were a therapeutic treat for those with limited mobility. The most seriously affected polio survivors, whose respiratory muscles were paralyzed, experienced severe breathing and swallowing difficulties, and for them life hung in the balance. From the 1930s, artificial respiration was provided by the 'iron lung', a large, cumbersome and noisy device in which the patient was placed horizontally, and which pushed and pulled the chest muscles to make them work. For some patients, the iron lung provided temporary assistance, giving them much needed time to recover their own respiratory muscle power. Others found themselves condemned to spend the rest of their lives in this fearsome and isolating machine. In Copenhagen, Denmark, in 1952, in one of the worst recorded polio epidemics in Europe, a shortage of iron lun inspired the invention of an alternative method of artificial respiration. This involved making a surgical cut in the patient's trachea or windpipe (tracheotomy) and ventilatin the patient using tubes and rubber bags. Some 1500 medic students assisted with the 'bagging method', devoting ove 165,000 hours to saving the lives of many small children during the course of the epidemic.

A NARROW ESCAPE FOR THE RESPONAUTS

Patients who were confined to iron lungs to aid them with their breathing were sometimes known by the term 'responauts'.

One patient vividly remembers a night in the early 1950s when suddenly the harsh hum of the iron lungs ceased. The night nurse had tripped over the cable that supplied power to the machines, and those encased within their iron lungs gasped for breath. The nurse quickly switched the power back on, and the 'swooshing and pulsing sounds' of the iron lungs returned.

SISTER KENNY

Iron lungs, tracheotomies, crutches, braces, splints and ca: were all used with the best of intentions, albeit immobilizi patients and restricting the use of their paralyzed limbs. In the 1930s Sister Elizabeth Kenny (1880–1952), a colourful and imposing lady from the Australian outback, pioneered alternative approach to try to get polio survivors back on their feet. The 'Kenny method', which combined physical and psychological techniques, involved hot packs, gentle 'retraining' of muscles, optimism and determination. For the lucky patients for whom this method worked it was close to a miracle, enabling them to reuse their weakened limbs with perhaps only the use of a walking stick, so giving them a new lease of life. Sister Kenny's methods were controversial but, until her death, she kept up her message that it was vital to 'remind the brain how to walk'.

A TALE OF TWO VACCINES

In the year of Sister Kenny's death in 1952, the USA was once more hit by a major outbreak of polio. Some 58,000 people were affected: 3000 died and another 21,000 were left paralyzed. Funds raised by Roosevelt's March of Dimes and the National Foundation for Infantile Paralysis had mostly been diverted to the care of survivors. Now the time was ripe to invest more into the search for a cure or vaccine. While antibiotics were revolutionizing the treatment of bacterial infections, attempts to find a remedy for viral diseases eluded the scientific community. There was, and perhaps never will be, a cure for polio. But in 1955 the USA celebrated the success of the first large-scale immunization of over 400,000 children with a safe and effective vaccine.

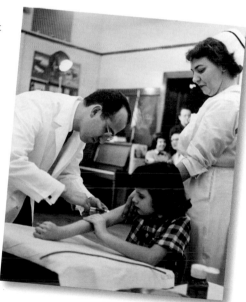

Jonas Salk injects a child with his inactivated polio vaccine during field trials in Pittsburgh, 1954. Although this was superseded by Sabin's oral vaccine, an inactivated polio vaccine is still used in some countries.

The man who had developed the vaccine, the American virologist Jonas Salk (1914–95), became a national hero overnight. His vaccine was based on an inactivated (i.e. dead) polio virus administered by injection and tested on nearly 1.8 million children (known as the 'Polio Pioneers') in a double-blind trial,

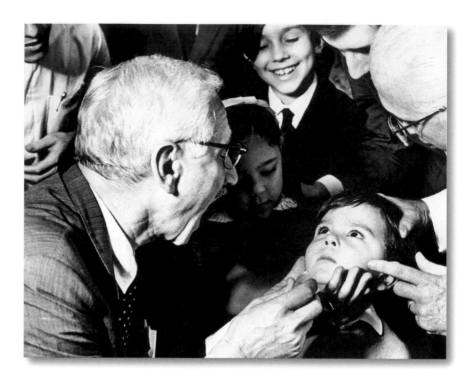

American scientist Albert
Sabin, seen here examining a
young patient at an anti-polio
hospital in 1967, developed
the form of polio vaccine that
was to become the accepted
standard in most countries.

with some receiving the vaccine, some a placebo and the rest acting as controls.
Another American scientist, Albert Sabin (1906–93), went on to develop a live-
attenuated vaccine, which was administered orally and offered some advantages
over the Salk vaccine. Rivalry between supporters of one or the other vaccine
flared up into one of the great feuds in medical history, with the players in the saga
either at each others' throats or not on speaking terms.

Sabin conducted trials on a range of subjects, including his own family and
prisoners in federal penitentiaries, followed by a large-scale immunization of
several million people in the Soviet Union. Eventually, by the early 1960s, it was
Sabin's oral vaccine that became the accepted standard in most countries. On
'Sabin Sundays', about 100 million Americans received the vaccine free of charge.
A simple lump of sugar impregnated with the live polio virus – now usually given
to infants – was subsequently instrumental in all but eliminating the disease in the
Western world. There are still occasional outbreaks among unvaccinated groups,
and rare cases of polio caused by the oral vaccine itself.

ON THE VERGE OF GLOBAL ERADICATION
While polio is no longer endemic in much of the Western world, it has remained
until recently a serious problem in parts of Africa and Asia. In the late 1980s 'wild'
polio was endemic in over 125 countries on five continents, paralyzing more than
1000 children every day. Its highest incidence was in the Indian subcontinent, and
children crippled by polio begging on crutches on the streets of Calcutta, Delhi
and other Indian cities were a common and haunting sight. Since then, there
has been a major international effort to combat polio. In 1988, following the

success of smallpox eradication in 1979 (see page 136), the World Health Organization, inspired by Rotary International, passed a resolution to eradicate polio by the year 2000 so that '*no child will ever again know the crippling effects of polio*'. Private donors supplemented the funds given by national and international agencies. Some 2 billion children around the world have been immunized since the resolution was passed and, notwithstanding the difficulties and costs of administering the vaccine, the incidence of polio has declined dramatically.

Although the goal of eradication was not quite reached by the turn of the millennium, polio could now be on the verge of worldwide eradication. It remains endemic in only four countries – India, Nigeria, Pakistan and Afghanistan – and the annual number of new cases is down to hundreds rather than thousands. Total eradication of polio could be possible if the disease is eliminated from these last remaining hot spots, and we can only hope that the spectre of 'The Crippler' will no longer haunt the dreams of the world's children.

In an Indian village in 2003 a puppet show helps to educate children about polio, whilst behind them a poster about oral vaccine explains the preventative treatment to their parents.

POST-POLIO SYNDROME

For those who survived but were seriously affected by polio in the pre-vaccination era, life has often been a struggle. Some polio survivors have been dependent on long-term care, but many faced the aftermath of this crippling disorder with resilience and strength. For them there was always the reassurance that, unlike diseases such as multiple sclerosis and muscular dystrophy, polio was not a progressive disorder.

In the late 1970s a disturbing and unexpected trend began to appear. A number of people who had suffered from polio in the past began to experience alarming symptoms of severe fatigue, muscle weakness and a range of debilitating polio-like symptoms. Some, who had been able to function with the aid of canes or crutches, now found their mobility severely limited. This is known as post-polio syndrome (PPS) or late effects of polio (LEP). Various theories have been proposed to explain PPS, though it is not believed to be related to persistence of the virus itself. The condition remains something of a mystery.

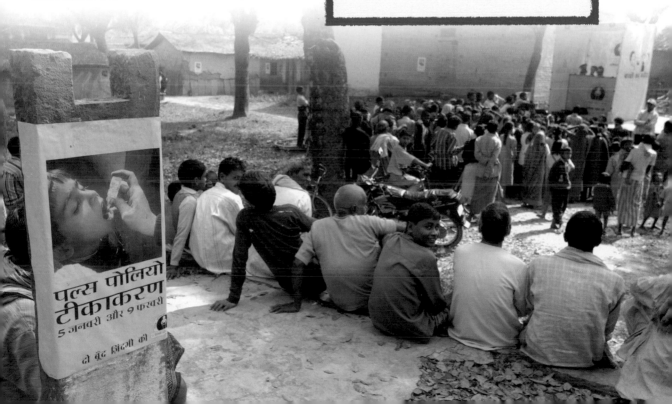

INFLUENZA – commonly referred to simply as 'flu' – is a highly

infectious viral disease that affects the respiratory tract. Many winter and spring outbreaks of influenza have been recorded over the past 500 or so years, but it is the pandemics – those epidemics that are global in scale – that have created the greatest mystery. The disease was called influenza in the 18th century because it was assumed that some heavenly 'influence' must be at work in striking so many people over such vast areas in such a short space of time. The 1918–19 pandemic (the so-called Spanish flu) killed some 50 million people across the globe – the highest death toll of any single pandemic in the annals of human history. Today, the world awaits anxiously to see whether a new and virulent strain, known as avian or bird flu, might result in a similar global catastrophe.

In 1918–19, as undertakers around the world worked to bury the millions of people who had died from influenza in *'the greatest single demographic shock that the human species has ever received'*, children sang this ditty:

'I had a little bird
And its name was Enza
I opened a window
And in-flu-enza.'

So often, when we feel ill, we say we have 'a touch of flu' and, until quite recently, a trip to the doctor with a bit of a fever might have been met with a shrug and the response, *'It's just a virus'*. A bout of flu, which is usually spread from person to person by coughing and sneezing or touching infected objects, can be miserable - involving aches and pains, a high fever, a head cold, a cough and sore throat - but may need no more than aspirin, a week in bed and a lot of handkerchiefs. But some types of influenza, as in 1918-19, can be much more serious and even deadly. And for centuries there was no cure, no vaccine and no real understanding as to how this complex disease could so quickly infect large numbers of people right across the world, with - at times - such catastrophic consequences.

During the 1918–19 influenza pandemic (the Spanish flu) all sorts of preventive measures were tried. This public-health worker wears a mask and is holding a so-called anti-flu spray pump for use on buses.

timeline

1173 *Possibly the first influenza epidemic in Europe.*

1493 *Native Americans on the island of Hispaniola are hit by an epidemic – now thought by* *some historians to have been a 'swine' influenza virus carried by pigs aboard Columbus's ships.*

1510 *An influenza epidemic 'attacked at once and raged all over Europe not missing a family and scarce a person'. Over the course of the next centuries other epidemics* *and pandemics of influenza spread far and wide..*

1878 *'Fowl pest', a disease causing high mortality in poultry, is first identified in Italy.*

1889–90 *Russian flu: the first well-documented human pandemic, with 1 million deaths.*

1892 *The German physician Richard F.J. Pfeiffer (1858–1945) mistakenly believes he has identified the flu 'bacillus'. In fact, flu is caused by a virus.*

1918–19 *Spanish flu: the greatest influenza pandemic ever, with possibly over 50 million deaths.*

1930-1 *American scientists transfer an influenza-like disease from*

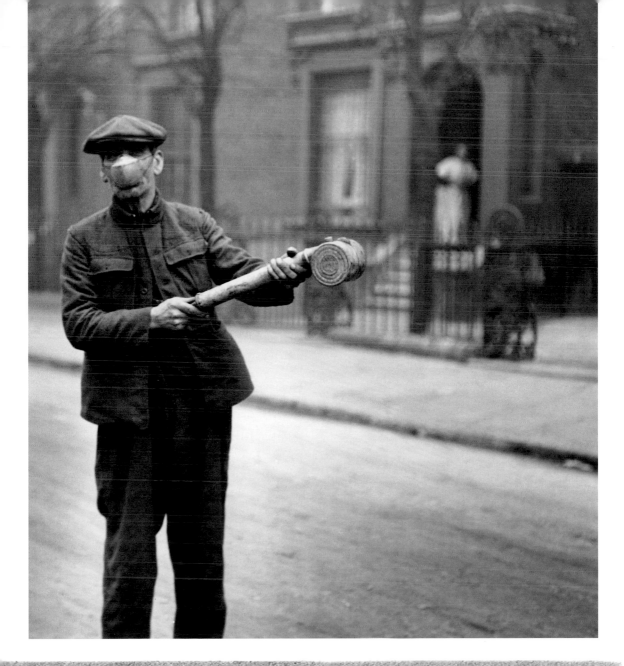

a sick pig to a healthy one, via nasal secretions.

1933 Scientists at the National Institute for Medical Research in London manage to transfer flu from humans to ferrets, enabling the virus to be studied and experimentally manipulated.

Mid-1930s The new electron microscopes enable scientists to see and photograph influenza viruses. In the following years the A, B and C types are isolated and identified.

1940s First mass production of influenza vaccines.

1948 The World Health Organization (WHO) sets up an international network for influenza monitoring and control, to identify suspected new strains and to recommend the appropriate vaccine composition to be used.

1957–8 Asian flu: the pandemic (eventually designated H_2N_2) spreads rapidly from China across the globe, with an estimated 2 million deaths.

1968–9 Hong Kong flu: another global pandemic, designated H_3N_2, with an estimated 1 million deaths.

(continued ...)

A BLAST FROM THE STARS

In April 1658, after an exceptionally cold winter, a 'distemper' suddenly arose in many parts of the world. The English physician Thomas Willis (1621–75) said it was as if

> ' … it was sent by some blast of the stars, which laid hold on very many together, that in some towns, in the space of a week above a thousand people fell sick together. The particular symptom of this disease, which invaded the sick, as a troublesome cough, with great spitting, also a catarrh falling down on the palate, throat and nostrils: also it was accompanied, with a feverish distemper, joined with heat and thirst, want of appetite, a spontaneous weariness and a grievous pain in the back and limbs … such as were indued with an infirm body, or men of a more declining age, that were taken with this disease, not a few died of it; but the more strong, and almost all of an healthful constitution recovered.'

The disease was widespread, and it was said that *'a third part of mankind almost was "distempered" with the same in the space of a month'*. An epidemic in the winter of 1732–3 was described as *'the most universal disease upon record'*. It visited every country in Europe and raged in America and the Caribbean. *'The uniformity of the symptoms of the disease in every place was most remarkable'*, wrote the Scottish physician, John Arbuthnot (1667–1735). And in 1781–2, within the short space of six weeks, some three-quarters of the British population were infected by another epidemic, which also reached the Americas and many parts of the known world.

This 'universal' distemper was called by a number of names, including 'the hot or epidemic catarrh', 'the fashionable cold', 'vernal' or 'spring fever'. To the French it was *la grippe*. The Italians, however, had come up with the name by which we now know the disease: influenza. It was, indeed, as if a blast of the stars, or some heavenly influence, could be the only explanation for such sudden and widespread global visitations.

A MYSTERIOUS BUT NOT VERY DANGEROUS DISEASE?

Equally striking to the physicians who documented some of these earlier outbreaks (which most historians agree probably were influenza) was the way it targeted

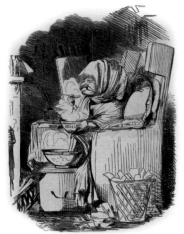

A cartoon entitled 'The Prevailing Epidemic', from an 1847 edition of the periodical *Punch*. Mr Punch, wrapped in blankets in front of the fire, eating gruel and suffering from influenza, complains: *'Ah! You may laugh, my boy; but it's no joke being funny with the influenza!'*

timeline

1976 In the USA, worry about a new strain of swine flu leads to 50 million Americans being vaccinated. The feared outbreak fails to materialize, but the vaccine causes a painful paralytic disorder in 500 people, leading to 25 deaths and extensive litigation.

1996 A new strain of flu, H_5N_1 – known as bird or avian flu – is detected in some geese in China.

1997 Bird flu spreads through live poultry markets in Hong Kong; the first documented human cases of H_5N_1 (18 cases and 6 deaths) occur in Hong Kong.

2003 Two further cases and one death of H_5N_1 in Hong Kong.

2005 Die-off of more than 6000 migratory birds infected with H_5N_1 begins at Qinghai Lake in central China. The virus spreads to poultry and wild birds in the Russian Federation and parts of Kazakhstan, with further outbreaks in late 2005 in Romania, Turkey, Croatia and Ukraine.

2007 By June 2007, 315 human cases of H_5N_1 avian flu have been reported over the previous decade from a number of countries, including Azerbaijan, Cambodia, China, Djibouti, Egypt, Indonesia, Iraq, Laos, Nigeria, Thailand, Turkey and Vietnam. Of these, 191 cases have been fatal.

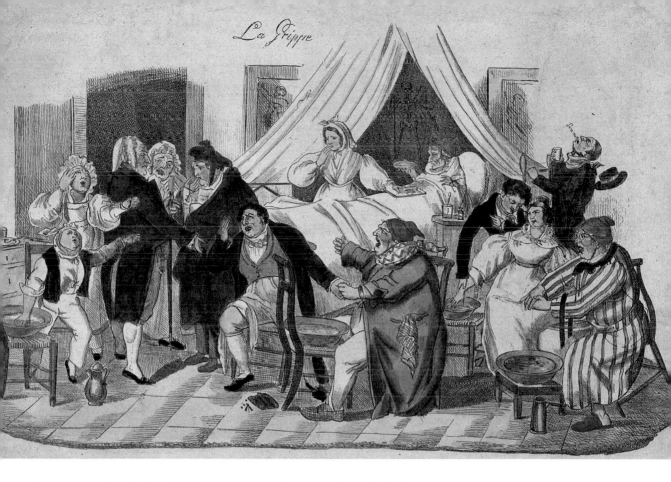

the weak, aged and infirm. While countless numbers were sick and the disease *'scarce spared any one family'*, it was noted that the infection was very often only fatal to *'consumptive old men, asthmatics, cachetic, phlegmatic, gross bodied, plethoric people'* or those recently afflicted with one of the many other fevers around at the time. The healthy and robust fell sick, but generally survived.

Over the course of the 19th century, further global pandemics of influenza rolled around the world. The most virulent and widespread of all these was the so-called Russian flu, which appeared in St Petersburg in December 1889 and by the following spring had laid low hundreds of millions of people worldwide. Although the total number of deaths was high – perhaps around a quarter of a million in Europe alone – the overall mortality rate was probably less than 1 per cent of all those who were infected. It tended to be only the very young and the very old who succumbed.

We do not know how old influenza is, but it was these first epidemics and global pandemics – from the 15th to the late 19th century – that gave rise to many puzzles about its origin and mode of transmission, especially in the days before people were able to travel around the world by rapid means of transportation. Influenza in its brief visitations caused misery, suffering and sometimes death, especially amongst the elderly, but overall it did not seem as dangerous or

A family threatened by a bout of influenza is prepared for a large-scale bleeding. Bleeding was a popular, if ineffectual, treatment for a variety of ailments in the days before the true nature of some diseases was known.

frightening as some of the other great plagues, poxes and pestilences of the past. This view was soon to be shattered as the 1918-19 pandemic erupted, destroying millions of people in their prime of life.

A FORGOTTEN PANDEMIC

In 1976 the medical historian Alfred Crosby wrote a book on the history of influenza called *Epidemic and Peace, 1918* (later reissued as *America's Forgotten Pandemic: The Influenza of 1918*). For historians it was a grim reminder that the 1918-19 flu pandemic was one of the greatest single mortality crises of all time.

The Black Death of the mid-14th century (possibly both bubonic and pneumonic plague; see pages 8–19) had killed around 25 million people over a period of four

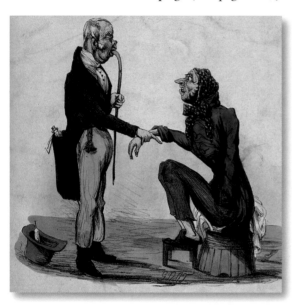

A humorous coloured lithograph from the 1840s with the caption: *'Well Pat – how's the influenza? Do you expectorate?' 'Expect-to-ate! How the devil should I expect-to-ate, widout a saxpence in my pocket?'*

or five years. The 1918-19 flu, or Spanish flu as it was known, resulted in the death of millions of people in about six months. Crosby and others put the figure at around 20 million - higher than the death toll from the First World War. Moreover, half of all deaths were among those aged between 20 and 40. Influenza on this occasion did not just kill the weak and elderly. It struck right at the heart of the most active sections of the population. Crosby's book was a wake-up call for historians to look more deeply at the great outbreaks of influenza of the past, in particular the 1918-19 pandemic.

But beyond scholarly and scientific circles, it was, as one newspaper has recently called it, *'a global calamity that the world forgot'*. This global calamity is now hot news. With the threat of bird flu and the fear of another major human influenza pandemic, there is every reason to revisit this historical case study. Indeed, it is now thought that up to 50 million people may have died in this single pandemic, and some have suggested that the toll was as high as 100 million.

Yet for the past century, it has been an episode 'sketched' rather than 'etched' in people's memory. As historians have pointed out, most people know more about the horrors of bubonic plague in Medieval Europe than they do about this awesome tragedy, which killed so many millions of their grandparents and great-grandparents. There are no memorials, few contemporary novels evoking the heartbreak, no remembrance services or lengthy lists of the deceased. Unlike the devastation and brutality of the two world wars, the unleashing of one of the most deadly pathogens of all times had almost been forgotten.

THE SPANISH FLU ERUPTS, CIRCULATES AND 'DISAPPEARS'

The recent interest in the 1918-19 influenza pandemic has brought to light startling new facts and figures, as well as scientific confirmation that the disease really was influenza. But this brief and deadly episode still holds many mysteries

THE MANY NAMES OF FLU

The phrase *una influenza* was first used by the Italians. Its Latin equivalent was *influentia coeli*, which literally meant 'heavenly influence', as it was thought that some ominous configuration of the planets and stars may account for this seemingly mysterious disease. The English adopted the word 'influenza' in the mid-18th century, while the French called it *la grippe*. There is also a similar-sounding Arabic phrase, *anfal-'anza*, which means 'the nose of a she-goat': female goats were thought to be carriers of disease.

By the time of the 1889 Russian flu epidemic, people began to attach place names to describe the major pandemics – in some cases this was done to denote where it was thought the disease had first started; at other times it was done in order to put the responsibility for the outbreak on another nation. The 1918–19 pandemic was called the Spanish flu because its ravages in Spain were not screened from world attention by government censorship.

In the second half of the 20th century, naming flu outbreaks and their causative organisms became more complex, as it was recognized that this group of viruses could constantly mutate into new forms. The three main types are A, B and C and there are many sub-types, including H5N1 (which stands for Haemagglutinin 5, Neuraminidase 1). Haemagglutinin and Neuraminidase are key molecular components of the virus.

for historians and virologists. The disease, at the time, was called the Spanish flu – not because it started in Spain but because Spain was not a belligerent country in the First World War and its press was not prevented by government censors from freely reporting its alarming impact when it struck there in May 1918. In fact, no one can say for certain where the disease began, or map precisely its route of dissemination. Some believe that it was first seen amongst the Allied troops in France (where it was known as 'Flanders grippe' or 'purulent bronchitis' by the British, and *Blitz Katarrh* by the Germans). Others speculate that it began in the military cantonments of the Midwest United States in the spring of 1918 when the Americans were preparing to join the Allied forces in Europe. More recently it has been suggested that, like the current bird flu outbreak, it may have originated in China or Hong Kong.

But whatever the origin of the first wave, in late August 1918 a second and far more virulent wave seems to have erupted simultaneously in three widely separated locations: Boston, Massachusetts, USA; Brest in Brittany, France; and Freetown in Sierra Leone on the west coast of Africa. These three ports were all engaged in dispatching troops and supplies to the trenches of the Western Front. By the time the Armistice was signed on 11 November 1918, ending the Great War,

In 1918, many American army bases were among the places hit by the flu epidemic. This is the influenza camp at Lawrence, Maine, where patients were given fresh air treatment. This measure was tried as a way of curbing the epidemic. The soldier in the centre of the picture is wearing a mask to avoid becoming infected.

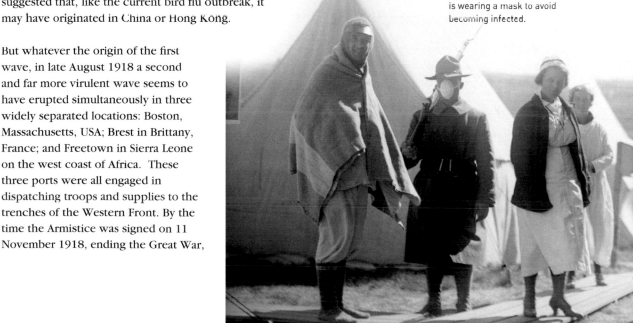

the disease had spread like wildfire around the entire world. From the bloody battlefields of Europe to the isolated islands of the South Pacific, from the Arctic Circle to Australasia, from the tropics to the tundra, north, east, south and west, the 'grim reaper' of the early 20th century felled soldiers and civilians, killed young men and women, healthy infants, pregnant mothers and the elderly.

It touched the lives of nearly every person on earth, leaving countless children orphaned or bereft of one or other parent. In India, one of the worst-hit places, at least 17 to 20 million people died, and in Western Samoa in the central Pacific, about 7500 out of a population of 38,000 died in November and December 1918. During the whole pandemic only St Helena in the South Atlantic, New Guinea and a few Pacific islands seem to have escaped infection. Australia, possibly through strict quarantine measures, was not as badly hit as other continents.

Contemporary descriptions of the disease paint a graphic and grim picture of its horrors. People died quickly – often 48 hours after onset, some seemingly

WHY WAS THE 1918–19 FLU SUCH A KILLER?

'She lay on a narrow ledge over a pit she knew to be bottomless ... as she climbed back from that depth pain returned, a terrible compelling pain running through her veins like heavy fire, the stench of corruption filled her nostrils, the sweetish sickening smell of rotting flesh and pus; she opened her eyes and saw pale light through a coarse white cloth over her face, knew that the smell of death was in her own body, and struggled to lift her hand ... '

This passage comes from the novella *Pale Horse, Pale Rider*, by the American writer Katherine Anne Porter (1890–1980), first published in 1939. Porter was one of the few contemporaries to write a fictional account of the horrors of the 1918–19 flu, during which her fiancé had died, and she herself had almost succumbed.

The symptoms of the Spanish flu were far more dramatic than any other human flu pandemic before or since. The worst symptom – signalling imminent death – was known as 'heliotrope cyanosis', when the lungs were starved of oxygen and the patient would turn purple, black or blue. Physicians at the time struggled to understand the cause of this terrible 'purple death'.

Since then various explanations have been put forward (or ruled out) to explain this unusually high influenza mortality. The First World War and the movement of troops may have played a key role in the initial dissemination of the virus. Associated complications caused by secondary bacterial pneumonia (for which, at the time, there were no antibiotics), or a massive immune response may explain why it was quite so deadly.

In recent years – partly prompted by fears of another major pandemic – scientists have been searching past records, examining stored tissues and even exhuming influenza victims preserved in permafrost in Norway and Alaska. From this evidence, it has been suggested that the 1918–19 pandemic may have been the H_1N_1 sub-type of influenza A virus (an avian or bird virus that adapted to humans). If it was disseminated, perhaps initially by birds, the little ditty about the bird called Enza has a strikingly ironic twist to it.

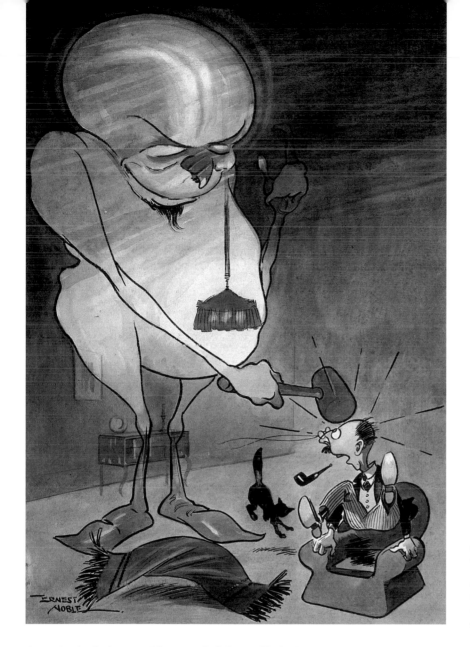

A cartoon from 1918 depicts a monster – representing influenza – hitting a man over the head accompanied by the caption, 'A-Tich-OO!! Good evening, I'm the new influenza!!'

drowning in their own phlegm as their lungs filled with fluid. Blood oozed from noses, ears and lungs. Some literally dropped down dead in the streets, slumped forwards while driving trams and streetcars, or toppled off horses and buggies. In the crowded military bases and troop ships, soldiers collapsed in feverish delirium. Everywhere undertakers worked round the clock to keep up. Nurses and doctors rapidly succumbed to the disease, and there were desperate requests for volunteers to help cope with the terrible burden of sickness and death.

Efforts to prevent the spread of the disease – especially once its severity was evident – included the prohibition of public gatherings, disinfecting streets and homes, sterilizing water fountains, banning spitting and shaking hands (which, in

'Never since the Black Death has such a plague swept over the face of the world; never, perhaps, has a plague been more stoically accepted.'

THE TIMES OF LONDON, 18 DECEMBER 1918

some places, became a punishable offence), quarantining ships and enforcing the wearing of gauze masks. Some invoked folk remedies, such as carrying garlic, sulphur, cucumbers or potatoes to ward off infection, and any number of quack remedies were sold as 'sure cures' – but they were mostly of little avail.

The Spanish flu exploded in late 1918, circulated the globe, briefly erupted again in the following winter, but by the spring of 1920 it had disappeared. It had done most of its brutal killing in little more than six months. The reaction throughout the world had varied from initial denial, censorship of newspaper reports, fatalism and inaction to shock, bewilderment and a world-wide attempt to 'get a grip on the grippe'. But, for reasons that are still puzzling, there was far less panic than during many other great plagues of the past – perhaps because it was overshadowed by the horrors of the First World War. Only one major literary work, *Pale Horse, Pale Rider* by Katherine Anne Porter (1890–1980), herself a survivor, was written in its aftermath (see Why Was the 1918–19 Flu Such a Killer?, page 178). The 1918–19 influenza pandemic 'disappeared' as quickly and as mysteriously as it had arrived.

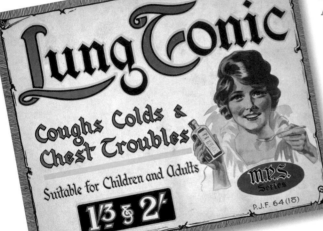

The influenza pandemic of 1918–19 resulted in the promotion of remedies such as Lung Tonic.

THE NEXT HUMAN FLU PANDEMIC?

Two further serious human influenza pandemics (in 1957–8 and again in 1968–9) and a number of minor epidemics (as well as many local seasonal outbreaks) occurred during the 20th century. The so-called Asian flu of 1957–8 spread across the globe, infecting around one-third of the world's population and, although there were large numbers of fatalities, the overall mortality rate was only around 0.25 per cent. The Hong Kong flu of 1968–9 was similarly widespread, possibly affecting as many as 30 million people in the USA alone, but the final death toll was, mercifully, not on the same scale as the 1918–19 pandemic. By the 1930s scientists had finally discovered that influenza was caused by a virus and, although there were no anti-viral drugs developed for influenza until recently, for those suffering from secondary bacterial pneumonia during the Asian and Hong Kong flu pandemics, antibiotics were available.

Once scientists had identified the influenza virus and produced the first mass vaccines in the 1940s, they also began to realize the complexities of the disease. Indeed, it is often said that influenza is not just one disease but a host of rapidly mutating pathogens. There are three main types – A, B and C. Type-A influenza is the one that causes most human sickness and the major pandemics. But there are

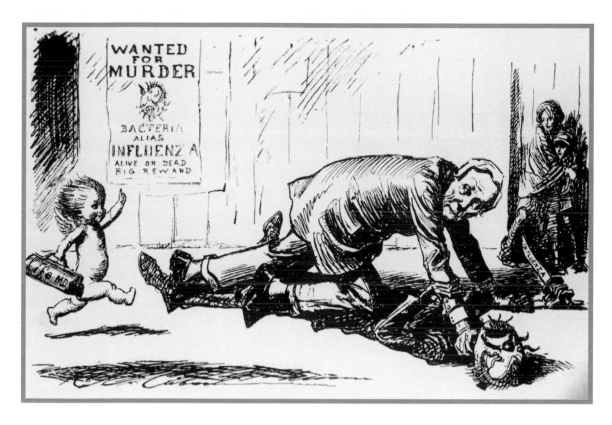

also many sub-types or different strains, some of which are 'mild' while others are labelled 'highly pathogenic' or just plain deadly. Exposure to one strain of influenza appears to provide no protection or immunity to another, and one of the most frustrating aspects facing the pharmaceutical industry in its efforts to produce vaccines is that, in any given year, we never know when a 'new' strain of influenza will emerge.

Across the world there are now experts identifying, monitoring and tracking new outbreaks of flu in the hope that the right vaccine can be produced each flu season in time to vaccinate vulnerable and high-risk sections of the population. The experts also hope that by being on constant alert they will be able to avert another major pandemic. Over the past two decades or so scientists have examined the historical record and concluded that another human influenza pandemic is now likely, and even overdue. When or if it will come, and whether or not it will be as deadly as the 1918–19 outbreak, are questions that are of great concern to health teams around the world.

Bird flu – H$_5$N$_1$ – arrives
That anxiety has increased over the last few years. In 1996, in the Guangdong province of China, a new influenza virus – H$_5$N$_1$ – was identified in some geese, and came to be known as bird or avian flu. It received little attention until it spread through the live-poultry markets in Hong Kong in May 1997 to

At the time of the 1918–19 influenza pandemic some, as illustrated in this cartoon, thought the disease was caused by a bacterium. We now know that influenza is a viral disease but it is likely that associated complications caused by secondary bacterial pneumonia may have contributed to its high mortality during this pandemic.

'The clock is still ticking. We just don't know what time it is.'

AN EXPERT'S OUTLOOK ON THE CURRENT AND FUTURE SITUATION, QUOTED IN JOHN BARRY, *THE GREAT INFLUENZA: THE EPIC STORY OF THE GREATEST PLAGUE IN HISTORY* (2004)

humans, killing six of 18 infected people. The authorities took drastic steps to stop the outbreak: disinfecting the bird markets, banning the sale of ducks and geese, culling millions of birds and destroying Hong Kong's entire poultry population.

By taking such quick action in this early wave, the authorities in Hong Kong may well have averted a global influenza pandemic. Since then, scientists have amassed a great deal more knowledge about the complexities of influenza. For centuries it has been realized that humans are not the only ones who catch flu: it can also affect wild birds, poultry, pigs, horses and other animals. Scientists now realize that birds and mammals such as pigs can also act as a reservoir for some sub-types of the virus – sometimes these sub-types exist in harmony with their hosts, but at other

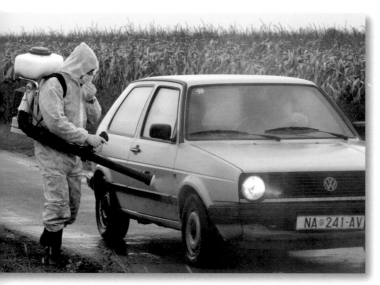

times they cause disease. And while in humans the virus replicates in the respiratory system, in birds it replicates in the intestinal tract so that it can be shed through bird droppings as well as in saliva and nasal secretions, and thus can easily contaminate cages, water and bird feed.

Since 2005, bird flu has spread more widely through domestic fowl and wild birds and has been devastating for poultry farmers in many parts of the world. For scientists, the knowledge they have acquired during the investigations of H_5N_1 bird flu has helped explain some of the mysteries of past human pandemics, in which the flu virus may have jumped from migrating or aquatic and domestic birds to humans, possibly with pigs acting as an intermediate reservoir.

A Croatian agricultural worker disinfects a car near a fishpond where bird flu was discovered in wild swans in the eastern Croatian village of Zdenci in 2005. In response, the country immediately banned the hunting and transport of wild fowl and poultry.

That knowledge has also led to the development of new drugs for influenza, which can, in principle, be used to treat any of the strains of bird, swine or human flu. But even with so much now revealed about the influenza virus, no one can yet say for sure if the H_5N_1 strain that is killing wild birds, chickens, turkeys and ducks will in the future become rampant in the human population.

So far, about 315 people have contracted H_5N_1 bird flu, and 191 have died as a result. In most cases, it is thought that the virus was caught by people handling infected birds or their droppings, and further human-to-human transmission has not occurred on a wide scale. But there are two scary scenarios for the future. First, once the bird flu virus enters the human body it might mutate so that it can then be readily passed from person to person – and with rapid air travel across the globe it may well descend 'like a blast from the stars'. A second, related possibility is that if a person has even a mild form of influenza (the '*it's just a bout of flu*' type) and then contracts H_5N_1 or one of the other nasty strains lurking amongst our feathered and farmyard friends, the two viruses may combine or cross-breed to become a 'new' lethal human strain.

These, of course, are worst-case scenarios. There are drugs that can treat the disease, and the World Health Organization (WHO) and those countries that can afford to do so have stockpiled millions of doses of Tamiflu (oseltamivir) and Relenza (zanamivir). A global network of 112 National Influenza Centres in 83 countries (the WHO Global Influenza Surveillance Network) is also keeping a very close eye on the current situation. Historians and scientists are combining their expertise to explore some of the mysterious patterns of past influenza pandemics, especially the now 'not-forgotten' great influenza pandemic of 1918–19 (of which the causative virus – H_5N_1 – appears to share some disturbing similarities with H_5N_1 avian flu). Quarantine restrictions are imposed on farms and markets to contain the disease in domestic flocks, and precautions such as face masks, disinfectants and airport controls (implemented during the SARS scare; see pages 202–7) are being made ready in the event of a human outbreak. Moreover, H_5N_1 has been around for some ten years, and so has had the time and opportunity to jump the species barrier and mutate into a pandemic strain. So far, it hasn't …

For the time being, we must just watch and wait – and hope that a little bird called Enza will not lead to another pandemic.

Romanian workers dispose of plastic bags containing dead domestic birds, culled on suspicion of harbouring bird flu disease, in a village east of Bucharest in 2005. In humans, H_5N_1 – or avian flu – can cause massive destruction of lung tissue. Most human deaths so far have been amongst people who have been in close contact with infected birds.

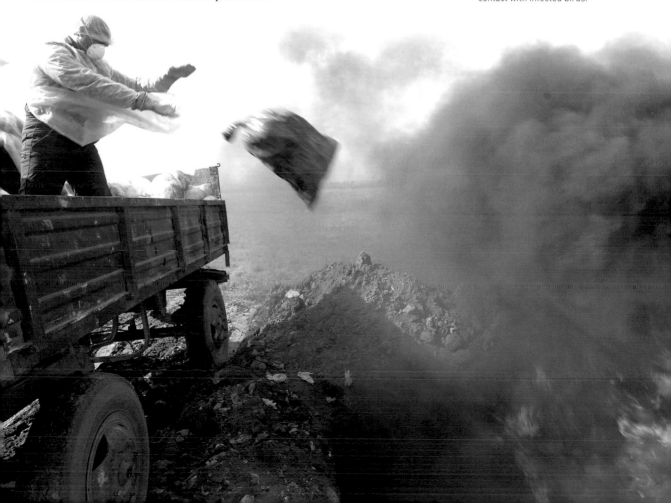

EBOLA haemorrhagic fever (EHF), commonly known simply as Ebola, is a highly infectious viral disease, and one of the deadliest diseases to have emerged in recent decades.

The first identified human case occurred in Africa in 1976, near the Ebola River in the Democratic Republic of the Congo (formerly Zaïre), and sporadic, localized outbreaks of the disease have since flared up in a number of countries in sub-Saharan Africa. Ebola is characterized by massive internal and external bleeding, and death from surgical shock and respiratory arrest occurs in some 50 to 90 per cent of all cases. The risk for anyone in contact with the Ebola virus is so great that the disease is classified as a 'Biosafety Level-4' pathogen, which requires the strictest safety precautions for laboratory investigation. There is as yet no approved vaccine or known cure for Ebola, and many mysteries about its origins remain unsolved.

In late August 1976 a schoolteacher called Mabalo Lokela living in Yambuku, a remote town in northern Zaïre (now the Democratic Republic of the Congo), developed a fever. At the local mission hospital they thought he might be suffering from malaria, but an injection of chloroquine failed to control his feverish symptoms. A week later he returned to the hospital, critically ill. He had begun to experience uncontrollable vomiting, acute diarrhoea and a blinding headache. He was also severely dehydrated, and had trouble breathing. Frighteningly, he then started bleeding from his nose, gums and eyes, and there was blood in his stools. There was no doctor in the hospital, but the Sisters who ran the mission did all they could to care for him. They had no idea what was wrong. Mabalo Lokela died on 8 September 1976.

FUNERALS, FAMILIES, FRIENDS AND HEALTH WORKERS
Lokela's body was cleansed and prepared in the traditional way for his funeral. Not long afterwards, many members of his family and friends who had attended

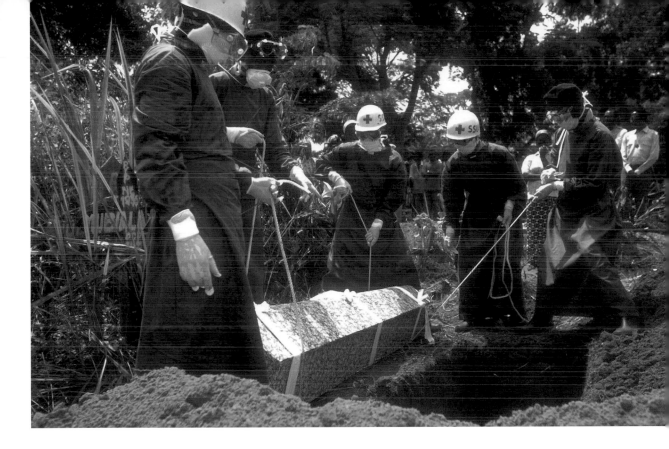

the ceremony succumbed to the same symptoms, and several of the staff at the mission hospital became desperately ill. Panic broke out: it seemed as if people were literally bleeding to death. The mission hospital at Yambuku was eventually closed on 30 September, and the whole area sealed off by the Zaïrian army. A microbiologist and epidemiologist were sent from the National University of Zaïre to investigate the epidemic at Yambuku. The disease ultimately spread to more than 50 villages in the vicinity of Yambuku, as well as to Kinshasa, the capital of Zaïre, resulting in a total of 318 cases and 280 deaths – a mortality rate of nearly 90 per cent.

Wearing protective clothing, officials bury a victim of the Ebola virus. Such extreme care is a necessity – Ebola can spread during the preparation of infected corpses.

1994 Several cases of Ebola in chimps discovered in the Tai Forest in Côte d'Ivoire, West Africa. A scientist performing an autopsy on an infected chimpanzee becomes sick. She is treated and recovers.

1994 Ebola is first documented in Gabon in gold-mining camps deep in the forest. It is initially thought to be yellow fever but subsequently identified as Ebola, with 52 cases and 31 deaths.

1995 Epidemic in Kikwit, Democratic Republic of the Congo, traced to a person who worked in the forest adjoining the city. The epidemic spreads through families and hospitals, with 315 cases and 250 deaths.

1996 A chimpanzee found dead in the forest in Gabon is eaten by people hunting for food: 19 of those involved become ill, with other cases in family members. In total, 21 people die.

A medical professional travels from Gabon to Johannesburg, South Africa, after having treated patients infected with Ebola. He is hospitalized and recovers. A nurse taking care of him contracts Ebola and dies.

1996–present Several further outbreaks of Ebola in Gabon, Uganda, the Democratic Republic of the Congo, the Republic of the Congo and Sudan. Since 1976 there have been some 1800 cases and 1200 deaths.

2004 Two cases – one fatal – of Ebola among laboratory workers, one in the Russian Federation and the other in the USA.

MONKEY ALARMS

In 1967 clinicians at a hospital for infectious diseases in Marburg, Germany, were shocked and mystified to see several severely ill patients whose fever was accompanied by agonizing pain and bleeding from multiple sites on the skin and the mucous membranes. It turned out that all the affected patients had worked for the same pharmaceutical company, and had acquired the virus from infected African green monkeys. The monkeys, half of which had been dead on arrival from Uganda, were used in the preparation of cell cultures for vaccines. Seven of the infected lab workers died. Further cases occurred in Belgrade, Serbia (then part of Yugoslavia) and Frankfurt, Germany. A 'new' deadly disease had arrived – Marburg virus or green monkey disease.

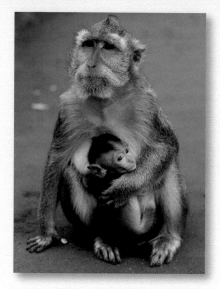

Shipments of the crab-eating macaque imported into the USA and Italy from the Philippines were found to be carrying the deadly Ebola virus.

In 1989 alarm bells rang again – this time in the USA. A shipment of 100 cynomolgus monkeys, also known as crab-eating macaques (*Macaca fascicularis*), was sent from Manila in the Philippines to a quarantine laboratory in Reston, Virginia, for research. The monkeys started dying. Officials of the US Army Medical Research Institute were called in and found that the monkeys were dying from a form of Ebola virus – which was labelled Ebola-Reston. While it was highly lethal to monkeys, no humans were infected, though four of the animal handlers developed specific antibodies to this form of Ebola. The remaining monkeys were destroyed and the lab decontaminated. But this wasn't the only scare. Several more times in the course of the next few years, both in the USA and in Italy, monkeys shipped from the same export facility in the Philippines were found to be infected and dying of Ebola-Reston.

While no locally acquired human cases of Ebola have been found outside Africa, the presence of the virus in monkeys in Asia is an extremely worrying aspect of this deadly and mysterious disease. Where else in the world is Ebola circulating in the wild, waiting to jump species?

Some two months earlier, an ominously similar disease had broken out in Nzara and Maridi in the south of Sudan, a country bordering Zaïre in the northeast. This outbreak had led to the deaths of 151 people out of 284 cases (a 53 per cent mortality rate). The local hospital soon turned into a morgue, and many of the patients, as well as relatives and hospital staff, succumbed to the disease.

As later in Zaïre, people were petrified – it is said that some of the fearful victims in the last stages of the dreadful disease threw off their clothes and staggered out naked into the streets, while the surviving medical staff panicked and simply ran off to escape.

IDENTIFYING THE CAUSE

The Sudan outbreak did not initially receive international attention. But when news of the terrible mortalities in Zaïre reached the World Health Organization (WHO) headquarters in Geneva, Switzerland, and at the same time reports of the Sudan outbreak arrived, alarm bells rang. Blood samples were sent to a number of laboratories in Europe and the USA. A major international investigation was launched into the causes of the outbreaks, to see whether there was a link, and whether further epidemics could be prevented.

In their maximum-security laboratories, peering down their electron microscopes at the blood of a patient from Yambuku, scientists were both shocked and puzzled. The disease initially appeared to be similar to another scary 'new' haemorrhagic fever – Marburg disease or green monkey virus. This had first been identified a decade earlier and named after the German town of Marburg, where a shipment of African green monkeys had infected laboratory staff at a pharmaceutical research company (see Monkey Alarms, left). Common features included the high mortality and the severe haemorrhagic fever (the word 'haemorrhage' comes from the Greek words *haima*, 'blood', and *rhēgnumai*, 'to break forth'). Both diseases seemed to be caused by viruses that looked like threads or spindly filaments. There were, however, serological differences between the two, and in early November 1976 the 'new' highly pathogenic virus was named 'Ebola' after a small river in the vicinity of Yambuku.

EBOLA SHOCKS THE WORLD

For Western medicine, the 1950s and 1960s had been decades of tremendous optimism. Books on the history of disease were published with titles that incorporated such promising phrases as 'the rise and fall of … ', 'the conquest of … ' and 'the eradication of … '. Epidemic infectious diseases seemed to be becoming a thing of the past. The eradication of smallpox in 1979 was an especially key moment in medical history (see page 136).

'Weak, emaciated men and women lay about the mud-and-stick chamber, staring out of ghost eyes at the white men. The virus was so toxic that it caused their hair, fingernails and skin to fall off. Those who healed grew new skin.'

A DESCRIPTION OF THE 1976 OUTBREAK IN SUDAN, FROM LAURIE GARRETT, *THE COMING PLAGUE: NEWLY EMERGING DISEASES IN A WORLD OUT OF BALANCE* (1994)

But from the 1950s through to the end of the 20th century, previously unknown and deadly diseases, including a number of haemorrhagic fevers, had begun to surface in various parts of the world. The real significance of these diseases was not fully recognized in the West until their impact began to be felt in Europe and the USA. Marburg fever (first identified in Germany in 1967), Lassa fever (recognized in Lassa, Nigeria, in 1969, when it struck down an American nurse), Lyme disease (first observed in the town of Old Lyme, Connecticut, USA, in 1975), Legionnaires' disease (which caused the deaths of 29 members of the American Legion attending a conference in Philadelphia in 1976), Ebola in 1976, and HIV/AIDS in the 1980s (see pages 192–201) – all these shattered the general mood of complacency. By the 1990s books had begun to

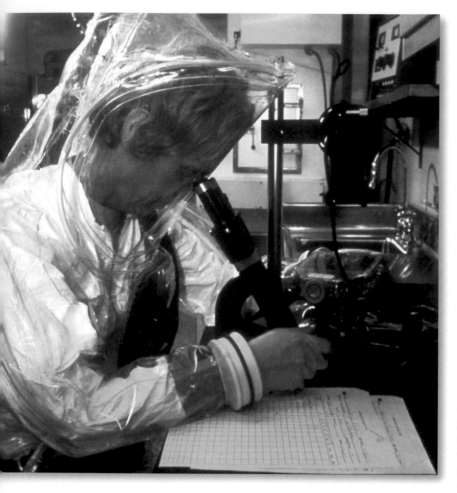

appear with such titles as *The New Killer Germs, Quest for the Killers* and *The Coming Plague*, reminding readers that poxes, pestilences and plagues were by no means vanquished. As the English chemist and physiologist John Mayow (1640–79) had observed in the 17th century: *'As a rule disease can scarcely keep pace with the itch to scribble about it.'*

Ebola was perhaps the grisliest of the new plagues, provoking, as one scientist has put it, *'convulsive shudders'* in the public imagination. Ebola made it not only into the news, but also into gruesome novels and movies, and images of scientists in protective spacesuits arriving in African villages and carrying lethal viruses back to high-security labs, not to mention graphic depictions of ghastly symptoms and agonizing deaths, scared many people witless. While reports of internal organs dissolving into mush and victims squirting blood from every

A scientist wearing protective clothing carries out tests for the Ebola virus in Atlanta, USA. Ebola is classified as 'Biosafety Level-4', meaning it is regarded as an extremely dangerous agent which poses a high individual risk of life-threatening disease. There is also a risk that such diseases might be harnessed as bioterrorist weapons.

orifice are exaggerated, there is no doubt that when Ebola hit the headlines in the late 1970s (a few years before HIV/AIDS), it was seen as the most frightening and lethal of the newly emerging diseases.

THE VIRUS HUNTERS

As scientists in high-security laboratories – such as those in Atlanta, Georgia, and Porton Down in England – wrestled to identify and understand the Ebola virus, others in remote parts of Sudan and Zaïre were tracking down the epidemiology of the disease and doing all they could to arrest its spread. These 'disease cowboys', as the medical detectives in Africa were called, faced almost insuperable difficulties as they tried to contain the nightmare of Ebola.

Joe McCormick and Susan Fisher-Hoch, in their 1996 book *The Virus Hunters: Dispatches from the Front Line*, narrate just how tragic it was to witness the impact of this deadly virus in parts of Africa where there were limited health facilities and few safety precautions, and where the population was consumed by grief and terror. Jonathan Mann (1947–98), in his preface to Laurie Garrett's book *The Coming Plague*, described the 'disease cowboys' – comprising both international and local teams of scientists and health workers – as:

> *'Heroes of a special kind: bonding science, curiosity and humanitarian concern combined with a practical attitude … who [went] into the field armed only with … will, intelligence, and confidence that a way forward would be found.'*

Their stories could have been written a hundred years ago by their predecessors in tropical medicine – men and women who had grappled to understand and control diseases such as malaria, yellow fever and sleeping sickness.

Many significant discoveries about Ebola were made during these first outbreaks. It appears that the Sudan and Zaïre epidemics of Ebola were coincidental and probably unrelated. Both, however, spread rapidly through personal contact, especially within hospitals and clinics, via infected bodily fluids, blood, tissues and organs. Funeral customs – handling and cleansing the corpses – were also instrumental in spreading the infection. A particularly rapid transmission of the virus occurred through the practice of using and re-using unsterilized syringes in medical centres. In Yambuku, following Mabalo Lokela's illness and death, it is thought that about 300 to 600 people a day were injected at the mission hospital with the same five hypodermic needles. Some patients came for a minor complaint, only to leave with the deadly virus now in their bloodstream.

BUSHMEAT AND THE GREAT APES

In some African countries political instability, a rising population and deplorable economic conditions have forced many people to become dependent on 'bushmeat' (the meat of wild animals), either by selling it or by consuming it themselves. Hunters usually either use wire snares to trap the animals, or simply shoot them.

While conservationists are concerned about over-hunting and the threat to wildlife, epidemiologists are worried about the risk of infected wild animals spreading diseases like Ebola to the human population, as well as the risk of Ebola for populations of great apes. Researchers in the region straddling the border between Gabon and the Republic of the Congo believe that some 5000 gorillas have been wiped out by Ebola, with suggestions that the disease is now passing from gorilla to gorilla through direct contact.

Since its first reported case in 1976, there have been around 1800 cases and 1200 deaths from Ebola, with fatality rates in each of the outbreaks varying from around 50 to 90 per cent. No locally acquired human cases have occurred outside Africa. Ebola has been placed, along with Marburg, in a new family of viruses, the Filoviridae or filoviruses (after the Latin word *filo*, 'thread').

Four sub-types of the Ebola virus have been identified: Ebola-Zaïre, Ebola-Sudan, Ebola-Côte d'Ivoire and Ebola-Reston. The first three have been found to cause haemorrhagic fever in both humans and animals. The last form was identified in a shipment of cynomolgus monkeys dispatched from the Philippines to laboratories in Reston, Virginia, USA, in 1989. Many of the monkeys died, generating a major global scare. However, Ebola-Reston is the only form that has not so far caused clinical illness in humans (see Monkey Alarms, page 186). The Ebola-Zaïre strain is the most lethal form, with death rates as high as 90 per cent, while the Ebola-Sudan

PREVENTING FUTURE OUTBREAKS

Since the 1980s health agencies have recognized the serious threat presented by 'new' diseases, as well as by re-emerging 'old' diseases such as malaria and tuberculosis. Quests to find either a vaccine or cure for diseases such as Ebola are of immediate priority, and one or two promising candidates are on the horizon.

In the meantime, various measures can be put in place to contain outbreaks. Immediate diagnosis is paramount, followed by strict isolation and the use of barrier nursing techniques – not only involving protective clothing and disposable gowns, masks, goggles, and gloves but also the sterilization of all contaminated medical equipment and soiled bedding and clothing. Patients have the best chance of survival if their fluid and electrolyte balance is maintained, and, in the case of the critically ill, if blood and plasma are given to those who are haemorrhaging. Also vital to prevent the spread of Ebola is the rapid and safe disposal of corpses and liquid and solid wastes. Warning local hunters about the dangers of contracting Ebola from forest animals is another part of the jigsaw. However, in many poor and remote parts of Africa, it is difficult to implement such measures.

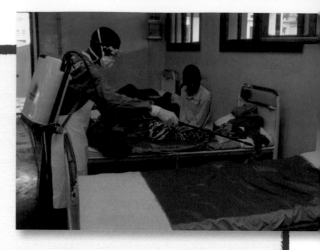

A worker uses spraying equipment to disinfect a hospital bed used by an Ebola virus victim at Kikwit General Hospital, Zaïre (now Democractic Republic of the Congo), during the Ebola epidemic of 1995. This Ebola outbreak killed 250 people in the city of Kikwit over a period of just a few months.

For the affected nations of Africa – including the Democratic Republic of the Congo, Sudan, the Republic of the Congo, Uganda and Gabon – Ebola is yet one more merciless microbe that has been tragically unleashed on a continent that already suffers the heaviest burden of old and new diseases on Earth. The incidence and impact of Ebola in Africa is currently not on anything like the same scale as that of malaria or HIV/AIDS. But Ebola – one of the most virulent diseases known to humankind – still has the ability to destroy lives and shatter families and communities, and the power to spread terror across the rest of the world.

strain kills about half of all known cases. The reasons for this varying mortality rate, and why some people survive the disease, are not fully understood.

Where did Ebola come from?

There are many other outstanding puzzles about the Ebola virus, especially regarding its origins. Where did it come from, and why did it apparently suddenly infect humans? During the first outbreaks, numerous species of animal were collected and tested by the virus hunters in an attempt to track down a non-human reservoir. Bedbugs, mosquitoes, pigs, cows, bats, monkeys, squirrels and other rodents showed no signs of the Ebola virus, in either Zaïre or Sudan. It has subsequently been shown, however, that a number of non-human primates – including monkeys, chimpanzees and gorillas – seem to be susceptible to the virus, along with forest antelopes and porcupines. These animals also appear to be able to transmit the disease to people. Mabalo Lokela had eaten antelope meat shortly before he showed his first symptoms, and he and another patient had also handled fresh monkey meat. In 1994 a scientist contracted the disease in the Tai Forest of Côte d'Ivoire while performing an autopsy on the carcass of an infected wild chimpanzee. In 1996, in the Mayibout area of Gabon in West Africa, a chimpanzee was found dead in the forest and eaten by hunters, 19 of whom became ill. Some of their relatives also came down with Ebola.

The high mortality among monkeys infected with the Ebola-Reston virus in the USA suggests that these non-human primates, may, like humans, be 'new' to the virus. The disease probably originated not with monkeys, chimps or antelopes, but with some as yet unidentified host.

One of the first cases in the 1976 Sudan outbreak was a man who worked in a local cotton factory. The factory was also home to a number of bats and, although none were found to be harbouring the Ebola virus at the time, bats have remained a possible, but not proven, suspect of other outbreaks. Laboratory observation has shown that fruit- and insect-eating bats experimentally infected with Ebola do not become ill or die, and this has raised speculation that these mammals may play a role in maintaining the virus in the tropical rainforest. Until scientists can track down its natural host or reservoir, understanding and breaking the transmission cycle of Ebola will be fraught with difficulties. Indeed, even if the true reservoir is ever discovered, there is still the intractable question of how to deal with Ebola.

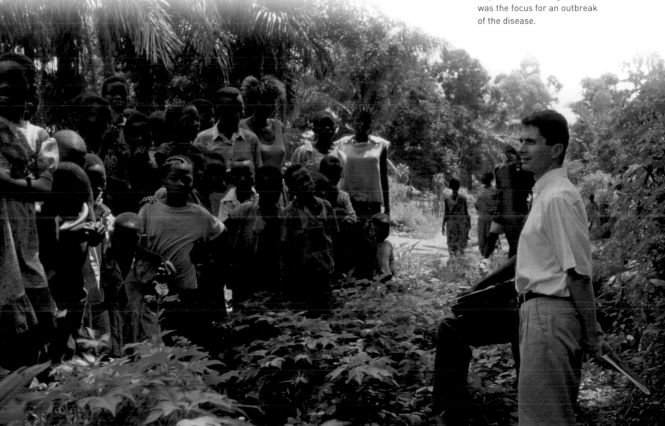

May, 1995. A World Health Organization official supervises the distribution of information about Ebola to residents of Kikwit – the city in Zaïre (now Democratic Republic of the Congo) which was the focus for an outbreak of the disease.

AIDS

AIDS

– acquired immune deficiency syndrome – is one of the leading causes of death in the 21st century. It is also one of the greatest tragedies of the modern era. First recognized and named in the early 1980s, its cause – the human immunodeficiency virus (HIV) – was identified in 1984. HIV is a retrovirus that is transmitted from one person to another through sexual intercourse, contaminated needles or infected blood products, and can also be passed from mother to unborn child across the placenta, or to infants via breast milk. HIV leads to a progressive breakdown of the immune system, which if left untreated eventually develops into AIDS. The origin of HIV/AIDS remains puzzling, but since its sudden emergence in the human population in the 1980s, over 25 million people have died of the disease. Today, its greatest impact is in the poorest parts of the world.

In 1980, Dr Selma Dritz of the San Francisco Department of Public Health gave a warning about the incidence of disease among the city's gay population: *'Too much is being transmitted, we've got all these diseases going unchecked. There are so many opportunities for transmission that, if something new gets set loose here, we're going to have hell to pay ... '*

In the late 1970s and early 1980s, physicians in the USA noted a rising incidence amongst young homosexual men of a rare skin cancer called Kaposi's sarcoma (see Kaposi's Sarcoma, page 199) and an increase in a number of infections, including rare forms of pneumonia. Alarmingly, physicians in clinics in San Francisco, Los Angeles, New York City and Miami found that some patients had very low levels of white blood cells, which play a key role in how the body fights disease. Something was destroying the immune systems of these men, leaving them prey to a host of rapidly fatal opportunistic infections. The syndrome was initially called GRID ('gay-related immune deficiency'), while some referred to it as the 'gay plague'. The Centers for Disease Control and Prevention (CDC) in the USA published their first description of five cases in the 'Morbidity and Mortality Weekly Report' of 5 June 1981.

timeline

1981 The Centers for Disease Control and Prevention in the USA report on five patients with an unusual immune deficiency.

1982 The term AIDS – acquired immune deficiency syndrome – is coined in the USA.

The San Francisco AIDS Foundation, the AIDS Project Los Angeles, the Gay Men's Health Crisis in New York and London-based Terrence Higgins Trust are launched.

1982–3 First reported cases of AIDS in haemophiliacs who have received Factor VIII from contaminated blood.

1983 An AIDS epidemic among heterosexuals is revealed in Africa.

1984 The causative virus for AIDS (later called HIV or the human immuno-deficiency virus) is identified in laboratories in the USA and France.

1985 HIV-antibody screening tests are licensed, and blood banks in the USA begin screening for HIV.

Hollywood star Rock Hudson (1925–85) dies from AIDS.

Zimbabwe is the first developing country to screen all blood before transfusion. But HIV/AIDS has still taken its toll in Zimbabwe: in 1990 life expectancy at birth was 52 years; by 2003 it was 34 years.

First International AIDS Conference takes place in Atlanta, Georgia.

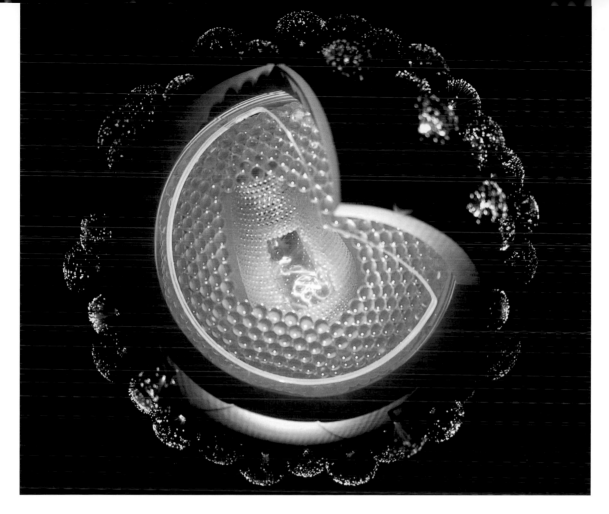

As further reports of this strange new syndrome cropped up in the USA, the Caribbean, Europe and in travellers from Africa, vague connections began to be made. Although scientists were still uncertain as to its cause, in 1982 the disease was officially named AIDS. The story of AIDS had begun, but it was a story that had been silently unfolding over several decades. Somewhere, at some time and somehow, a lethal virus had entered the human population (see The Mysterious Origin of HIV/AIDS, page 196), and had been slowly smouldering until it was ready to unleash its devastating effects on the whole world.

A cutaway model of the human immunodeficiency virus (HIV), the cause of AIDS. HIV is a retrovirus, which means that genetic information for its replication becomes permanently integrated into the cells of its host.

1986 The International Committee on the Taxonomy of Viruses recommends use of the term HIV.

President Reagan first mentions the word AIDS in public.

In the UK, a cabinet committee on AIDS is set up, and the UK's first needle exchange is opened.

A blood sample collected in 1959 in Zaïre (now the Democratic Republic of the Congo), tests positive for the presence of HIV.

1987 71,751 cases of AIDS reported by 1987 to the World Health Organization (WHO); 47,022 of these are in the USA.

The WHO launches its Global Programme on AIDS, estimating that 5 to 10 million people could be infected with HIV worldwide.

'Stop AIDS' campaigns are initiated in

the USA and Europe.

AZT (azidothymidine), the first antiretroviral drug for HIV/AIDS, is approved by the US Food and Drug Administration (FDA).

American scientist Robert Gallo (b.1937) and French scientist Luc Montagnier (b.1932) are recognized as co-discoverers of HIV.

1988 AIDS cases jump by 56 per cent worldwide.

The WHO declares the first World AIDS Day on 1 December.

1991 Freddie Mercury (1946–91), of rock band Queen, dies from AIDS. The same

[continued …

STIGMA AND SCIENCE

Over the past quarter of a century, individuals, families and communities around the world have been shattered by the AIDS pandemic, and millions have died. Few could have predicted the coming AIDS crisis, especially given its long incubation period of up to ten years, during which time most people show few symptoms.

In 1979 the World Health Organization (WHO) announced the eradication of smallpox (see pages 136–7). Life expectancies, even in some of the poorer countries of the world, were rising. It was a time of great optimism and faith that infectious diseases could be conquered, if not entirely eradicated. When the first AIDS cases were identified, the syndrome was thought to be rare, affecting only certain high-risk groups, primarily homosexuals and intravenous drug users (IDUs). Politicians were slow to grasp the enormity of the impending crisis. Activist groups in the USA and Europe took the centre stage, lobbying for more public funding, overcoming prejudices and demanding a greater awareness of the gravity of the disease.

'If human civilization lasts, if it continues to spread, infectious diseases will increase in number in every region of the globe. Exchanges and migrations will bring the human and animal diseases of all regions to every country. The work is already well advanced; its future is assured.'

CHARLES NICOLLE, *THE DESTINY OF INFECTIOUS DISEASES* (1932)

When a number of haemophiliacs were diagnosed with AIDS in 1982–3, having received Factor VIII (a clotting factor) prepared from contaminated blood, some began to distinguish between such 'innocent victims' and the so-called 'guilty perpetrators'. Collectively, all of the sufferers became known as the '4-H Club': homosexuals, Haitians (originally targeted and, erroneously, blamed for having introduced the disease to the USA), heroin users and haemophiliacs. Blaming, shaming and discriminating against these marginalized groups was one of the most regrettable responses in the early days.

Scientists were quick to start searching for an explanation of the disease. The bizarre manifestations, the dramatic effect on the immune system and the likely transmission through sexual intercourse or blood products provided some early clues. Between 1983 and 1984, scientists at the National Cancer Institute in the USA and the Institut Pasteur in Paris discovered the AIDS virus independently of

timeline

] year the red ribbon becomes the international symbol of AIDS awareness.

1992 AIDS becomes the foremost cause of death for US men aged 25–44.

1993 Arthur Ashe (1943–93), African-American tennis player, dies of complications from AIDS, having contracted HIV during blood transfusions for heart surgery.

1995 In the USA the highly active anti-retroviral therapy (HAART) is approved for use.

The WHO announces that one million cases of AIDS have been reported and 19.5

million people have been infected with HIV since the epidemic began.

1996 Joint UN Programme on HIV/AIDS (UNAIDS) is established to advocate global

action on the AIDS pandemic.

The 11th International AIDS Conference in Vancouver, Canada, adopts the theme: 'One World, One Hope'.

The International AIDS Vaccine Initiative is set up in New York to speed the search for a vaccine. By this time, 90 per cent of all people infected with HIV live in the developing world.

1997 AIDS-related deaths in the USA decline by more than 40 per cent compared to the previous year, largely due to HAART.

1998 The first full-scale trial of

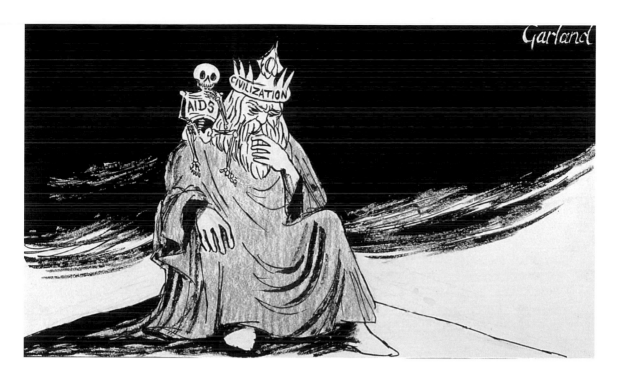

each other. It was indeed a completely 'new' virus – a retrovirus that had not hitherto been seen in the human population. The virus was labelled HIV (the human immunodeficiency virus) in 1986. A fierce and bitter wrangle ensued over which of the two labs could claim priority for the discovery of the AIDS virus and who should own the patent of an HIV-antibody blood test. But at the same time there was a groundswell of hope that, with the causative agent known, and a diagnostic test and a method of screening blood products available, science would soon come up with a means of curing or preventing the disease.

News of the discovery of the AIDS virus slowly filtered into the public arena in the mid-1980s. The death in 1985 of Hollywood star Rock Hudson from AIDS made the headlines. In 1987 the WHO launched its Global Programme on AIDS, and in a number of countries various self-help and charity organizations were set up to deal with the epidemic and to combat the prevailing stigmatization of HIV/AIDS.

An allegorical cartoon from 1988 shows AIDS sitting on the shoulder of civilization. The long incubation period of HIV, during which time most infected people show no symptoms, is one of the key reasons why the shock of AIDS came some years after the HIV virus had silently and slowly disseminated itself across much of the world.

a vaccine for HIV begins in the USA.

2000 The 13th International AIDS Conference is held in South Africa (the first in a developing nation) raising awareness of the pandemic's global nature.

The Millennium Development Goals include the aim of reversing the spread of HIV/AIDS, malaria and tuberculosis.

2002 Launch of the Global Fund to fight AIDS, TB and malaria.

2003 On World AIDS Day WHO and UNAIDS launch an initiative to provide 3 million people in the developing world with antiretroviral treatment by 2005.

2004 UNAIDS launches the

Global Coalition on Women and AIDS to raise visibility of the impact on women and girls around the world.

2005 UK hosts the G8 summit in Edinburgh with a focus on development in

Africa, including tackling HIV/AIDS.

'Live 8' concert held in London to raise awareness of HIV/AIDS.

At a historic joint press conference WHO, UNAIDS, the US government

and the Global Fund to Fight AIDS, TB and Malaria announce the results of joint efforts to increase the availability of antiretroviral drugs in developing countries.

2006 United Nations secretary general Kofi Annan urges the international community to continue to 'fight to bring the global AIDS epidemic under control'.

THE MYSTERIOUS ORIGIN OF HIV/AIDS

Attempting to trace the origins of the HIV virus has occupied the minds of many people for a number of years. One of the first and most controversial theories was the 'out of Africa' hypothesis, which led many to object that Africa was being 'blamed' for unleashing a deadly microbe on the world. In the early days, others also pointed the finger at people from the Caribbean island of Haiti. Some investigators even claimed to trace the disease to 'Patient 0' (also known as 'Patient Zero') – a Canadian flight attendant called Gaetan Dugas who had crisscrossed the world supposedly infecting numerous sexual contacts with the HIV virus.

In his 1999 book, *The River: A journey back to the source of HIV and AIDS*, Edward Hooper shifted the blame onto Western scientists. He suggested that the origins of HIV/AIDS began in US laboratories in the late 1950s, when researchers trying to develop a polio vaccine inadvertently used infected kidney cells from chimpanzees to culture the polio virus. The vaccine was given to 1 million people in what were then the Belgian colonies of the Congo and Rwanda-Urundi between February 1957 and June 1960.

Hooper's hypothesis has since been undermined by the discovery of some of the original polio vaccine, which showed no evidence of either the simian or human forms of the virus. However, the widespread use of hypodermic needles (often unsterilized and re-used time and again), both in the polio and smallpox eradication campaigns and for other purposes may, along with blood transfusions, have played a critical role in the early dissemination of the virus.

The current consensus as to the origin of HIV/AIDS – based on examination of accounts

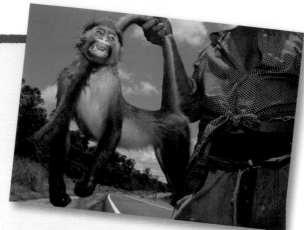

Bush meat offered for sale by the roadside in Gabon, Africa. HIV/AIDS researchers are investigating how the AIDS virus may have moved from animals like this monkey to humans, via hunting, butchering or consumption of bush meat.

of unusual clinical syndromes in the mid-20th century, testing of blood stored from the 1950s, and computer-generated 'evolutionary trees' of the HIV virus – is that the human disease did probably originate in the western equatorial region of Africa, possibly between the 1930s and the 1950s. HIV-1 (the first of the human viruses to be identified) is closely related to a harmless virus (SIV or Simian Immunodeficiency Virus) of chimpanzees. HIV-2 (a less aggressive form of the human disease identified in West Africa) is more closely related to a virus found in the sooty mangabey, a monkey found in the region, and is possibly the older of the two sub-types. How, when and why either of these two viruses crossed the species barrier is a mystery. It is possible that hunters slaughtering chimpanzees or monkeys may have become infected either through cuts, or by eating the meat.

Maybe we will never know. What is becoming clear is that, if the disease did originate in Africa some decades before the first identified cases of AIDS in young homosexual men in the USA in the early 1980s, then it had already been silently evolving and erupting in its new human hosts before anyone knew of its existence or imagined what its future impact would be.

But by then, for many, it was already too late. The HIV virus had already seeded itself in populations of people from all walks of life and in many parts of the world. Complacency, denial and recrimination were succeeded by shock, fear, hysteria and further confusion about how to deal with this unforeseen epidemiological crisis. HIV/AIDS was no longer a disease to be marginalized or ignored. It was a global problem.

AIDS EMERGES IN AFRICA

Recorded cases of HIV/AIDS in the USA had jumped from zero in 1980 to 7699 in 1984, and of these 3665 had died. In Europe there were some 762 cases by the end of 1984, with 108 cases and 46 deaths in the UK. Over this period, AIDS remained predominantly a disease of homosexuals and IDUs (and their children), with the poor urban minority groups and, increasingly, women taking the brunt of the impact.

> 'It all started as a rumour. Then we found we were dealing with a disease. Then we realized that it was an epidemic. And, now, we have accepted it as a tragedy.'
>
> AN EPIDEMIOLOGIST IN KAMPALA, UGANDA, QUOTED IN JOHN ILIFFE'S *THE AFRICAN AIDS EPIDEMIC* (2006)

As the number of people with AIDS (known as PWAs) continued to rise in the USA and Europe, its worldwide incidence became increasingly apparent. Especially worrying was its slowly evolving impact amongst the heterosexual population of sub-Saharan Africa. In Uganda, people were dying of a mysterious disease, dubbed 'Slim', which caused severe weight loss. Doctors in Uganda and Zambia then began to notice cases of Kaposi's sarcoma and wondered if there was a connection with AIDS. In 1985 a number of patients with 'Slim' tested positive for HIV.

In its early stages in Africa, as in the West, there was denial, blame-mongering and a hybrid of moralistic and scientific explanations. Governments were slow to grasp the scale of the emerging crisis, and the long incubation period and lack of distinctive symptoms made it difficult to detect cases and see what was really happening. But within a few years in sub-Saharan Africa the disease had spread east, west, north and south along the truck routes (the 'AIDS Highways'), out of the commercial overnight sex stops and into the heterosexual population, from cities to villages, from men to women, women to men, old to young, and from mothers to babies. By the end of the 20th century HIV/AIDS in sub-Saharan Africa was on a scale unimaginable in the early 1980s, and by the start of the 21st century the infection had spread even further, to North Africa, Asia, the Middle East, eastern Europe and the Pacific, causing nearly 3 million deaths a year worldwide.

STOP AIDS: THE WORLD REACTS

As the world reacted to the realization of the enormity of this newly emerging global disease, many questions were posed and dire predictions made. Where had the disease come from? What could be done to control and prevent its spread? What would be its long-term impact on the world?

The questions surrounding HIV/AIDS raised important medical, racial, political and ethical issues. Trying to unravel its origins – probably in Africa, possibly jumping

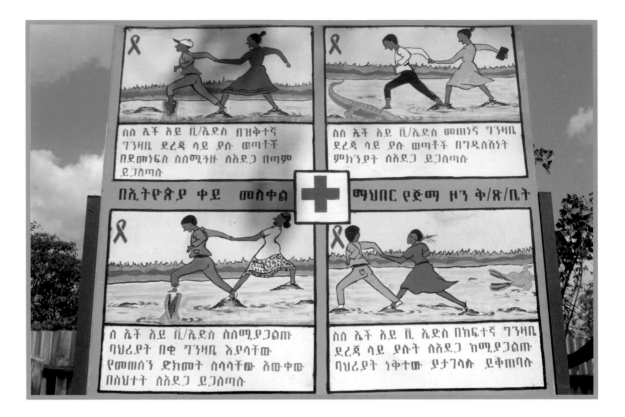

An AIDS awareness poster in Ethiopia illustrates the risk of acquiring the disease. It shows young couples crossing a river, trying to avoid crocodiles as an analogy for trying to avoid AIDS. There is a red cross in the centre of the poster and red AIDS ribbons in the corners.

species from chimpanzees to humans, maybe sometime between the 1930s and the 1950s – led to more recriminations. As with syphilis four centuries earlier (see pages 28–30), no country wanted to take the blame. Moreover, pondering over the origins of AIDS distracted many from the urgent need to do something about it.

Likewise, comparing AIDS to past plagues and pandemics led to endless debates as to how to stop its spread. Mandatory testing of young adults and quarantining of HIV-infected people were experimented with in Cuba, but most activist groups and governments, as well as the WHO, lobbied against coercive measures, which, given the long incubation period (one to ten years), would mean isolating the infected for long periods. In fact AIDS quickly proved to be so different from any other disease known in history (except possibly syphilis in its first wave from the late 15th to the 16th centuries) that what had been tried before was unlikely to work, or be acceptable, in the late 20th century. The importance of acknowledging individual human rights, the realization that a 'police-style' approach to the control of disease was not appropriate or likely to be successful, and the need to enlist the support of those most at risk led to a liberal consensus (in some but not all countries) as to how to approach the new epidemic.

But amidst the doom and gloom of the AIDS crisis in the second half of the 1980s there was a clamour for action, and campaigns for prevention and behavioural changes became key targets of national and global health organizations. Around the world people were advised about the risks of contracting HIV/AIDS and the ways of avoiding or spreading it. Posters, media voices and images dropped through letterboxes spelt out the messages of 'safe sex' or abstinence, and the use of condoms and clean needles. The 'Stop AIDS' campaign became one of the biggest health-education drives the world had ever seen.

DRUGS AND DILEMMAS

As the Stop AIDS campaign got under way, a therapeutic breakthrough came in 1987 with the licensing of the first antiretroviral drug, AZT (azidothymidine). AZT was not a magic bullet, but it was a start. However, it soon became apparent that the drug would be extremely expensive and thus beyond the reach of most of the world's population. It also caused severe side effects. Moreover, while it prolonged the life of some HIV-positive people and could prevent transmission from mother to child, epidemiologists argued that its use would mean a rise in the number of infectious people able to transmit the virus to others. There were heated debates in scientific circles about the rights of the individual versus the dictates of public health.

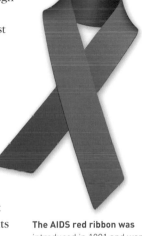

The AIDS red ribbon was introduced in 1991 and worn as a symbol of solidarity with HIV-positive people.

Almost a decade later, a 'cocktail' of three or more powerful antiretroviral drugs (known as HAART – highly active antiretroviral therapy) was given the go-ahead. In North America and Europe, the efficacy of this combination therapy became known as the 'Lazarus effect'. People infected with HIV, who would once have died from AIDS, were now returning to normal life. In the USA and Canada, death rates from HIV/AIDS dropped significantly between 1996 and 1997. Similar success stories were evident in parts of western Europe. The drugs do not cure the disease, but by slowing the progress of the virus, suppressing its replication and preventing it from rapidly destroying the immune system, the combination therapy was a breakthrough. Other drugs, including antibiotics and painkillers, combined with vaccines and long-term medical care, also help to prevent opportunistic infections from taking their deadly toll. In wealthier nations, by the close of the 20th century, HIV was no longer an inevitable death sentence.

But the cost of the drugs is exceptionally high, and they have to be taken daily for life. People with HIV, whether in cities or remote villages, need to be tested, diagnosed, counselled, treated and monitored. The drugs can make an amazing difference to people's lives – for example, they prevent the infection passing to unborn children from pregnant mothers who are HIV-positive. But how could these drugs reach those in the poorer nations?

In 1996 UNAIDS (Joint United Nations Programme on HIV/AIDS) was set up – the first UN organization entirely dedicated to confronting the AIDS crisis.

KAPOSI'S SARCOMA

Moritz Kaposi (1837–1902), an Austrian physician, made a number of original contributions to the understanding of skin diseases. In 1872 he published an article on the strange case of a man from Burma who was tattooed on almost every part of his body, including his genitals. In 1876 he described the form of skin cancer that still bears his name: Kaposi's sarcoma. The disease remained relatively rare until a number of cases began cropping up amongst gay men in the USA in the late 1970s and early 1980s. Kaposi's sarcoma became one of the diagnostic markers of AIDS. Over the past few years, the incidence of HIV-associated Kaposi's sarcoma has declined for reasons that remain uncertain.

In the year 2000 several thousand scientists from 189 nations signed a Declaration of Commitment, in which they expressed the hope that through international efforts *'Science will one day triumph over AIDS, just as it did over smallpox … '*

The tragedy of HIV/AIDS

A decade after the founding of UNAIDS – in 2006 – a tenth-anniversary volume was published. Its stark statistics summarize the tragedy of HIV/AIDS over the past quarter of a century: more than 65 million people have been infected with HIV, nearly 40 million (half of them women) are currently living with HIV/AIDS, and over 25 million have already died from the disease, making it one of the most destructive pandemics in recorded history. There are nearly 3 million deaths every year (half a million are children), and around 6000 people become infected with HIV every day. A parallel rise in tuberculosis fatalities has also occurred – HIV and TB are a lethal combination – and people with latent TB are six to eight times more likely to develop clinical TB once infected with HIV. This interaction has led to a five to tenfold increase in TB over the past two decades, and in some parts of the world 10–15 per cent of the adult population have dual infections.

The impact of these parallel pandemics has been most devastating in the poorer countries of the world. In sub-Saharan Africa, some 25 million people are living with (or, as some say, 'dying from') HIV, 12 million children have lost a parent, and over 13 million have already died from HIV/AIDS. Sub-Saharan Africa also has as many as 2 million – 90 per cent – of the world's HIV-positive children. In some of the worst affected countries, such as Botswana and Swaziland, between one-quarter and one-third of the young adult population live with the threat of AIDS. Life expectancy in many places has dropped by as much as ten years (to below 40 years in nine African countries), primarily as a result of AIDS. In South Africa, where influential figures tried for some time to deny that HIV causes AIDS, the death toll has been massive, with 5.3 million currently infected. Countries most recently hit by the pandemic are counting their losses. India

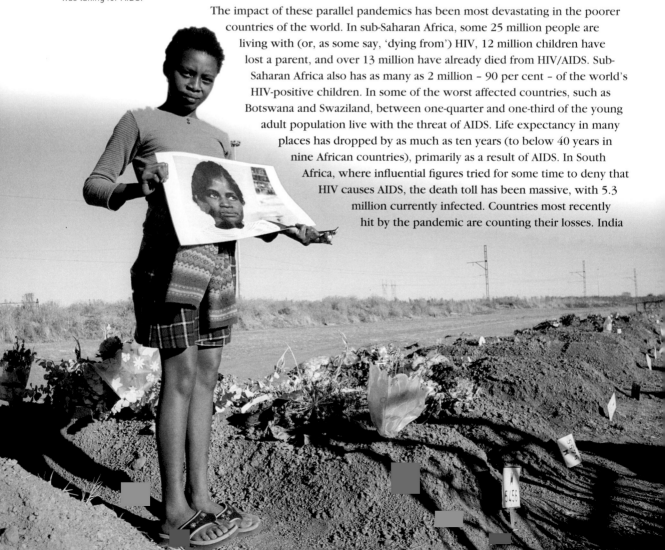

Looking AIDS in the face. Puleng Hlalele holds a portrait of her mother, Sarah Hlalele, at her graveside in South Africa. Sarah Hlalele was an activist with the Treatment Access Campaign, but she died tragically after suffering a very rare side effect from the drugs she was taking for AIDS.

now ranks third in terms of the numbers infected with HIV, after South Africa and Nigeria.

Behind the figures are countless tragic stories: a generation of productive people of child-bearing age decimated; scarce resources used to pay for long-term care, expensive drugs and funeral costs; farms, houses and schools abandoned; orphans with no hope; impoverished grandparents trying to cope with the children left behind; households headed by teenagers; relatives queuing up at the mortuaries to collect and bury loved ones; the burden of care for families and health workers; and – in both the developed and developing world – millions of needy, victimized, lonely people living with a death threat.

ONE WORLD, ONE HOPE

At the 11th International Conference on AIDS held in Vancouver, Canada, in 1996 the theme 'One World, One Hope' was adopted. There is always hope. In the last few years, pharmaceutical companies have reduced the costs of the drugs for poorer countries, and there are cheaper generic alternatives available. Global funding, especially for antiretroviral drugs in low- and middle-income countries, has trebled since 2000, and some 1.3 million people in developing countries are now benefiting from these drugs – though this is still only a small fraction of those in clinical need. Private charities, including the Bill and Melinda Gates Foundation, are providing substantial funding for AIDS research; rock stars such as Bono have raised awareness of the AIDS crisis; and concerts, like the 2005 'Live 8' event organized by Bob Geldof, have helped to raise awareness of AIDS. Possibly the best hope of ending the AIDS pandemic is vaccination. Trials of various vaccines are under way, but, in spite of the endeavours of immunologists over the last 25 years, an effective vaccine has so far eluded scientists, partly because of the rapidity with which the HIV virus can mutate, so evading both detection and destruction.

When Dr Selma Dritz warned in 1980 that *'if something new gets set loose here, we're going to have hell to pay'*, her words were prophetic. Something new was set loose, and its consequences have been catastrophic. As Kofi Annan, former secretary general of the United Nations, has said:

> *'What was first reported as a few cases of a mystery illness is now a pandemic that poses among the greatest threats to global progress in the 21st century … We need a far greater commitment of political will, courage and resources; we need united action on a new scale.'*

THE FIGURES

ESTIMATES FROM UNAIDS 2006 DATA

- People living with HIV/AIDS globally in 2006: 39.5 million.
- People newly infected with HIV/AIDS in 2006: 4.3 million.
- AIDS-related deaths in 2006: 2.9 million.
- By 2006 more than 25 million people had died of AIDS since 1981.
- By the end of 2006 women accounted for 48 per cent of all adults living with HIV worldwide.
- Young people (under 25 years old) accounted for half of all new HIV infections worldwide.
- Around 63 per cent of people living with HIV are in sub-Saharan Africa.
- Africa has 12 million AIDS orphans.
- In sub-Saharan Africa 24.7 million are living with HIV/AIDS.
- In 2006 in sub-Saharan Africa 2.8 million became infected with HIV/AIDS.
- In North America, 1.4 million are living with HIV/AIDS.

'I do not mind dying, but to die without having a child is most painful because I shall go to my grave knowing that nobody will remember my name.'

YOUNG WOMAN FROM A SMALL VILLAGE IN UGANDA, SPEAKING SHORTLY BEFORE HER DEATH FROM AIDS, QUOTED IN JOHN ILIFFE'S THE AFRICAN AIDS EPIDEMIC (2006)

SARS

In the spring of 2003 the World Health Organization (WHO) issued an emergency global alert. Reports had come in from Asia of a potentially lethal new disease known as severe acute respiratory syndrome – SARS for short. There was a worldwide panic. Airports began screening passengers, and international trade and travel were disrupted. People everywhere held their breath (or put on masks) as this mysterious pneumonia-like disease travelled rapidly to every continent of the world, infecting over 8000 people in 29 countries, with more than 700 deaths. By July 2003 the SARS pandemic – identified as a coronavirus, spread primarily via airborne droplets – was apparently over. Whether it will re-emerge at some time in the future remains to be seen.

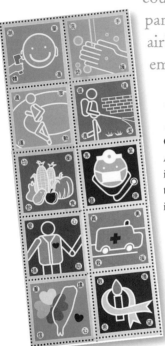

Funds from the sale of these special stamps issued in Taiwan in 2003 were used to help fight SARS.

In mid-February 2003 a small notice in the WHO's *Weekly Epidemiological Record* mentioned a mysterious respiratory infection that was cropping up in Guangdong province, southern China. It had caused the deaths of five people. A week later, Dr Carlo Urbani (1956–2003), an Italian-born WHO specialist in infectious diseases based in Hanoi, Vietnam, rang the WHO regional office for the Western Pacific. An alarming and unidentifiable disease was breaking out in the French Hospital in Hanoi, causing severe pneumonia-like symptoms and deaths, especially amongst the hospital staff. One key patient in this story was the Chinese-American businessman Johnny Chen, who had been admitted to the hospital on 26 February. After three weeks of dealing with the crisis round the clock, on 11 March Dr Urbani travelled to a medical conference in Bangkok, Thailand. On arrival he felt unwell and told a waiting friend not to touch him but to call an ambulance. He was put into an isolated intensive care unit and died on 29 March.

Between the time of the first notice from China of an unusual 'atypical pneumonia' and Dr Urbani's death, the WHO had become suspicious. Reports of a strange new disease had begun to surface from Hong Kong, Singapore, and Toronto, Canada, as well as China and Hanoi. On 15 March the director-general of the WHO, Gro Harlem Bruntland (b.1939), took the unprecedented step of alerting the world to the threat of a new disease, and at the same time issued an emergency travel warning.

SUPER-SPREADERS

SARS had probably begun not in February 2003 but in China in November 2002. In the intervening period, the newness and potential global severity of the disease had gone unrecognized. The first case was probably a young man from the town of Foshan, China. He was admitted on 16 November 2002 to Foshan No. 1 People's Hospital with an unusual respiratory illness. How and why he contracted the disease remains a mystery. The young man recovered and was discharged from hospital, but, like many cases that were to follow, he set up a trail of infection that was to spread rapidly through China, including Hong Kong, and then around the rest of the world.

The complex sequence of subsequent events was pieced together by the WHO in the spring of 2003. What emerged is that while in many individual cases the spread of the infection to others was limited, a number of so-called 'super-spreaders' were capable of transmitting SARS at an alarming rate and to a disproportionately large number of people, who then carried the virus around the world.

In China the first super-spreader was Zhou Zuofeng, a seafood trader who contracted the disease in late January 2003 in the city of Guangzhou in Guangdong province. He not only infected staff and patients in three local hospitals (health workers in the end accounted for 20 per cent of all SARS cases), but also transmitted the disease to Liu Jianlun, an elderly professor of nephrology. The professor and his wife travelled to Hong Kong on 21 February and stayed at the Hotel Metropole, on the ninth floor. Ten days later the professor was dead.

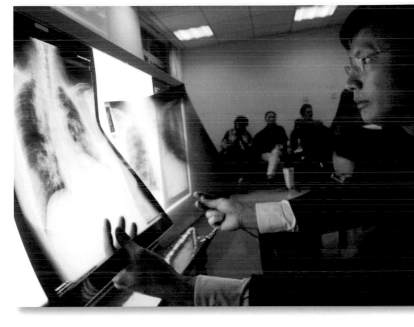

A Chinese expert examines X-rays of SARS patients during a meeting with the World Health Organization (WHO) in Guangzhou, capital city of Guangdong province in southern China, 5 April 2003, in the hunt for clues to the disease which was first reported in the area.

---

en route to Hanoi. The disease spreads to hospital staff.

5 March *A woman who stayed at the Hotel Metropole in February dies of what later turns out to be SARS in Toronto, Canada. Her son also contracts SARS and dies, setting up a chain*

of cases across Ontario.

11 March *WHO specialist Carlo Urbani travels to Thailand and is admitted to hospital.*

12 March *Hong Kong health officials report an outbreak of 'acute respiratory syndrome' to the WHO.*

15 March *The WHO alerts the world to the threat of a possible new infectious disease of unknown origin. The disease is named SARS (severe acute respiratory syndrome).*

By this time cases have also appeared in Indonesia and the Philippines.

17 March *The WHO sets up a worldwide collaborative effort to find the cause of SARS and to develop reliable diagnostic tests.*

(continued ...)

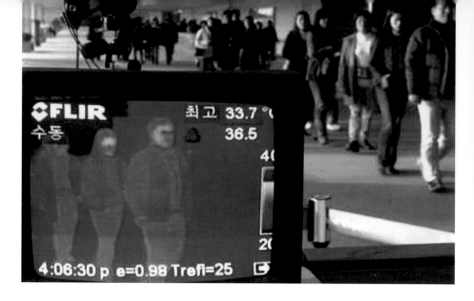

A special camera at Inchon International Airport, South Korea, measures the body temperature of travellers arriving from China as a way of detecting possible infection with SARS during late 2003. Control measures were clearly instrumental in containing the disease and breaking the chains of transmission, although luck or the quirkiness of the SARS virus also probably played a role in its rapid disappearance.

By the end of February a number of visitors to the ninth floor of the hotel had become infected. Some had been admitted to hospital in Hong Kong but some, unaware that they were ill, visited family in the Amoy Gardens housing estate of Hong Kong, while others flew to Vietnam, Singapore or Toronto.

Johnny Chen was one of the unlucky 'super-spreader' victims. A Chinese-American businessman from Shanghai, Chen was en route to Hanoi when he stopped over at the Hotel Metropole – on the ninth floor. When he reached Hanoi he was taken ill with pneumonia-like symptoms, and on 25 February was admitted to the French Hospital. Staff and patients at the hospital were subsequently infected. Among them was Dr Carlo Urbani, who first alerted the WHO as to the potential seriousness of this new disease. Johnny Chen was taken back to Hong Kong by his relatives, where he died on 13 March in an isolation facility.

The race to identify the new disease

When the WHO issued its emergency global travel alert on 15 March, no one had any idea what this deadly disease was. It did not even have a name – other than 'atypical pneumonia'. The first reaction was that it might be an influenza virus. The initial symptoms (a high temperature, muscle aches, chills and a cough) were similar to flu, but tests soon disproved this theory. In severe and fatal cases there was overwhelming damage to the lungs, and while some suggested it might

timeline

2003: 19 March SARS spreads to the USA and Europe, with the UK, Spain, Germany and Slovenia reporting cases.

26 March Ontario, Canada, declares SARS a provincial emergency.

29 March Dr Carlo Urbani dies of SARS.

8 April Hong Kong scientists publish a paper identifying a new coronavirus as the causal agent of SARS. Their work is the result of an international collaboration.

May–June Peak of the epidemic, with some 200 new cases reported every day.

17–18 June The WHO sponsors a global conference on SARS in Kuala Lumpur, Malaysia, with over 900 participants from 44 countries.

23–4 June China and Hong Kong are given the all clear by the WHO.

2 July Toronto, Canada, is declared SARS-free after 20 consecutive days without new cases. It had prematurely

been declared SARS-free in April.

5 July The WHO announces that all countries touched by SARS are now free of the disease.

be pneumonic plague, the disease did not respond to antibiotics – ruling out a bacterial infection. It took, however, only a few weeks to identify the cause of this mysterious infection and to discover that it was the first serious 'new' disease to emerge in the 21st century.

The disease was labelled 'severe acute respiratory syndrome' – SARS. On 17 March the WHO set up a worldwide collaborative initiative bringing together some of the leading microbiologists, virologists, clinicians and epidemiologists. The scientists corresponded daily using tele-conferences and a secure website on the internet. They shared their findings and swapped ideas. By early April the lethal pathogen was shown to be an entirely new 'coronavirus' – never before seen in humans or animals. Ironically, SARS is of the same family as one of the world's most widespread and harmless diseases – the common cold. How and why one human coronavirus has been around as a mild irritant for centuries and a new and deadly one suddenly emerges is a troubling question.

CONTROLLING THE SPREAD OF SARS

At the peak of the epidemic in early May 2003, when over 200 new cases were being reported every day, there was still no specific antiviral drug and no vaccine. Controlling the spread of SARS relied on classic epidemiological methods of patient isolation, contact tracing, quarantine, travel restrictions, screening at international borders, and infection-prevention measures in hospitals.

Tracking down those who might be incubating the virus, often in distant parts of the world, involved trying to establish who had been in contact with SARS patients in the previous ten to 20 days, and precisely where and when. In Singapore those suspected or known to have been in contact with a SARS patient were issued with home-quarantine orders, and web cameras were installed in their houses to detect violators. Severe penalties were imposed on anyone breaking the regulations. In Hong Kong, where 320 people fell sick from SARS in one of the blocks on the Amoy Gardens estate, the residents were at first quarantined in the building and then evacuated to isolation camps for ten days. Following the first death (at the time, of unknown cause) in Toronto on 5 March, hospitals across Ontario were quarantined for months, and a number were closed altogether in an effort to contain the disease. The WHO advised against all but essential travel to Toronto.

A SHRINKING WORLD

SARS has demonstrated how quickly infectious diseases can be spread around the globe.

In the late 18th century it took a year to travel by ship from Britain to Australia, with the result that many outbreaks of infectious disease had died out by the time the first settlers reached their destination. With the advent of steamships from the later 19th century, the voyage to Australia was reduced to three months, with passengers often arriving carrying or incubating a number of communicable diseases. By the 1950s, passenger ships took less than six weeks to make the passage.

Air travel has, however, significantly increased the speed with which diseases can spread. In 1925 it took 16 days to travel by air from England to Australia. Today it takes about a day. Most of the world's great cities are now within a few hours of each other. As SARS showed, a virus that is in Hong Kong one day can be carried by an infected traveller to any point in Southeast Asia within three or four hours, to Europe in 12 hours and to North America in 18 hours. Nearly 1.5 billion passengers travel by air every year, creating many opportunities for diseases to spread quickly across the globe.

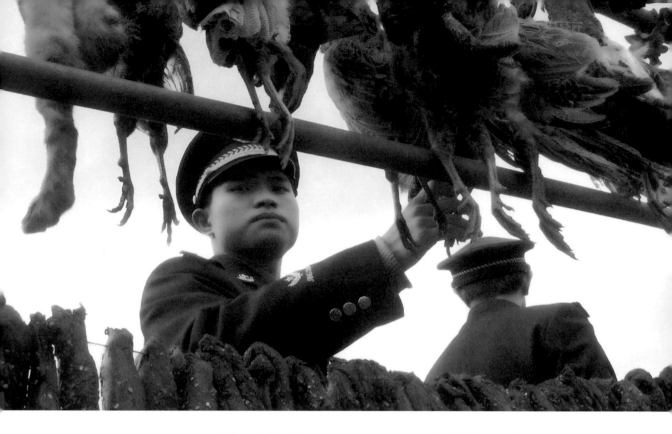

Chinese police with wild animals confiscated at a market. Following the suggestion that the SARS virus entered the human population from civets or from animals eaten in restaurants and butchered in live animal markets in southern China, the Chinese embarked on a culling programme, killing over 10,000 civets as well as other animals suspected of harbouring SARS.

In hospitals strict preventive measures included the use of masks, gloves, eye protection, disposable gowns and of footwear that could easily be decontaminated. Hospital staff were advised to wash their hands before and after contact with an infected patient, and to use disinfectants and disposable equipment. In many airports sophisticated temperature scanners were set up alongside the metal detectors to check for passengers with a fever. The fear of SARS was as great as the fear of terrorism.

In China, once the government had recognized the enormity of the problem – especially following a major outbreak in Beijing that in the end accounted for over a quarter of all SARS cases worldwide – they too responded with amazing speed to try to bring the disease under control. Schools, internet cafés, discos, cinemas and theatres were closed, and marriages suspended. Spitting in public places was prohibited. Nevertheless, the impact on the hospital system was immense – hundreds of doctors, nurses, ambulance drivers and other health workers contracted the disease. On 27 April work started on a new 1000-bed hospital for SARS patients on the outskirts of Beijing – it took 7000 construction workers just eight days to build it, at a cost of US $170 million.

The new Xiaotangshan Hospital treated 680 patients, of whom only eight died and by the end of June it was no longer needed for the treatment of SARS victims. China was given the all-clear by the WHO on 24 June 2003, and on 5 July 2003 the WHO announced that all 29 countries that had been touched by SARS were free from the disease. The deadly virus had mysteriously 'vanished'.

THE MYSTERIES OF SARS

One possible clue to the origin of the epidemic
was found in a market in southern China. In some
animal species, including the masked palm civet, the
raccoon dog and the Chinese ferret badger, scientists
found a genetically identical virus to the human SARS
virus. Antibodies in those handling and selling these
animals for human food or medicinal purposes were
found to be higher than in the general population.
One-third of the early cases of SARS in southern
China also involved food handlers, suggesting that
the disease may have jumped the species barrier
from animals to humans. On the other hand, the
animals could have been infected by contact with
humans. It is also possible that the animals sold in
the markets were originally infected in the wild by
some other species (see Sars and Bats, right).

A FOOTNOTE IN MEDICAL HISTORY?

The panic associated with SARS is over – at least
for the time being. Some epidemiologists have
wondered whether the short-lived epidemic will
simply go down as a footnote in medical history. The WHO maintains global
surveillance of probable and suspect cases: there have been a few isolated cases
since July 2003, mostly associated with accidental laboratory transmission. As
the world braces itself for a possible outbreak of bird flu (see pages 172–83), who
knows whether or when SARS will re-emerge on a global scale in the future.

Many lessons have been learnt from the SARS experience. As experts at the WHO
have noted: *'SARS dramatically
showed the wide-ranging impact
that a new disease can have in a
closely interconnected and highly
mobile world. It also underscored the
importance of a co-ordinated global
response characterized by close
collaboration and open sharing
of data and experiences'.*

While increasing global contact can
prove deadly, worldwide scientific
collaboration can prove vital. At
present it is not known whether SARS
is lying dormant, or whether the chain
of infection has actually been broken.
Is this really the end of the story? Only
time will tell us the answer.

SARS AND BATS

Bats have been
implicated in the
transmission cycle for a
number of diseases, most notably rabies.
There is also a possibility that bats are a
natural reservoir for the SARS virus. Fruit-
eating bats chew fruit to extract the sugar
and then spit out the rest, which falls to
the ground. Insect-eating bats get rid of
the hard body parts of the insect. Scientists
have suggested that these undigested
bits might harbour viruses that can then
be picked up by foraging animals on the
ground, such as the masked palm civet,
and then potentially passed on to humans.
The Chinese horseshoe bat has been
considered a suspected source of SARS.

'The analogy of war echoed throughout
the SARS crisis. This was an attack by
an unseen invader to which nations had
to respond as they would to any other
attack – by mobilizing the resources to
repel the invader. For many countries
it became clear that the real threat to
security would come not from invading
armies, but from unknown microbes.'

THOMAS ABRAHAM, *TWENTY-FIRST CENTURY PLAGUE: THE STORY OF SARS*
(2005). (THE SARS EPIDEMIC COINCIDED WITH THE LEAD-UP TO AND THE
BEGINNING OF THE IRAQ WAR.)

SCURVY When European seafarers began to embark on long voyages of exploration and

trade in the late 15th century, they met with many new hazards. One of the most insidious of these was scurvy, which we now know is caused by a lack of vitamin C. Away at sea for weeks or even months on end, sailors had to put up with filthy, cramped living conditions, and a monotonous and barely nutritious diet of foul water, rations of rum, rancid salt meat, seabirds, 'mouldy maggoty biscuits' and the occasional rat. Afflicted with bleeding gums, livid spots on the skin and fetid breath, the 'scurvy sailor' was not a pretty sight – and if the disease went unchecked, the result was an agonizing death. In the mid-18th century James Lind (1716–94) came up with compelling evidence that a daily dose of orange and lemon juice (which contain the critical vitamin C) prevents the disease. Fortunately, scurvy is now a rare disease in most parts of the world.

Of all the hazards of life at sea – storms, shipwrecks, battles and infections – none claimed as many lives as scurvy. Between the 15th and 19th centuries, it is estimated that as many as 2 million European sailors succumbed to this hideous and painful disease. Scurvy, or scorbutus, became the scourge of the sea.

The disease started slowly and insidiously. The first signs were aching joints and lethargy – sailors showing such symptoms were often flogged for 'laziness'. Then, some weeks later, the visible omens of death would spread over the body: black, bloody patches under the skin, wobbly teeth, spongy and swollen purple gums, seething sores. By the time the disease had taken hold, the afflicted emitted an intolerable stench of putrefaction – just one more stink to add to the cocktail beneath decks of rotting food, urine, faeces and vomit. When death eventually came the victim was sewn into his hammock. The Dutch and the English buried their dead at sea by slipping the corpse overboard, but the French and Spanish took their deceased comrades home for burial.

timeline

1405–33 The Chinese admiral Zheng He makes several long voyages around the Indian Ocean, without suffering from scurvy. His sailors carry mung beans on board which, when sprouted, are a good source of vitamin C.

1492 Christopher Columbus (1451–1506) sails across the Atlantic. Scurvy was less of a problem on the shorter Atlantic voyages.

1497–8 The Portuguese navigator Vasco da Gama (c.1469–1524)

sails round the Cape of Good Hope to Asia. Scurvy costs the lives of 100 men from a crew of 160 sailors.

1519–22 During the first circumnavigation of the world, the sailors commanded by Ferdinand

Magellan (1480–1521) attempt to stave off scurvy by eating rats and wild celery – but only 18 out of 218 survive the voyage.

1535–6 A French expedition led by Jacques Cartier (1491–1557) overwintering

in Canada is badly affected by scurvy. They try a concoction recommended by the local Iroquois, which is made from the 'annedda' tree (possibly the white cedar), and are cured.

1541 Dutch physician Johannes Echthius first uses the word 'scorbutus', referring to scurvy, but believes it to be an infectious disease.

1577–80 Francis Drake (c.1540–96) records cases of scurvy during his circumnavigation of the globe.

1593 First recorded use of lemons to cure scurvy, on Pacific voyage of Sir Richard Hawkins (1562–1622).

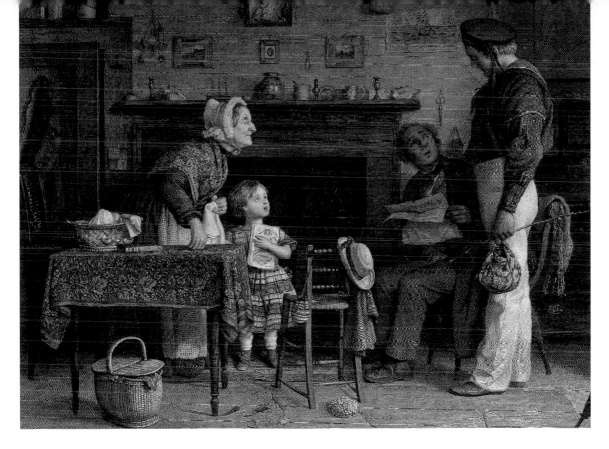

Scurvy occasionally occurred on land, but it was particularly rife on long sea voyages. In 1593, Admiral Sir Richard Hawkins (1562–1622), the English seaman and explorer, wrote:

> 'In twentie years that I have used the sea I dare take upon me to give an accompt of ten thousand men consumed with this disease.'

In 1596 the English naval surgeon William Clowes (1544–1604) described the symptoms thus:

> 'Their gums were rotten even to the very roots of their teeth, and their cheeks hard and swollen, the teeth were loose neere ready to fall out …

Many sailors died or suffered from scurvy in the days before a cure was found. This sailor, returning home, was one of the lucky survivors.

1601 *Of four English East India Company vessels sailing for the Spice Islands, only one escapes devastation by scurvy. The exception is the Red Dragon, commanded by Sir James Lancaster (c.1554–1618), who has* provisioned his sailors with oranges and lemons.

1740–4 *Voyage to the Pacific of a British fleet under Commodore George Anson (1697–1762). Sickness eliminates most of the ships' companies.*

1747 *James Lind (1716–94) conducts his clinical trial and confirms the importance of oranges and lemons in the diet to prevent scurvy. He publishes his findings in 1753 in A Treatise of the Scurvy, and in 1762 publishes An Essay on the* Most Effectual Means of Preserving the Health of Seamen in the Royal Navy.

1756–63 *During the Seven Years' War, nearly ten times more men die from disease, primarily scurvy, than are killed in action.*

1768–71 *James Cook (1728–79) loses no men to scurvy during his circumnavigation of the world, having ensured a constant supply of fresh fruit and vegetables.*

1795 *Gilbert Blane (1749–1834), commissioner of the Board of Sick and Wounded Sailors, advises the British Admiralty to provide a daily dose of lemon juice for each sailor. As a result, Nelson's fleet in the Mediterranean* consumes over 50,000 gallons of lemon juice. Over the next 20 years, scurvy virtually disappears from the British fleet.

(continued …)

their breath a filthy savour. Their legs were feeble and so weak, that they were not scarce able to carrie their bodies. Moreover they were full of aches and paines, with many blewish and reddish staines or spots, some broad and some small like flea-biting.'

Admiral Hawkins went on to express his wish that:
'Some learned men would write of it, for it is the plague of the sea and spoyle of mariners.'

ORANGES AND LEMONS AND A PECK OF SCURVY GRASS

Hawkins, from his experience of scurvy during his 1590s expedition to the South Seas, astutely recommended *'Sowre Oranges and Lemmons'* as *'the most fruitfull remedy for this sickness'*. He was not the first or only person to point to fresh fruit as a possible remedy. Indeed, by the beginning of the 17th century there was an increasing number of reports commending orange, lemon or lime juice as 'an infallible prophylactic and cure' for scurvy. In practice, however, it was all but impossible to carry perishable provisions such as fresh fruit on long voyages. Occasionally, if a ship landed at a port, the officers might enjoy the savours of fresh produce for a short while, but for the bulk of the crew, the taste of citrus fruit would have been a rare, and probably unknown, treat.

Another popular remedy, grown in Medieval physic gardens, was a plant known as scurvy grass (*Cochlearia officinalis*). William Clowes described *'the cure of two seafaring men that fell sicke at sea of the Scorby'*: the cure was a mug of new ale spiced with pepper, cinnamon, ginger, saffron, watercress and *'a peck of scurvy grass purely picked and cleane washed'*. A story from the 17th century tells of a ship ravaged by scurvy just off Greenland. One sailor was so close to death that his shipmates put him ashore to die, where he *'grazed like a beast'* on scurvy grass. He survived.

Scurvy grass, we now know, pales in comparison with fresh fruit as a remedy for scurvy. But it was a lot better than some of the other alternatives tried out

In the 16th and 17th centuries, nutmeg was believed to be a cure for the plague. The round trip to the Bandas, in the Spice Island Group west of New Guinea, to obtain the plant took two years. It also exacted a heavy toll on sailors' health, with scurvy being one of the main afflictions suffered.

timeline

1808 *The US Navy begins issuing lemon juice on long voyages.*

1845–7 *The Irish potato famine is accompanied by widespread scurvy.*

1846 *American sailors blockading Mexico during its war with the USA suffer badly from scurvy.*

1848–50 *During the Californian Gold Rush, scurvy strikes those in remote gold fields.*

1854–6 *British and French soldiers suffer badly from scurvy during the Crimean War.*

1861–5 *Many soldiers die from scurvy during the American Civil War, especially in prisoner-of-war camps.*

1867 *In Britain, Lauchlan Rose patents his method for preserving citrus juice without using alcohol, and launches Rose's lime juice.*

1870–1 *Many suffer from scurvy during the Siege of Paris.*

1912 *The term 'vitamine' is coined, later shortened to 'vitamin'.*

1928 *Discovery of vitamin C.*

to cure scurvy. Bleeding, purgatives, sulphuric acid, vinegar, mercury paste – this last 'cure', smeared on to oozing sores, often proved as dangerous and deadly as the disease itself.

Meanwhile, physicians puzzled over the real cause of this horrifying disease. Was it the salted and smoked meats, the mouldy and maggoty ship's biscuits or the absence of fresh food? Or perhaps it was the cold damp air of the sea, the lack of exercise, the 'slothfulness' of the sailors, the foul vapours of the air below decks, an excess of 'black bile' or some mysterious miasma?

THE FIRST CLINICAL TRIAL

In 1734 Johann Friedrich Bachstrom (1686–1742), a Polish pastor living in Holland, wrote his *Observationes circa scorbuticum*, in which he noted:

> *'Its causes have been generally, though wrongfully, supposed to be, cold in northern climates, sea air, the use of salt meats, etc., whereas this evil is solely owing to a total abstinence from fresh vegetable food, and greens; which is alone the primary cause of the disease.'*

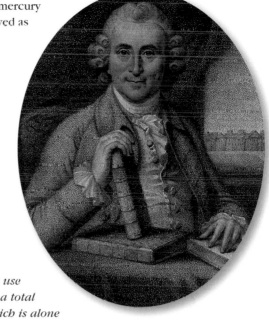

James Lind, an early pioneer in the treatment of scurvy, helped prove the importance of fresh fruit in combating the disease.

With so many pointing their finger at the importance of a 'missing factor' in the diet, and suggesting that fresh fruit and vegetables might act as a remedy, historians have wondered why it took so long for the medical profession to act on this hypothesis. But how to turn speculation into proof? James Lind (1716–94), recently qualified as a doctor from Edinburgh, and appointed as surgeon's mate on HMS *Salisbury* in 1747, was able to do just that (at least in part).

In the early 1740s, shortly before Lind's appointment, the curse of scurvy was dramatically highlighted when 997 out of 2000 sailors died of scurvy during a voyage to the Pacific of a British fleet under Commodore George Anson (1697–1762). When Lind joined HMS *Salisbury*, then patrolling the English Channel, many of the mariners aboard were already seriously sick with scurvy. Lind decided it was time to test some theories and to base his work on 'observable fact'. He took 12 men with similar symptoms, sent them down to the ship's sick bay and conducted his now famous trial. For 14 days each pair of men was to be given an addition to their usual diet, ranging from cider, sulphuric acid, vinegar, seawater, oranges and lemons, to a paste of garlic, horseradish, 'balsam of Peru' and 'gum myrrh' washed down with barley water. The results were astonishing. Those receiving two oranges and one lemon daily recovered rapidly – even before the meagre supply of fruit had run out after six days. Lind had, or so he hoped, found the remedy for scurvy.

'But of all the articles, either of medicine or diet, for the cure of scurvy, lemons and oranges are of much the greatest efficacy ... they are the real specifics in that disease ... this was first ascertained and set in a clear light by Dr Lind.'

GILBERT BLANE (1749–1834)

FAMINES

FAMINES Throughout human history famines have caused millions of deaths. Today, PEM (protein energy malnutrition) remains one of the world's great killers. Two of the most serious forms are marasmus (meaning 'wasting away') and kwashiorkor (a Ghanaian word meaning a disease suffered by a child displaced from the breast). Infectious diseases acting in combination with hunger and starvation lead to premature deaths of millions of children and young adults in the developing world.

A RECIPE FOR 'ROB'

Lind wrote up his results in his 1753 book, *A Treatise of the Scurvy*. But while he had produced convincing evidence that a daily dose of citrus fruit was a remedy for scurvy, even Lind remained confused about the actual cause of the disease. He favoured the idea that the disease was a result of damp unwholesome air and 'putrefaction' on board ships. Lind was, moreover, realistic about the practicalities of taking fresh fruit on long voyages, and so came up with a recipe for 'rob' of oranges and lemons, a syrupy concoction, which would not spoil over time.

When James Cook (1728–79) and the young naturalist Joseph Banks (1743–1820) were sent on a voyage by the Royal Society of London and the British navy to the South Pacific in 1768, they took with them a number of possible 'anti-scorbutics' – barrels of malt, sauerkraut, carrots, mustard and a small quantity of Lind's 'rob' of oranges and lemons. They stopped wherever possible to supplement their supplies with fresh fruit, plants and water. When they eventually returned to Britain in 1771 they were able to report that almost none of the crew had died of scurvy. It was not clear, however, to Cook or those reading his earlier reports, which of the various 'anti-scorbutics' were actually effective – but there was no doubt that the supplements provided to the sailors' diet (as well as Cook's insistence on cleanliness and ventilation) were radical improvements.

BRITISH 'LIMEYS'

Some have suggested that had the British heeded the advice of James Lind and the practice of Captain Cook, the American Revolutionary War (1775–83) might have turned out differently. The British lost many men at sea in the skirmishes, but more to scurvy. By contrast, it has been mooted that during the Napoleonic Wars (1804–15) the British had the upper hand over the French at sea partly because they had begun to tackle scurvy. In 1795 the British Admiralty, following the recommendation of the naval physician Sir Gilbert Blane (1749–1834), imposed a regulation that after two weeks at sea every sailor should be provided with a daily allowance of an ounce of lemon juice with one and a half ounces of sugar.

Lemons from the Mediterranean were expensive, and difficult to obtain in the required quantities, so the Royal Navy then turned instead to limes from the British West Indies – hence British sailors subsequently

'My gums swelled and some small pimples rose on the inside of my mouth which threatened to become ulcers. I then flew to the lemon juice … the effect was surprising … In less than a week my gums became as firm as ever …'

JOSEPH BANKS, NATURALIST ON BOARD CAPTAIN COOK'S SHIP, *ENDEAVOUR*, WRITING IN 1769

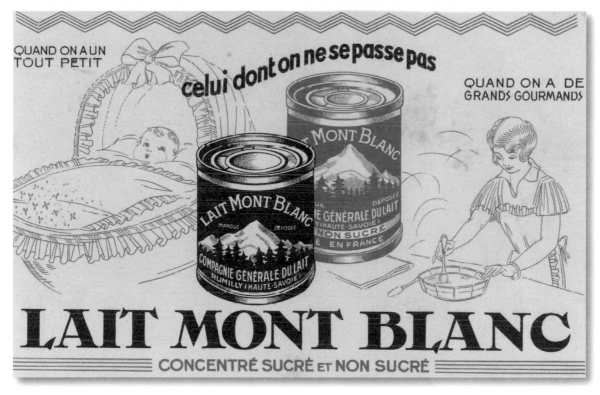

QUAND ON A UN
TOUT PETIT

celui dont on ne se passe pas

QUAND ON A DE
GRANDS GOURMANDS

LAIT MONT BLANC

MARQUE   DÉPOSÉE

COMPAGNIE GÉNÉRALE DU LAIT
RUMILLY (HAUTE-SAVOIE)

LAIT MONT BLANC
ie GÉNÉRALE DU LAIT
(HAUTE-SAVOIE)
NON SUCRÉ
É EN FRANCE
DÉPOSÉE

LAIT MONT BLANC
CONCENTRÉ SUCRÉ ET NON SUCRÉ

became known as 'limeys'. Unfortunately, the juice of the lime was far less effective than that of the lemon, and the whole debate was, for a time, thrown open again. Even Lind's long-lasting 'rob' of oranges and lemons (which, because of the preparation process, actually lost some of its potency) was less than ideal. Some physicians began to doubt the efficacy of the citrus-fruit remedy. However, by the middle of the 19th century, and several million gallons of citrus juice later, scurvy had virtually disappeared from the British fleet.

Scurvy continued to occur in other environments, causing many deaths in prisons, workhouses and orphanages in Europe and America. During the Irish famine of the 1840s, following the failure of the potato crop, scurvy was rife (potatoes are a good source of vitamin C), and in the same decade it severely affected the 'Forty-niners' of the Californian Gold Rush. Elsewhere it debilitated armies, especially during sieges, and was a constant problem for polar explorers. In the late 19th and early 20th centuries, 'infantile scurvy' hit the upper classes of Europe and the USA: mothers who eschewed breast-feeding, preferring to feed their babies with preserved milk products, unwittingly deprived their offspring of vitamin C, which is present in breast milk.

THE DISCOVERY OF VITAMIN C
For some decades following the emergence of the 'germ theory' from the 1870s, scientists looked for a bacterial cause of scurvy. One naval surgeon proposed that the benefit of citrus juice was simply that it acted as an anti-bacterial mouthwash.

The first preserved milk for babies, promoted during the 1920s as a popular breast-feeding substitute, contained products such as cows' milk, wheat and malt. However, it lacked vital elements such as vitamin C.

Albert von Szent-Györgyi, the scientist responsible for isolating vitamin C, photographed in 1955. Inset: crystalline vitamin C viewed under a light microscope using polarized light.

It was not until the biochemical studies of the 1910s onwards that scientists such as Frederick Gowland Hopkins (1861–1947) and Christiaan Eijkman (1858–1930) became convinced that the key to poor nutritional health lay in the absence of crucial elements or 'accessory food factors' in the diet.

It gradually became clear that nutritional deficiencies of one kind or another were responsible for a number of diseases, including scurvy (a deficiency of vitamin C), pellagra (a deficiency of niacin, a B-complex vitamin), beri-beri (also a deficiency of vitamin B), rickets (a deficiency of vitamin D in the diet or caused by lack of sunshine) and iron-deficient anaemia. The word 'vitamin' itself (originally 'vitamine', combining Latin *vita*, 'life', and 'amine', a chemical substance) was coined in 1912 by Casimir Funk (1884–1967), a Polish-born biochemist working at the Lister Institute, London. (The final 'e' was dropped in 1920 when it became clear that not all vitamins were amines.)

Vitamin C was isolated by Albert von Szent-Györgyi (1893–1986), a Hungarian scientist working at Cambridge University. In 1928 he found an unknown compound in adrenal-gland tissue, as well as in cabbages and oranges. Szent-Györgyi thought it was a sugar, but he wasn't sure what kind of sugar it was. The chemical names of sugars (like glucose, fructose, sucrose, etc.) end in the suffix '-ose', so, professing his own ignorance, he called the mystery compound 'ignose'.

When the editor of the *Biochemical Journal* received a copy of his paper describing his discovery (which was to earn him a Nobel Prize in 1937), the editor sent it back suggesting Szent-Györgyi rename it. He returned his manuscript calling the compound 'godnose'. Eventually, the frustrated editor named it 'hexuronic acid' (because it contained six atoms of carbon). It was subsequently called 'ascorbic acid', and is now widely known as vitamin C.

It has since been shown that a deficiency of vitamin C interferes with the synthesis of collagen (a substance found in the body's connective tissues and bones), giving rise to bleeding, bruising, poor healing and the eventual onset of scurvy. Since the 1930s the sales of manufactured vitamins and the addition of vitamins to food have been big business.

AN EPIDEMIC OF OBESITY

The story of scurvy is not quite over. The disease can still occur in areas of the world where fresh fruit and vegetables are in short supply, or in people who, for various reasons, have little vitamin C in their diets.

The Western world, by contrast, is now facing what the newspapers call 'an epidemic of obesity'. Nutritionists and scientists continue to remind us that children and adults alike need a daily dose of fresh fruit and green vegetables, and warn us about the over-consumption of sugar and fatty foods, the dire consequences of being overweight, the dangers of high cholesterol levels, the problems associated with lack of physical exercise, and the heightened risk of developing diabetes and heart disease. Chips and burgers may taste better than maggoty biscuits and salt beef, but a balanced and nutritious diet remains vital for the future health of all of us.

FILTH PARTIES

Pellagra (from an Italian word meaning 'rough skin') is a nutritional-deficiency disease, characterized by the 'three Ds' – dermatitis, diarrhoea and dementia – followed in over half of all cases by a fourth D: death. It occurs especially in societies where maize (corn) is eaten to the virtual exclusion of most other foods, and was especially common in the poor rural south of the USA in the early 20th century.

In 1916 Joseph Goldberger (1874–1929), a Hungarian-born epidemiologist working in the Hygienic Laboratory of the US Public Health Service, was determined to prove that pellagra was a dietary disorder rather than an infectious disease, as most people believed. Following a number of experiments he was still unable to convince his critics – so he tried one last, dramatic experiment.

Goldberger and his assistant, George Wheeler, injected blood from a pellagra sufferer into their own arms. They then swabbed out the secretions of a patient's nose and throat and rubbed them into their own noses and throats. They even swallowed capsules containing scabs and rashes from people with pellagra. Others volunteered to join what Goldberger called his 'filth parties'. None of the experimenters 'caught' pellagra.

In 1937 it was eventually proved that pellagra was, as Goldberger suspected, caused by a dietary deficiency – now known to be deficiency of the B vitamin niacin, along with reduced levels of the essential amino acid tryptophan.

KURU & CJD

Kuru is the name associated with a mysterious and fatal disease that was first observed by scientists in Papua New Guinea in the mid-20th century. Their investigations suggested a link between the disease and the ritualistic practice of eating the brains of deceased kinsfolk. Creutzfeldt-Jakob disease (CJD) is a very rare degenerative brain disorder that occurs sporadically throughout the world and was originally described in the 1920s. Scientists have recently proposed that both kuru and CJD are caused by infectious agents known as 'prions', which are also linked to a number of animal diseases, including bovine spongiform encephalopathy (known as BSE or 'mad cow' disease) in cattle, scrapie in sheep and chronic wasting disease in deer and elk. In both humans and animals, prion diseases can cause devastating and deadly symptoms, with the tissues of the brain becoming 'spongiform' in appearance – riddled with holes, like a Swiss cheese.

In the early 1950s, J.R. McArthur, an Australian government patrol officer working in the South Fore region of the highlands of Papua New Guinea, came across a strange medical condition amongst the local inhabitants. In a diary entry for 1953 he noted:

> *'Nearing one of the dwellings I observed a small girl sitting down beside a fire. She was shivering violently and her head was jerking spasmodically from side to side. I was told that she was a victim of sorcery, and would continue thus, shivering and unable to eat, until death claimed her within a few weeks.'*

The Fore people used the word *kuru*, which translated means 'trembling' or 'fear', to describe what McArthur had witnessed and what they believed was the outcome of sorcery. This group of tribespeople had been virtually isolated from the rest of the world until the late 1940s. They claimed that the untreatable condition, which they attributed to the malevolent activities of Fore sorcerers in their midst, was a relatively new affliction and had spread slowly within living memory. McArthur realized that he had stumbled upon an important new mystery – and one that needed a solution.

timeline

1750s *First report in the* London Journal *of the House of Commons of scrapie among sheep. Its regional names include the 'shakings', 'goggles' and 'the rubbers'.*

1920–1 *CJD- (Creutzfeldt-Jakob disease) is first described by the German physicians Hans G. Creutzfeldt (1885–1964) and Alfons M. Jakob (1884–1931).*

1935 *A vaccine for 'louping ill' in sheep is made in Scotland from the brains of sheep later presumed to have had scrapie, as two years later the inoculated sheep develop the disease.*

1938 *Experimental transmission of scrapie is first convincingly demonstrated.*

1950s *Researchers, including Carleton Gajdusek (b.1923), begin to investigate a mysterious condition known as kuru – attributed to sorcery amongst the Fore tribe in Papua New Guinea. It is initially thought to be an inherited genetic disease.*

1954 *The Icelandic virologist Björn Sigurdsson (1913–59) formulates the concept of a 'slow virus' for the agent of scrapie.*

DEADLY FUNERAL FEASTS

From the late 19th century it had become a custom among the Fore people of Papua New Guinea to prepare their dead kinsfolk for burial by cooking and eating parts of their dismembered bodies at a funeral feast. It was the women, assisted by their children, who took the main role of cutting up the corpses, and scooping out and eating the brain tissue. Scientists and anthropologists suggested that it was in this way that kuru was passed from person to person, and the predominant role of women in this practice explained why they were far more commonly infected than men. This ritualistic cannibalism was stopped in the late 1950s, leading to a rapid decline in the number of newly acquired cases.

However, not everyone agrees that kuru was the direct result of eating human brains. Some suggest that the infection could have been acquired by handling the corpses, the infectious agent entering the body through skin lesions, sores or cuts, or via nose-picking or eye-rubbing. The origin of kuru, however,

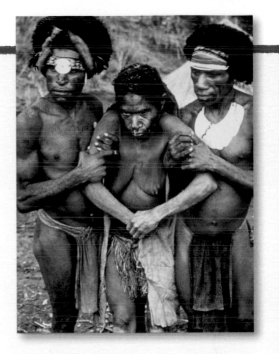

One of the Fore people from Papua New Guinea suffering from the disease known as kuru. It quickly declined following the cessation of ritualistic cannibalism.

remains a mystery. It is possible that a case of sporadic CJD, known to occur at random in all populations, occurred in a member of the Fore people, and was subsequently transmitted through consumption or handling of brain tissue.

KURU – THE TREMBLING DEATH

Over the next few years Vincent Zigas, district medical officer in the Australian Public Health Service, together with the American virologist Carleton Gajdusek (b.1923), worked to uncover the mystery of kuru. Initially they suspected that it was an inherited genetic disorder. They and others trekked across hundreds of miles of remote mountain and jungle, mapping and documenting the villages

1959 *The American veterinary scientist William Hadlow publishes his observations on the pathological similarities between scrapie and kuru.*

Late 1950s *The kuru epidemic in the Fore region of Papua New Guinea reaches its peak.*

Mid–late 1960s *Carleton Gajdusek and colleagues in the USA conduct experiments to* show that kuru is an infectious disease – possibly a 'slow virus'. Other researchers, including Michael Alpers, Robert Glasse and Shirley Lindenbaum, who have also studied the Fore people in Papua New Guinea, establish a link between an infectious agent for kuru and the practice of ritualistic cannibalism.

1967 *Tikvah Alper (1909–95) and colleagues in London develop the theory that scrapie is caused by an infectious agent made solely of protein and lacking nucleic acid. The* idea provokes immediate scepticism, but is taken up at the time by Cambridge mathematician J.S. Griffith.

1976 *Carleton Gajdusek wins the Nobel Prize for his discovery of a 'new mechanism for the origin and dissemination of infectious diseases'.*

(continued ...)

'The principal symptoms of the first stage of this distemper are a kind of high headedness. The affected sheep appear much wilder than usual … In the second stage the principal symptom of the sheep is his rubbing against trees, posts, etc. … with such fury as to pull off his wool and tear away his flesh … The third and last stage … the poor animal appears stupid … till death follows.'

AN ACCOUNT BY THOMAS COMBER OF 'SHEEP DISTEMPER' IN LINCOLNSHIRE IN THE 18TH CENTURY

afflicted by kuru. They observed its symptoms – which included involuntary tremors, jerks, uncontrollable outbursts of laughter, loss of co-ordination, wasting and eventual death. They listened and talked to the Fore people, watching their eating patterns, customs and rituals. They collected specimens of blood, cerebrospinal fluid and urine and sent them to research laboratories in Australia and the USA for examination. Women and children seemed to die from kuru far more often than men. But it was invariably a man who was accused of being the sorcerer responsible for the 'bewitched' victim's death, and who might subsequently be hacked to death by his fellow tribesmen in a ritual known as *tukabu*. The combination of kuru and *tukabu* was beginning to destroy whole villages and break up the entire fabric of Fore society.

THE SCRAPIE CONNECTION

On the other side of the world, in Britain, Iceland and the USA, a number of scientists who had been trying to elucidate the cause of a disease of sheep known as scrapie (or sheep distemper) were struck by its similarities with kuru. Scrapie had been described in Europe since the early 18th century, and is so called because the intense itching that accompanies the disease causes the sheep to rub themselves against walls, trees, rocks or fences.

Scrapie was, like kuru, also known as 'the trembles'. Sheep and goats affected by the condition begin to lose control, staggering around and eventually dying from a slow wasting disorder. An Icelandic scientist, Björn Sigurdsson (1913–59), suggested in 1954 that a 'slow virus' might be the causative agent of scrapie. As chance would have it, a few years later an American veterinary scientist, William Hadlow, who was also studying scrapie, visited an exhibition in London at the Wellcome Museum of Medical Science that told the story of kuru.

timeline

1979 Edinburgh-based researchers suggest a 'new' type of infectious agent for scrapie, which they call a 'virino'.

1982 Stanley Prusiner (b.1942) publishes a paper in the journal Science, suggesting scrapie is caused by a hitherto unknown kind of infectious agent – the 'prion'.

1984 The first 'mad cow' is seen in the UK; the disease is first identified as BSE in 1986.

1988 The British government bans the use of animal-derived feed supplements for cattle. All cattle that could possibly be affected by BSE are to be slaughtered.

1992 Peak of BSE cases in UK.

1996 Epidemiologists suggest a possible link between BSE in cattle and a new variant form of CJD (vCJD) in humans.

The European Union bans all exports of British beef.

1997 Prusiner is awarded the Nobel Prize for his discovery of prions: 'a new biological principle of infection'.

21st century The British BSE epidemic comes to an end and the ban on the export of British beef is lifted, but occasional cases of BSE occur in other parts of the world including Canada and the USA, causing concern and prompting constant vigilance. By 2007, 203 cases of human vCJD have been reported, 165 of them in the UK.

It suddenly hit him: *'The kuru brains had holes ... just like those in scrapie brains.'* In 1959 he published a paper suggesting that scrapie and kuru had distinctly similar pathologies.

Carleton Gajdusek, inspired by such ideas, began to look for evidence of the 'slow virus' hypothesis for kuru. He took brain tissue from people who had died of the disease in Papua New Guinea and injected it into chimpanzees in the USA. Within two to three years the chimps developed very similar symptoms to kuru, suggesting that the agent causing kuru was infectious, like a virus, but that the disease had a long incubation period, with symptoms in humans taking many years to develop. In 1976 Gajdusek was awarded the Nobel Prize for his discovery of a *'new mechanism for the origin and dissemination of infectious diseases'.*

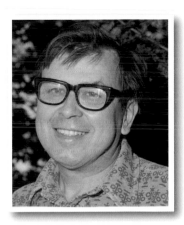

Dr Carleton Gajdusek, photographed in 1976 after learning he was to share the Nobel Prize in Physiology or Medicine for his work on the transmission of kuru.

While Gajdusek and colleagues were following up their ideas of a slow virus, other researchers also working in the Fore area in the 1960s, concluded that kuru was related to the consumption of the brains of relatives who had died of the disease (see Deadly Funeral Feasts, page 217).

The number of cases of kuru reached its peak in the late 1950s, and by the mid-1960s few if any children were contracting the disease. The decline was attributed to the end of ritualistic cannibalism in the mid- to late 1950s, which had come about as a result of government and missionary intervention. (There have, however, even recently, been a number of cases of kuru among people who were presumably infected decades ago.)

CJD AND THE DISCOVERY OF PRIONS

This might have been the end of the story, but it proved to be only the beginning of one of the most intriguing medical discoveries of the late 20th century. At the University of California, San Francisco, a physician and research scientist called Stanley Prusiner (b.1942) had been shocked by the symptoms of a patient who died of CJD in 1972. CJD is named after two German doctors, Hans G. Creutzfeldt (1885–1964) and Alfons M. Jakob (1884–1931), who had first described a strange form of dementia in humans in the 1920s. CJD is an extremely unusual neurological disease (with only one or two cases a year per 1 million population), but for those afflicted it proves devastating. In its

> **'The story of prions** is truly an odyssey that has taken us from heresy to orthodoxy.'
> STAN PRUSINER, NOBEL BANQUET SPEECH, STOCKHOLM, 1997

classic form, the patient begins to show early signs of dementia, which is followed by the destruction of the brain. Prusiner was told that the possible cause of CJD was a 'slow virus'. Intrigued, over the next decade Prusiner began exploring the possible link between CJD, scrapie and kuru.

In 1982 Prusiner published a paper in the prestigious journal *Science* that *'set off a firestorm'.* Using experimental hamsters, he produced evidence to show that the cause of these diseases was not, as suspected, an *'unconventional slow virus'* but in fact a very different kind of infectious agent. It was an aberrant form of protein, or, as he called it, a prion (short for 'proteinaceous infectious particle'). Although able to self-replicate, prions – unlike other conventional infectious agents such as bacteria, viruses, parasites and fungi – are apparently devoid of nucleic acids. In 1997 Prusiner was awarded the Nobel Prize for his discovery of prions – '*a new biological principle of infection*'.

MAD COWS AND ENGLISHMEN

Between the time that Prusiner put forward his prion ('protein-only') hypothesis and the award of his Nobel Prize, another intriguing and alarming part of the puzzle unfolded – the outbreak of BSE (bovine spongiform encephalopathy) in cattle, primarily in the UK.

In 1984 a farmer in Britain noticed that his cows were acting strangely: staggering around and behaving aggressively. When one of the cows died, an autopsy revealed that the animal's brain had sponge-like holes in it. The symptoms and signs were alarming, and very much like scrapie and kuru. Across Britain, more and more cows began to show similar abnormal symptoms – eventually dying. Scientists quickly set to work to find out what was causing this 'mad cow' disease.

The destruction of infected cow carcasses on fiercely burning pyres became a common sight during the BSE crisis in Britain in the 1990s.

The origins of BSE remain puzzling. It has been suggested that one possible source of the infection was the consumption by cows of contaminated feed. Cows are herbivores, but by the 1970s intensively reared cattle were being fed all sorts of other substances, such as proteins derived from sheep and cattle offal, including brain and spinal cord. Scrapie, the prion disease in sheep, had, it was speculated, jumped the species barrier to become BSE in cows. Once within the cattle population, the disease spread rapidly throughout herds in the UK. It was, according to some, reminiscent of kuru, but in this case the cannibalism involved was 'high tech'. In spite of the politicians saying otherwise, there was a very real fear: if cattle might have been infected by consuming sheep tissue, could people have been infected by eating 'mad cow' meat?

NEW VARIANT CJD

In 1996 an article in the British medical journal *The Lancet* voiced the first serious concerns about the implications of BSE for human health. Over the previous years the CJD surveillance centre in Edinburgh had monitored cases of patients dying of CJD. In a small number of cases they noticed significant differences from those with 'classic' forms of the disease. They were younger (with a median age of death of 28 years, compared to 68 years in the classic cases), the course of the disease was different – usually beginning with personality and behavioural changes before progressing to dementia – and the clinical course from first symptoms to death was more protracted.

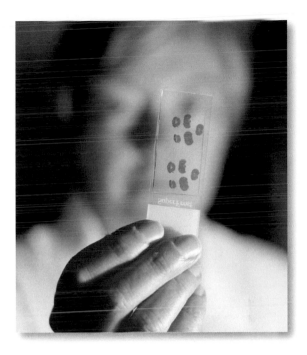

Research into new variant CJD. A scientist at Edinburgh University, Scotland, carries out research in a specialized department.

It was postulated that this new 'variant' form of human CJD (vCJD) had come from eating beef prior to the UK ban on using offal in cattle feed in the late 1980s. The official report cautiously stated that the theory that vCJD *'is due to exposure to the BSE agent is perhaps the most plausible interpretation'*. The press picked up the story as *'Mad Cow Disease Kills Humans'*.

With the fear that an 'epidemic' of vCJD was about to explode amongst people who had eaten contaminated beef products, more and more cattle were slaughtered. British beef was banned from export, and tighter regulations were imposed to prevent any infected meat ending up either within cattle feed or on supermarket shelves. Several hundred thousand cases of BSE in cattle occurred in the UK, and another 2 million or so cows were slaughtered as a preventative measure. To date, there have been about 200 cases of human vCJD, mainly in the UK but small numbers in several other countries. Surveillance continues in order to determine whether cases of vCJD have peaked since BSE-infected cattle were removed from the human food chain – or whether, given its long incubation period, there is still the possibility that new cases of vCJD will surface.

Thus, what began as a mysterious disease in Papua New Guinea and an esoteric discussion in scientific circles about the cause of a rare class of animal and human neurological disorders led to the revolutionary discovery of *'a new biological principle of infection'* – which, with the BSE crisis, has become one of the major public-health issues of the 21st century.

CANCER is a generic term for a group of some hundred or so related disorders.

It can develop in many parts of the body and can result from many different causes, some known, others still unknown. Its unifying feature is a loss of control of normal cell division, which results in a proliferation of abnormal cells often forming tumours. Cancer is not a new disease – it was known to the ancients. Over the centuries people have tried to remove, cure or control cancerous tumours, and scientists continue to search for ways to destroy rogue cells or 'switch off' the underlying mechanisms that lead to their proliferation. In the past century or so there have been some remarkable developments in diagnosing and understanding the disease, as well as the discovery of new therapies. But in spite of the successes of modern medicine, cancer remains a serious global disease in both advanced and, increasingly, in developing nations, accounting for 7.6 million deaths worldwide every year.

In 1811 Fanny Burney (1752–1840), the English novelist, underwent a mastectomy for cancer of the breast. Her account of the trauma of her operation – which she was lucky to survive – is a chilling reminder of the pain and suffering caused by cancer (see Fanny Burney's Mastectomy, page 226). In the early 19th century there were few effective therapies or treatments for cancer, and the cause and nature of the disease was baffling. And as Fanny Burney's case illustrates, it was only as a last resort, when the disease had spread and clearly manifested itself, that surgeons would attempt the removal of a tumour. Patients were offered little in the way of anaesthetics to help dull the pain of such a drastic operation.

THE MODERN RISE OF CANCER

While there are now far more effective ways of treating cancer than in Fanny Burney's day, the disease nevertheless continues to take a terrible toll on modern societies. Cancer has become increasingly 'visible' over the past century, touching

timeline

3000–1500 BC Eight cases of tumours or ulcers of the breast are described in an Egyptian document (the Edwin Smith Papyrus) – the oldest known descriptions of cancer.	**5th century BC** The Greek physician Hippocrates (c.460–c.370 BC) is thought to be the first person to recognize the difference between malignant ('bad') and benign ('good') tumours.	**c. AD 1** In his work De medicina, the Roman encyclopaedist Aulus Cornelius Celsus (25 BC–AD 50) describes superficial cancers of the face, mouth, throat, breast and penis, as well as cancers of the liver, spleen and colon.	**1st century AD** Galen (AD 129–c.210) writes a book on tumours, describing 61 kinds. His humoral theory that attributes cancer to an excess of black bile persists for the next 1500 years.	**16th century** Paracelsus (1493–1541), the Swiss physician and chemist, recommends that cancer be treated with simple or compound chemicals, including mercury and arsenic. **1543** The Flemish anatomist Andreas	Vesalius (1514–64) publishes De humani corporis fabrica libri septem, with illustrations of the structure of the human body, based on dissection of human corpses. **1622** The Italian anatomist Gaspare Aselli	(1581–1625) discovers the lymphatic system – leading to the end of the old theory that black bile is the cause of cancer. **1665** British natural philosopher Robert Hooke (1635–1703) coins the term 'cell' to describe minute

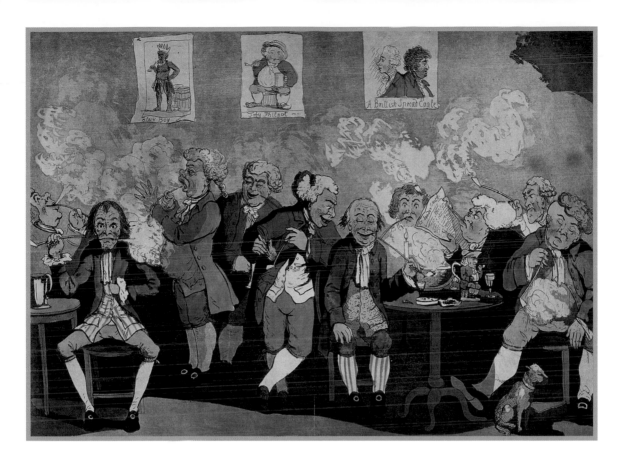

many people's lives, whether as sufferers, carers or through bereavement. In the Western world, one in three or four of the population will develop cancer at some time. Cancer is today more common than it was in the past for many reasons. Partly this has to do with the age-related spectrum of cancer. As life expectancies have risen in recent times in Western societies, so cancer has become one of the leading diseases of middle and older age groups (although a number of cancers affect young children). The process of ageing is also a fundamental factor in the development of many cancers – as people age their cellular repair-and-control

Gentlemen in the 18th century smoking in their club. Smoking in such confined places – even private clubs – is now banned by law in Britain and many countries and some US states.

structures in cork he has seen under the microscope.

1775 The British surgeon Percivall Pott (1714–88) establishes a link between cancer of the scrotum and chimney sweeps, blaming the soot.

1776 Bernard Peyrilhe (1735–1804) proposes that cancer is transmitted though air, saliva and other bodily secretions.

1824–7 The British surgeon Sir Astley Cooper (1768–1841) advocates breast mastectomy in

certain cases. American surgeon William Halsted (1852–1922) follows this practice using aseptic techniques.

1830 Joseph Jackson Lister (1786–1869) makes microscope lenses that lead to the beginnings of

histology (study of tissues) and making it possible to differentiate cancer cells from normal cells.

1832 Thomas Hodgkin (1798–1866), the English physicist and pathologist, describes cancer of the lymph nodes.

1838 The German physician Johannes Müller (1801–58) analyses the microscopic features of benign and malignant tumours, attributing cancer to the formation of new cells inside a diseased organ, with a potential to spread to other parts of the body.

German scientists Theodor Schwann (1801–82) and Matthias Jakob Schleiden (1804 81) suggest that cells are the basic unit of life.

1858 In Die Cellularpathologie, German pathologist Rudolf Virchow (1821–1902) proposes

that the cell is the smallest unit of life and that every cell is generated from another cell.

1895 Wilhelm Röntgen (1845–1923) discovers X-rays – these are used to diagnose and treat cancer.

(continued ...)

mechanisms tend to be less effective. Modern lifestyles and environmental as well as genetic factors have played their part, and infectious agents are now also known to be associated with a number of cancers. There has, too, been a great improvement in diagnosis. Oncology - the scientific study of cancer (from Greek *onkos*, 'tumour') - is very much a product of modern medicine.

A huge, malevolent claw pierces the breast of a naked sleeping woman, whilst another women swoops down to stab the claw with a knife. This early 20th-century watercolour symbolized science's fight against cancer.

CANCER — A DISEASE DATING BACK TO ANTIQUITY

Cancer is probably as old as the human race. It was known to the ancient Egyptians, Greeks and Romans and, indeed, was named by the Greeks in the fifth century BC. The Latin word *cancer* means 'crab', and originally came from the Greek word for the same creature: *karkinos*. One possible reason for the name is that the pain of the disease was like being pinched by a crab. Or perhaps the allusion was to the way in which tumours grasp the tissues in which they grow. Another possibility is that the swollen blood vessels around a malignant tumour looked like the claws of a crab, as the Greek physician Galen (AD 129-*c*.210) suggested:

> *'For just as in that animal the feet extend out from both sides of the body, so also in this disease the distended veins call to mind the picture of a crab.'*

'It is better not to apply any treatment in cases of occult cancer; for, if treated, the patients die quickly; but if not treated they hold out for a long time.'

THE HIPPOCRATIC CORPUS, *c.*FIFTH CENTURY BC

BLACK BILE AND CUTTING-EDGE DISCOVERIES

The ancients sought explanations as to why cancer occurred, and why certain types of people were most at risk. Cancer was clearly very different from the epidemic plagues and pestilences that would arrive suddenly from time to time and rapidly strike many down with grisly symptoms and a quick death. Malignant tumours were relatively rare, less visible and slower to kill their victims. In line with Galen's humoral theory - in which health depended on the proper balance of four 'humours' within the body - Greek and Roman physicians held that cancer was the result of an excess of black bile

timeline

1898 *Marie (1867–1934) and Pierre Curie (1859–1906) discover the radioactive elements polonium and radium – the latter used for treating deep cancers.*

1902 *The British Imperial Cancer Research Fund is set up, followed*

By similar non-profit-making organizations in Europe and USA.

1909 *The German physician Paul Ehrlich (1854–1915), using his ideas of specific drugs to target specific diseases, publishes the first book on chemotherapy.*

1923 *A German study suggests that an increase in lung cancer might be connected to an increase in smoking. The significance of this was appreciated only recently.*

1931 *The American pathologist James Ewing (1866–1943)*

publishes The Causation, Diagnosis and Treatment of Cancer, stressing that cancer is a disease with multiple forms and multiple causes.

1937 *Geoffrey Keynes (1887–1982) at St Bartholomew's*

Hospital, London, claims good results from the simple removal of breast tumours (lumpectomy), followed by radiation, rather than radical mastectomies.

1938 *American biologist Raymond Pearl (1879–1940) links smoking*

with decreased longevity. His and other studies receive little attention until the early 1950s.

1942 *American scientists study nitrogen mustard as a possible chemotherapeutic agent.*

1948 *Marie Curie Cancer Relief Fund created to support home care for the terminally ill.*

At Boston Children's Hospital Sidney Farber (1903–73) uses folic acid antagonists for treating leukaemia – the

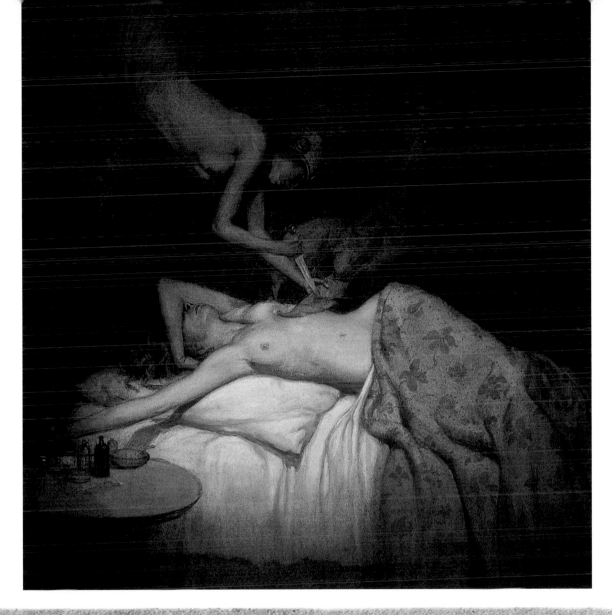

first evidence that chemicals can interfere with malignant cell growth.

1950 Reports of the possible link between cigarette smoking and lung cancer are published in the UK and USA.

1951 Richard Doll (1912–2005) and Austin Bradford Hill (1897–1991) set up a study to look at a possible link between lung cancer and smoking.

1953 Francis Crick (1916–2004) and James Watson (b.1928) describe the structure of

DNA, paving the way for the study of the role of genes in cancer development.

1955 The Cancer Chemotherapy National Service Center in the USA starts screening thousands of compounds for anti-cancer activity.

1971 The National Cancer Act in the USA commits an initial $500 million to wage a 'Crusade Against Cancer'.

1972 CT scans are developed, followed in the 1980s by MRI scans – important diagnostic cancer-detecting tools.

1982 American oncologist Robert Weinberg (b.1942) and others discover the first human oncogene (a gene causing normal cells to form tumours) and identify the first known tumour-suppressor gene.

1990 The Human Genome Project is

set up to map the genetic make-up of the human species.

1992 The European Prospective Investigation into Cancer and Nutrition (EPIC) is established to look at the interplay of different

contributory factors in cancer. Similar large-scale studies are set up in Estonia, China, Mexico and the USA.

2005 The World Health Assembly adopts a resolution to develop a Global WHO Cancer Control Strategy.

(*melan cholos*). People with a 'melancholic' disposition, accordingly, were seen as more susceptible to cancer. A wide range of treatments was tried for visible cancers, such as applying cabbage juice, or a mixture of honey, salt and egg white, or caustic creams and pastes, often containing arsenic. Purging and blood-letting were also tried, but most people with deep-seated or 'occult' malignant growths were thought to be incurable.

The tumours that were seen by the ancients were usually those that were apparent at the surface, especially breast cancers. The human body was deemed

FANNY BURNEY'S MASTECTOMY

In 1811 the English novelist Fanny Burney (1752–1840) was in France when she was 'cut', without anaesthetic, for cancer of the breast by the famous military surgeon Dominique-Jean Larrey (1766–1842). She was lucky to survive, and later recalled her excruciating experience:

'… when the dreadful steel was plunged into the breast – cutting through veins – arteries – flesh – nerves – I needed no injunctions not to restrain my cries. I began a scream that lasted unintermittingly during the whole time of the incision – & I almost marvel that it rings not in my Ears still! so excruciating was the agony. When the wound was made, & the instrument was withdrawn, the pain seemed undiminished, for the air that suddenly rushed into those delicate parts felt like a mass of minute but sharp & forked poniards, that were tearing the edges of the wound, – but when again I felt the instrument – describing a curve – cutting against the grain, if I may so say, while the flesh resisted in a

manner so forcible as to oppose & tire the hand of the operator, who was forced to change from the right to the left – then, indeed, I thought I must have expired … I attempted no more to open my eyes … The instrument this second time withdrawn, I concluded the operation over – Oh no! presently the terrible cutting was renewed – & worse than ever, to separate the bottom, the foundation of this dreadful gland from the parts to which it adhered … yet again all was not over … '

In the end the operation lasted a full 20 minutes – but it nevertheless saved her life.

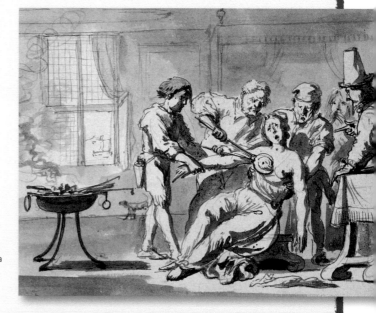

A gruesome and all-too-graphic depiction of a 17th-century mastectomy of the kind endured by Fanny Burney.

sacred in most ancient cultures in the West, and few physicians investigated internal human organs either of the living or the dead. From the 14th century AD, however, anatomical dissections of cadavers (mostly of executed criminals or the unclaimed corpses of paupers) began to be permitted in Europe. From the 17th century dissections were also increasingly conducted on those who had died in hospital, and the correlation of clinical and post-mortem examinations began to raise questions about Galenic models of cancer, opening the doors to new understandings of the disease.

'OMNIS CELLULA E CELLULA'

The real breakthrough in our understanding of the pathology of cancer came with the ability to study human cells under the microscope, whereby abnormalities could be seen not just in organs and tissues but at the cellular level. The German scientists Theodor Schwann (1801–82), Matthias Jakob Schleiden (1804–81) and Johannes Müller (1801–58) paved the way for the development of the cellular theory proposed by Rudolf Virchow (1821–1902), the German pathologist. Virchow placed slivers of flesh and smears of blood under the microscope and noticed that a mass of flesh that looked undifferentiated to the eye was, in fact, made up of millions of microscopic cells. He realized that cells were fundamental to life, and is best known for the theory he proposed in 1858: *'Omnis cellula e cellula'* – all cells come from cells. Virchow also recognized that the condition that he named leukaemia (from the Greek *leukos*, 'white', and *haima*, 'blood') was characterized by a proliferation of abnormal white blood cells. We now recognize leukaemia as cancer of the blood. Disease, Virchow argued, arose from abnormal changes within cells, and these could multiply out of control through division and spread to the rest of the body. This was the beginning of the modern science of oncology.

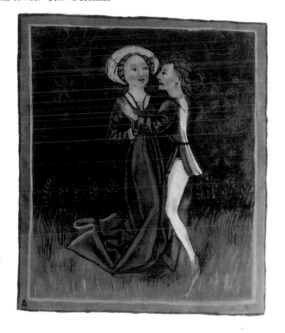

TUMOURS, SURGERY AND THE FIRE DRILL

Virchow published numerous studies on the cellular dimensions of cancer, urging his students *'to think microscopically'*. But when presented with a clinical case of cancer, the question always arising was: should the tumour be excised? Whether or not to wield the surgeon's knife is a quandary that goes back to antiquity.

Hippocrates (*c*.460–*c*.370 BC) and Galen, followed by the Persian physician Rhazes (ar-Razi, AD *c*.865–925/32) and the French military surgeon Ambroise Paré (1510–90), were generally against excision of deep tumours. In their view the risk of death far outweighed the likelihood of cure, as incisions were likely to turn gangrenous and putrefy. In some desperate cases, however, cutting out a tumour does seem to have been tried, and attempts were made to cauterize the incision using a red-hot iron known as the 'fire drill'. The pain from both procedures, with no anaesthetics to put the patient to sleep apart from the soporific effects of

The melancholic humour, one of the four classic 'humours' or temperaments once thought to balance the health of the body, as depicted in a Medieval manuscript. For centuries it was believed that persons with excessively melancholic dispositions were more likely to be predisposed to cancer.

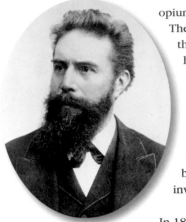

The German physicist Wilhelm Conrad Röntgen. His chance discovery of X-rays was a landmark in the detection and treatment of tumours.

opium or alcohol, must have been horrific, as Fanny Burney's account attests. The successful outcome of her operation was very much the exception rather than the rule. The introduction of anaesthetics and antiseptics by the second half of the 19th century (see pages 76–79) made some surgical operations for cancer less horrendous, but for the most part patients still preferred not to yield to the terrors of the surgeon's knife.

X-RAYS AND RADIOTHERAPY — A RAY OF HOPE

The success of surgery was, moreover, limited, especially since it was usually only those patients with advanced stages of cancer who were seen by the physician and operated on by the surgeon. The early stages of cancer invariably went undetected.

In 1895 the chance discovery of X-rays by the German physicist Wilhelm Röntgen (1845–1923) changed the whole outlook for cancer detection and treatment. X-rays were immediately used for non-invasive diagnostic purposes, and tumours could be detected long before the ominous signs and symptoms of cancer appeared. X-rays also proved to have a therapeutic function – it was noticed that they caused burns and could be used to treat minor skin problems such as moles, acne, ringworm and excessive hairiness. The potential for destroying cancerous cells was quickly picked up. The discovery of X-rays was followed in 1898 by the discovery in France of the radioactive elements polonium and radium by the wife and husband team, Marie (1867–1934) and Pierre Curie (1859–1906). With refinements in the technology of radiotherapy over the next few decades there was, at last, a way of treating cancer, albeit an expensive one. In the early days there was also a human cost, with some patients as well as radiographers dying as a consequence of excessive doses of radiation.

Luminous Watch Faces

In the early decades of the 20th century, watches that glowed in the dark became highly fashionable. The dials were painted with a luminous paint containing uranium – a radioactive element. Some of the young women who worked at the watch-painting studio of the US Radium Corporation in New Jersey took to decorating their fingernails and eyelids with the luminous paint – one young woman even went so far as painting her teeth, to impress her date. By 1927, 13 of the workers had died from a mysterious illness, found to be due to chronic radiation poisoning, which caused bone cancer.

Radiotherapy did not replace surgery, but was initially often used to reduce inoperable tumours to operable size, and also to reduce pain and to help stop recurrence after the operation. The longer-term implications and dangers of radiation were not readily appreciated until after the atomic bombs were dropped on Hiroshima and Nagasaki in 1945. Debates about the effects of even low doses of radiation – for example, on children or pregnant women – continue to this day.

MUSTARD GAS AND CHEMOTHERAPY

Over the centuries numerous 'cures' for cancer had been tried, including various chemicals. Mercury was often employed both externally and internally, while it was claimed that arsenic prevented cancers from ulcerating. Itinerant quacks often sold supposedly 'infallible' remedies for any disease you cared to name – for example, in the late 19th century 'Hamlin's Wizard Oil' (containing camphor, ammonia, chloroform, turpentine and herbs)

was said to cure everything from constipation to cancer. By this time
a range of alternatives to orthodox medicine – such as homeopathic remedies,
water therapy, mesmerism and electrical cures – had also been taken up by
cancer sufferers. By the early decades of the 20th century, many orthodox doctors
and surgeons had become concerned that such 'treatments' were preventing
people from seeking early diagnosis, radiotherapy and surgery. It was not,
however, until after the Second World War that chemotherapy became an added
and vital component of cancer treatment.

The term chemotherapy was first used by the German bacteriologist Paul Ehrlich
(1854–1915) in the early 20th century to refer to the treatment of infectious
diseases by drugs ('magic bullets') that killed the infective organism but left
the patient unaffected. Ehrlich went on to propose that cancerous cells could
be destroyed by chemicals without harm to the healthy host tissue. The first
breakthrough in cancer
chemotherapy was the
recognition that mustard gas,
used as a deadly chemical
weapon in the First World War,
decreased the number of white
blood cells in soldiers who
had been exposed to it. Some
reasoned that it might also be
used therapeutically to destroy
cancer cells. In the 1940s the
Americans Louis Goodman
(1906–2000) and Alfred Gilman
(1908–84) tested a number
of related nitrogen mustard
agents. One was administered
to a mouse with a lymphoma (a
tumour of the lymph cells) and,
amazingly, the tumour shrank.
A number of patients with
advanced lymphomas were

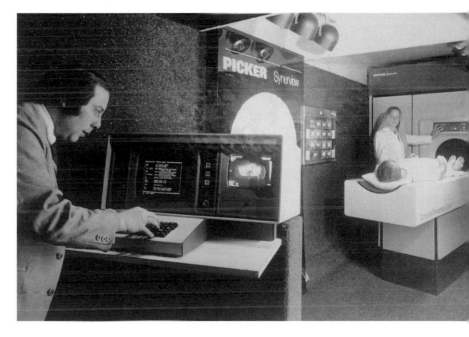

injected with the compound. Although successful in the short term, the effect
proved only temporary. These experiments did, however, stimulate further
research into new cytotoxic drugs – drugs capable of destroying rapidly
proliferating cells in tumours.

There were some successes in the 1950s and 1960s, and with the introduction
in the mid-1960s of combination therapy (using a number of drugs, each with
a different action) there was optimism that further research would yield the
answers to cancer. Hundreds and thousands of different chemicals were tested
for anti-cancer activity in the USA under the slogan 'Nothing too stupid to test',
and in 1971 the US Congress passed the National Cancer Act, which committed
more funds and resources to cancer research. In other countries, too, substantial

**A patient undergoing a
CAT** (Computerized Axial
Tomography) scan. A rotating
X-ray machine produces
images of a patient's internal
organs in a few seconds.
Such modern techniques have
aided cancer diagnosis. In
addition, drugs developed as a
result of recent understanding
of the molecular basis of the
disease are beginning to have
dramatic effects in some
types of cancer.

resources were directed towards universities and research institutes, and a huge industry, involving pharmaceutical and biotech companies, grew up around what had become known as the 'war against the Big C'.

Three types of previously incurable cancer – childhood leukaemia, Hodgkin's disease and testicular cancer – are now responding well to various recently discovered drugs. And with the increasing use of new diagnostic and computerized imaging techniques such as CT (computerized tomography), PET (positron emission tomography) and MRI (magnetic resonance imaging), as well as mass screening for some common cancers such as those of the breast and cervix, early diagnosis often ensures a greater chance of survival. For breast-cancer patients surgeons now try to limit surgery to the initial removal of just the tumours (lumpectomy), followed by radiation and chemotherapy, rather than radical mastectomies, which involve removing the whole breast and the surrounding lymphatic system. For many cancers, especially those in advanced stages, however, there is still a long way to go to find effective treatments.

ENVIRONMENTAL AND LIFESTYLE CANCERS

Over the past centuries scientists and physicians have tried to work out why cancer occurs in the first place. The older Galenic idea that certain people with 'melancholic' temperaments were predisposed to cancer persisted for many centuries. Some physicians additionally suggested that cancer was hereditary, while others believed it was contagious. Medical and domestic health books advised people to avoid activities that might 'excite' the onset of cancer, such

The devastation caused by the nuclear reactor explosion at Chernobyl, Ukraine, in 1986. Radiation from the accident killed workers in the immediate aftermath, blighted the surrounding area and produced a radiation cloud over many parts of Europe. More deaths as well as birth defects occurred in the years that followed.

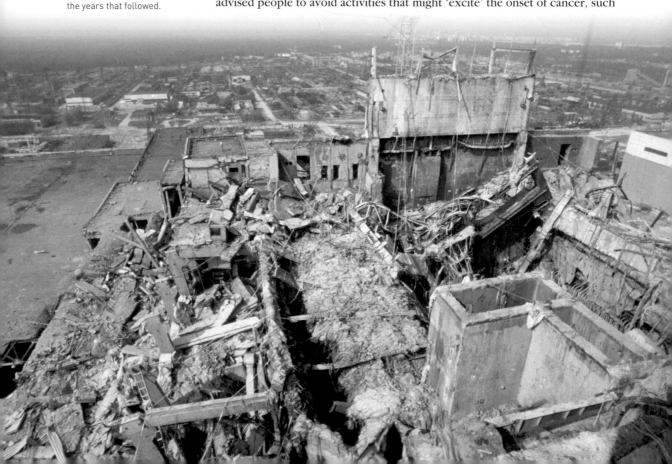

as the wrong diet, the wearing of corsets by women, incorrectly fitted dentures or insufficient exercise.

Environmental associations were also considered. One of the earliest studies to suggest a link between cancer and an external environmental agent dates back to the second half of the 18th century, when a British surgeon called Percivall Pott (1714–88) observed that men with cancer of the scrotum at St Bartholomew's Hospital in London had been chimney sweeps as boys, where they had been *'thrust up narrow, and sometimes hot chimneys where they are bruised, burned and almost suffocated; and when they get to puberty, become peculiarly liable to a most noisome, painful, and fatal disease'*. Pott hypothesized that cancer of the scrotum was linked with the irritation caused by soot.

By the 20th century, scientists began to re-examine some of these ideas and to speculate that external and 'lifestyle factors' – something in the air people breathed, the food they ate, the alcohol or tobacco they consumed, the conditions in which they worked – might be part of the cancer story. The list of possible carcinogenic (cancer-causing) agents that came under scrutiny was endless. Some of them were highly speculative, but others – such as tar on the roads, traffic fumes, industrial pollutants, smog, chemical dyes, viruses, radiation and pesticides – were more plausible.

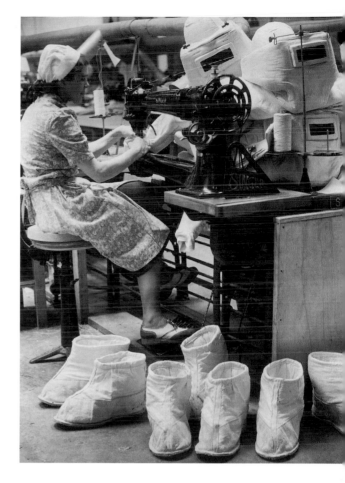

Making asbestos fire-fighting equipment in 1940. Before its links to cancer were realized, the use of asbestos was widespread, and safety precautions for both its manufacture and applications were far less rigid than today.

With better statistics on the incidence and causes of death in the 20th century, it became possible to examine long-term trends of cancer mortality and to map the distribution of various cancers with a view to finding environmental associations or behavioural risk factors. One of the most startling of all the findings came in the late 1940s as epidemiologists discovered that a dramatic increase in lung cancer had emerged over the course of the previous few decades: deaths from lung cancer in the USA had escalated from fewer than 400 recorded cases in 1900 to over 11,000 in the mid-1940s – and in Britain they had shot up six-fold between the 1920s and the 1940s. What was the cause of this alarming trend?

A number of studies were set up to find an answer, both in the USA and in Britain, and by the early 1950s there emerged one key factor – smoking. One of the most thorough investigations was the study initiated by the British epidemiologists Austin Bradford Hill (1897–1991) and Richard Doll (1912–2005) in the early 1950s. They wrote to all doctors in Britain to enquire about various aspects of their lives, including their smoking habits. Many doctors at that time smoked – often quite heavily – not perceiving any particular risk in the highly addictive habit. Over a number of years 40,000 male doctors were tracked, and

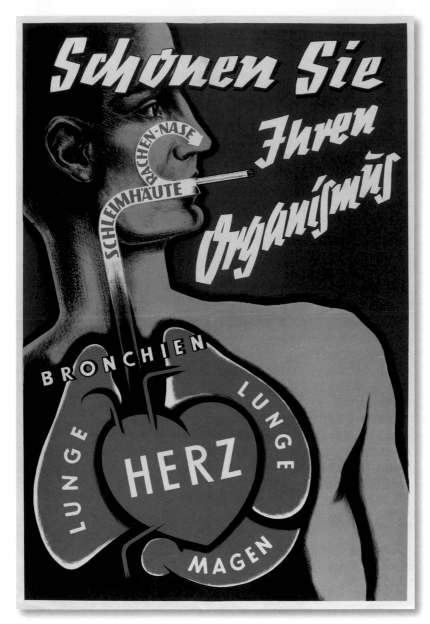

it quickly became apparent that heavy smokers ran a significantly higher risk of lung cancer than non-smokers. Mortality fell if individuals stopped smoking (though still remaining higher than the group of lifetime non-smokers), thus highlighting for the first time a possible way of preventing a major form of cancer.

Further studies supported these findings, and from the 1970s, with increasing fears about passive as well as active smoking, anti-smoking lobby groups, supported by governments, began to take up the cause. 'Smoking kills' has become one of the biggest health-education messages of the late 20th and early 21st centuries, with many countries introducing bans on advertising and smoking in enclosed public places, and imposing high taxes on tobacco and warnings on cigarette packets.

Over the course of the 20th century it is estimated that 100 million people died worldwide from smoking-associated diseases. Lung-cancer incidence and mortality has, however, now fallen for men in the USA and Europe, although the figures for women continued to rise through the 1990s, reflecting the more recent uptake of smoking

A German anti-smoking poster in the early 20th century shows the route through which the smoke passes to the heart and lungs.

amongst young women and the time lag between exposure and disease. In other parts of the world the message is only slowly having an impact. In China, annual cigarette consumption rose from 100 billion in the early 1950s to over 1800 billion in the 1990s. It is predicted that over the coming years, smoking-related mortality (including 15 other types of cancer besides lung cancer, as well as heart and respiratory diseases) will rise in many parts of the world.

CANCER – IS THERE A WAY FORWARD?
Smoking is one of the clearest lifestyle risk factors, but cancer is a complex and varied disease with many causes – some known, others still to be identified. Every day the media report on the latest scare story, or the most recent scientific

breakthrough. Diet is now thought to account for one-third of all cancers, though while some of the messages are clear (fresh fruit and vegetables are good, high salt intake and too much alcohol are bad), it is very much a multi-faceted and complex issue. Excessive exposure to the sun's ultraviolet light is a key factor in the increase of skin cancer, and, like smoking, is avoidable. Viruses, bacterial organisms and chronic infections have been implicated in some cancers, notably cervical cancer, liver cancer, Burkitt's lymphoma and stomach cancer. In developing countries 25 per cent of malignant cancers are linked to infectious diseases, compared to less than 10 per cent in developed countries. These could, in time, become preventable with vaccines and antibiotics.

'Horrible Stygian Smoke'
In 1604 King James I of England (1566–1625) published A Counterblaste to Tobacco, *in which he described smoking as 'a custom loathsome to the eye, hateful to the nose, harmful to the brain, dangerous to the lungs, and in the black stinking fume thereof, nearest resembling the horrible Stygian smoke of the pit that is bottomless'. King James organized the first public debate on the effects of tobacco at Oxford and, to make his point, he displayed black brains and black viscera, allegedly from the bodies of smokers.*

Since the discovery of the structure of DNA in 1953, there has been an explosion in our understanding of human biology at the molecular level – especially with the success of the Human Genome Project, an international collaborative effort to identify all the estimated 20,000 to 25,000 human genes in our genetic make-up. We now know that certain genes (oncogenes) predispose certain individuals to cancer, and we also know that environmental factors (such as radiation) can bring about genetic mutations leading to cancer. This understanding brings with it the promise of novel ways of targeting molecular abnormalities in cancer cells.

With earlier detection, greater use of specialist surgery, screening programmes and advances in chemotherapy and radiotherapy, cancer survival rates have doubled in many Western countries in the past 30 years. The incidence of cancer, probably due to reduced risk factors, has also recently declined in some Western countries.

Many aspects of cancer still remain a mystery. 'Why me?' is a typical reaction to cancer, and one that it is often difficult to answer. The cost of cancer – whether in terms of lives lost, personal and family tragedies, research, health-promotion campaigns, screening, funding for high-tech diagnostic tools, drugs and palliative care – is greater than it ever has been in the past. Once considered a 'Western' disease, cancer is also now emerging as a major problem in developing countries. It is estimated that

> **'We are so close to a cure for cancer. We lack only the will and the kind of money and comprehensive planning that went into putting a man on the moon.'**
> SIDNEY FARBER (1903–73) IN 1970

more than 70 per cent of all cancer deaths now occur in low- and middle-income countries where resources available for prevention, diagnosis and treatment are limited or virtually non-existent. As the WHO reminds us, *'Cancer is a global problem, and it's growing'*. There is, however, great hope that cancer-prevention strategies, early diagnosis and more effective therapies will provide a way forward.

HEART DISEASE is the term applied to a

diverse range of problems affecting the heart and its related blood vessels. Coronary heart disease, congenital heart disease, rheumatic heart disease, aortic aneurysm, angina and arrhythmia are among the commonest conditions – each of which may have different underlying causes, symptoms, prognoses and outcomes. Heart disease has become increasingly prevalent over the past century and is the single biggest cause of death in Western countries today. Although major advances have been made to prevent and repair or even replace an ailing heart over the last 50 years or so, heart disease, together with stroke (the two are collectively known as cardiovascular disease), account for 17 million deaths globally each year and are now also a serious problem for developing countries.

The beating of the heart is a fundamental sign of life. A baby's heart starts to beat in the uterus usually a month after conception. The heart beats about once a second for our entire lives, without taking a single rest. Over the course of 70 years it will beat over 2 billion times. When the heartbeat stops, unless reversed within a very few minutes, life comes to an end.

The heart has played a key role in shaping our understanding of the vital physiological forces of the human body and has also, metaphorically, been a central concept in an understanding of our emotions. Indeed, prior to the 20th century, more emphasis was given to the cultural, philosophical and scientific ideas concerning the role of the heart than to the incidence of heart disease itself. It is only in the last century or so that death or disease associated with a malfunctioning heart has become a critical issue, and it is only in the very recent past that major advances have been made to prevent and repair this vital organ when it goes wrong.

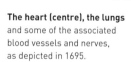

The heart (centre), the lungs and some of the associated blood vessels and nerves, as depicted in 1695.

timeline

2nd century AD *The Greek physician Galen (AD 129–c.210) puts forward a number of theories about the anatomy of the body (based on animal dissections), and the role of the heart, brain and blood.*

c.1000 *An Old English manuscript describes remedies for 'heartache', lung disease, tumours and liver disease. For heartache the patient is advised to take 17 different herbs, 'pound them all together; make an ale, and* drink it when you have need'.

Late 15th century *Leonardo da Vinci (1452–1519) observes that the 'vessels in the elderly, through the thickening of the tunics, restrict the transit of the blood' – an early* description of what we would now call 'arteriosclerosis. He produces beautiful and remarkably accurate drawings of the heart, based on post-mortem dissections of animal and human cadavers.*

1628 *The English physician William Harvey (1578–1657) proposes that the heart is a pump that circulates the blood around the body. Harvey's views on blood circulation are generally accept-ed by the 1660s. His* account of the movement of the heart as a 'living pump' remains controversial until the 19th century.*

1761 *The Austrian physician Joseph Auenbrugger (1722–1809) describes percussion, a* method of tapping lightly on the chest to discover pathological changes in the heart.*

1768 *The English physician William Heberden (1710–1801) describes 'angina pectoris' and differentiates it from other*

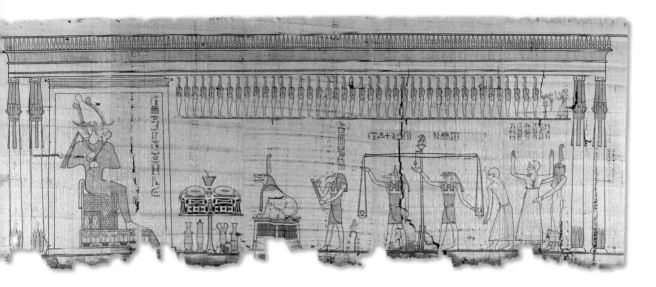

THE HEART OF THE MATTER

In ancient times, the heart, brain and liver were ascribed varying degrees of importance, which differed from culture to culture. The Babylonians considered the liver to be the seat and mirror of the soul, while for the ancient Egyptians the heart was the source of wisdom, the emotions, memory and personality. When Egyptian embalmers mummified their dead, major internal organs – the liver, the intestines, lungs and stomach – were removed, dried, wrapped in linen and placed in special containers known as canopic jars to be buried alongside the mummified corpse. The brain was considered to be unimportant – its only function was to pass mucus to the nose. It was removed from the skull through the nose using long hooked tools, and probably thrown away. The heart was given special significance. It was generally left in the body and would, in the afterlife, be weighed against the feather of truth in the hall of Ma'at during the divine judgement of the deceased. An unburdened heart would balance with the feather and enjoy eternal life. To help the heart on its voyage to the afterlife, a heart scarab or amulet, with an inscription from *The Book of the Dead*, would be placed on the chest of the mummy.

An illustration from an ancient Egyptian papyrus of *The Book of the Dead*, depicting the weighing of the heart of the deceased in the Egyptian afterlife.

chest pains.
1785 *The English physician William Withering (1741–99) recommends digitalis (from foxglove) for 'dropsy of the heart' (congestive heart failure).*

1816 *The French physician René Laënnec (1781–1826) invents the stethoscope, which is used to investigate heart sounds and murmurs.*

1902 *Willem Einthoven (1860–1927) of the Netherlands develops the electro-cardiograph for diagnosing abnormal cardiac rhythms.*

1908 *The Scottish physician James Mackenzie (1853–1925), along with others including French physiologist and founding father of cinematographic techniques, Étienne-Jules Marey (1830–1904), pioneers the use of the* polygraph for recording the pulse and its relationship to cardiovascular disease.

1911–12 *British physician Thomas Lewis (1881–1945) is first to master the use of the electrocardiograph and to use it as a* diagnostic tool to measure the heart's disturbances.

1912 *James Herrick (1861–1954), the American cardiologist, describes heart disease resulting from hardening of the arteries, and* later shows the value of the electro-cardio-graph for diagnosing myocardial infarction.

(continued ...)

BLOOD TRANSFUSIONS

For centuries doctors had been taking blood out of their patients, supposedly to cure them (a custom known as blood-letting). In the 1660s, scientists at the Royal Society of London looked at ways of putting blood back into people (blood transfusions).

In 1669 Richard Lower (1631–91) wrote his *Tractatus de Corde* (Treatise on the Heart). In 1666 he had begun experiments transfusing blood between dogs. At a meeting of the Royal Society of London in 1667 (witnessed by Samuel Pepys) he also transfused blood from a sheep into a *'poor and debauched man … cracked a little in the head'* that it might *'have a good effect upon him as a frantic man by cooling his blood'*. The recipient, Arthur Coga, survived but further experiments in France to carry out blood transfusions from animals to humans led to the death of one subject, setting back blood transfusion for another 150 years.

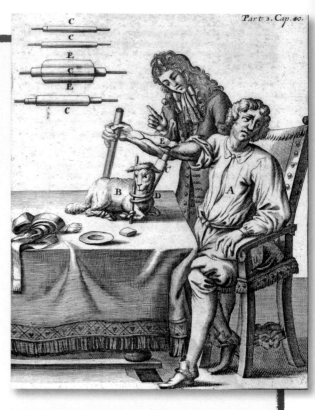

An early depiction of a blood transfusion, in which blood is passing from a lamb to a human.

The classical Greeks and Romans generally prohibited dissection of the human body, so their ideas about human anatomy and physiology were largely speculative, or based on animal dissection. Like the ancient Egyptians, the majority, including the philosopher Aristotle (384–322 BC), believed that the brain had no psychological significance, while it was the heart that was the primary source of intelligence, emotions and sensations. Expressions that are still with us today – 'heartbroken', 'disheartened', 'sweetheart', 'heart-to-heart', 'heartfelt', 'hard-hearted' and 'from the bottom of my heart' – all reflect the close link that was assumed to exist between emotions and the heart.

The Greek philosopher Plato (427–*c*.348/7 BC) challenged the 'cardio-centric' view. He favoured a tripartite explanation of the soul and the body in which parts of the soul – mind, spirit and desire – were located respectively in the brain, heart and liver. The Greek-Roman physician Galen (AD 129–*c*.210) reinforced Plato's view that the heart had no cognitive significance and that it was the brain that was the centre of sensation, speech, intellect and consciousness. Galen also explained how to take the pulse, how to classify its rhythm and differentiate between abnormalities – whether it was languid, racing, regular or erratic. In other parts of the ancient world, physicians would feel the pulse with the finger and often remark on the regularity or abnormality of the pulse in a sick patient. It was, however, many centuries before it was fully understood that the arterial pulse was the product of the impulse of the heart, and it is difficult to gauge to what extent heart disease or heart failure affected the populations of the ancient world.

BLOOD AND GUTS

While the ancient writers debated whether the brain or the heart was the fundamental core of the individual, most acknowledged that blood was the 'liquid' or, indeed, the 'very essence' of life, nourishing the body in health or causing disease when disordered, in excess or 'bad'. Galen, furthermore, proposed an influential theory on the movement of the blood through the body. He held that the veins, which carried the 'venous blood', originated in the liver. Dark blood was 'cooked' or 'concocted' in the liver and supplied with nutrients from the intestines; it then flowed through the veins carrying nourishment and was 'consumed' (used up) in various parts of the body. Venous blood also reached the lungs and the right ventricle of the heart, where it was imbued with 'vital spirits'. 'Arterial' or red blood stemmed from the left ventricle of the heart, flowing

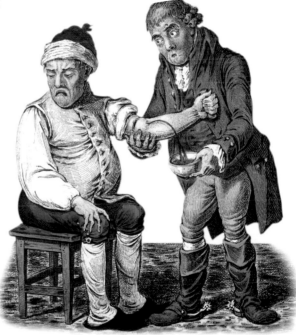

Blood-letting, depicted in 1804. The discovery of the circulation of the blood actually increased the popularity of blood letting. The practice was used on the sick (to get rid of 'bad' blood) as well as on the healthy (mostly as an annual 'spring-cleaning' venture). The task was often carried out by barber-surgeons; the red-and-white striped poles still seen outside many barbers' shops are a reminder of the service they once provided.

Town, South Africa.

Argentinian surgeon Rene Favaloro (1923–2000) performs a coronary bypass operation at the Cleveland Clinic, USA.

1968 American surgeon Norman Shumway (1923–2006) is first to carry out an open-heart transplant operation in the USA. The recipient dies 14 days later. Shumway and colleagues go on to find ways of preventing

transplant rejection, leading to the advent of cyclosporin.

1970s Heart transplantation leads to a change in the legal definition of death in various countries, from cessation of

heartbeat to the absence of brain function, enabling surgeons to remove a donor heart before it stops beating.

1980s Introduction of cyclosporin, an immuno-suppressive drug

that prevents transplant rejection.

1995 Pioneering heart surgeon Sir Magdi Yacoub (b.1935) sets up a British component to the French 'Chain of Hope' charity (begun in 1992) which sends

medical teams to the developing world to treat children suffering from heart disease, free of charge.

2000 First World Heart Day, now a global event.

2004 The World Health Organization (WHO) publishes The Atlas of Heart Disease and Stroke, 'graphically detailing a global epidemic that is the single leading cause of death worldwide'.

A Fit of Anger

Galenic theory held that anger was the result of a rush of choler, or bile, to the heart. Centuries later, the Scottish surgeon John Hunter (1728–93), who described disorders of the coronary arteries, declared, after performing an autopsy on a person who had died *'in a sudden and violent transport of anger: "My life is in the hands of any rascal who chooses to annoy me"'*. His words proved true. In 1793, he collapsed and died of a ruptured aortic aneurysm soon after a violent argument with a hospital colleague.

through the arteries to give 'life and motion', but did not return to the heart. It was the arteries, and not the heart which, according to Galen, propelled the blood around the body.

There was, though, a missing piece in this theory: how did the blood flow from the right to the left ventricle of the heart - from the veins to the arteries? Galenic theory suggested that there were 'invisible' pores that allowed the blood to seep across the septum (wall) of the heart (in fact it is quite solid). Galen's ideas about the heart and the circulation of the blood persisted for nearly a millennium and a half.

THE HEART — A LIVING PUMP

It was not until human anatomy began to be practised in Europe from the 14th century that the old Galenic theories were questioned and new discoveries were made about the human body. In 1628, the English physician William Harvey (1578-1657), by observation and experiment, proved conclusively that the blood continuously circulates through the body. He demonstrated that the blood, rather than simply flowing outward from the heart and liver to the extremities to be consumed and then somehow 'regenerated', actually remains constant in volume. It circulates through the veins and arteries, continuously returning to the heart. Dark venous blood flows towards the right ventricle of the heart and bright red arterial blood flows away from the left ventricle of the heart. The blood passes through the lungs (rather than 'invisible pores' in the septum as Galen had speculated) in its passage between the right and left ventricle of the heart. The heart, Harvey recognized, acts as a pump, keeping the blood circulating. It was, he said, the *'foundation of all life, and author of all'*.

'All things do depend upon the motional pulsation of the heart: so the heart is the beginning of life … by whose virtue, and pulsation, the blood is mov'd, perfected, made vegetable, and is defended from corruption, and mattering; and this familiar household-god doth his duty to the whole body, by nourishing, cherishing, and vegetating, being the foundation of all life, and author of all.'

WILLIAM HARVEY, *EXERCITATIO ANATOMICA DE MOTU CORDIS ET SANGUINIS IN ANIMALIBUS* (1628)

Other scientists of the time added further insights into Harvey's theory of the circulation of the blood. But, as exciting and revolutionary as these ideas were - and initiating the beginnings of modern scientific medicine - they made little impact on either the diagnosis or the treatment of human heart disease.

DYING OF A BROKEN HEART

On 18 January 1796 a young servant girl in Southeast England dropped down dead while reading a letter. She had apparently

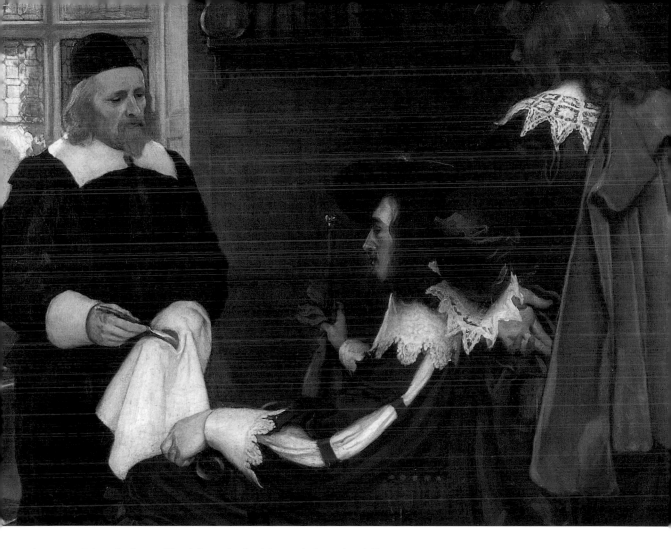

English physician William Harvey proposed in 1628 that the heart was a 'living pump', keeping the blood circulating around the body. He is shown here demonstrating his theory of the circulation of the blood to the monarch, Charles I.

discovered that the love of her life – who had formerly been her fellow servant – had married another. Her story was reported in the *Gentleman's Magazine*. The poor young woman had tragically 'died of a broken heart'.

Descriptions of diseases and causes of death in the 17th, 18th and 19th centuries – whether in journals, mortality records, doctors' case books, or diaries and letters – contain many 'diagnoses' that might suggest a heart problem.

Some, like the servant girl, were said to have died 'heartbroken' or from a 'broken heart'. Others were said to have died 'sad', 'weak', 'infirm', or suffering from an 'oppression of the spirits', a 'pining sickness' or an 'iliac passion'. Some died 'suddenly' or 'untimely', while others were 'planet-struck', inflicted by the 'visitation of God' or 'the work of the Devil'. Some died simply because they were 'worn out', 'frenzied', 'distracted' and 'short of breath', or declined through 'exhaustion', 'grief' or 'old age'. 'Decay' or being 'bedridden' were typically given as causes of death for the elderly. How many such sudden or slow deaths were related to heart disease is impossible to tell.

RECOGNIZING AND TREATING SYMPTOMS OF THE HEART

One of the first clear descriptions that we can now recognize as a heart-related condition was by the English physician, William Heberden (1710–1801). In 1768, he coined the term 'angina pectoris' and differentiated it from other pains in the chest:

'They who are afflicted with it, are seized while they are walking, (more especially if it be uphill, and soon after eating) with a most disagreeable sensation in the breast, which seems as if it would extinguish life, if it were to increase or continue; but the moment they stand still, all the uneasiness vanishes … In all other respects, patients are, at the beginning of the disorder, perfectly well … Males are most liable to this disease, especially such as have passed their fiftieth year.'

Another recognized condition was dropsy. Dropsy may have included those suffering from congestive heart disease. The discovery of digitalis as a remedy for 'dropsy of the heart' in the 18th century was one of the first drugs of value for treating heart conditions (see Beating the Heart: Blockbusters & Clot Busters, right).

PREVENTION IS BETTER THAN CURE

While there were a few specific recognizable clinical descriptions of heart disease prior to the 20th century, there was no shortage of possible 'predisposing' causes of disease and death (which, today, might be known as risk factors). It was frequently noted that *'gross'* individuals of *'corpulent living, ruddy complexion, hard drinking and overindulgence'* ran a high risk of disease and death, as did those who had *'a want of fresh fruit and greens and the disadvantages of a low diet'*. George Cheyne (1671–1743), the foremost British physician of his day, spent much of his time eating and drinking with his patients – at one point he weighed 32 stone (448 lb or 204 kg) and feeling *'excessively fat, short-breath'd, lethargic and listless'*, required a servant to walk behind him carrying a stool on which to recover every few paces. He eventually converted to vegetarianism and took to exercise and fresh air, vigorously riding a chamber horse when bad weather prevented outdoor exercise.

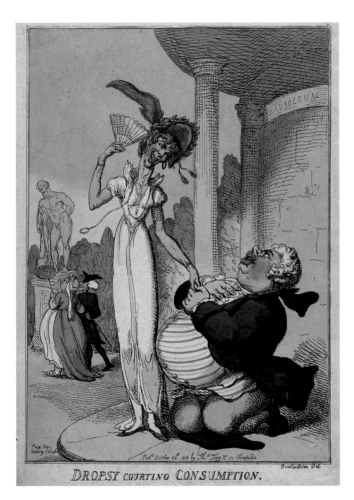

DROPSY COURTING CONSUMPTION.

An obese man woos a tall, lean woman outside a mausoleum, in this coloured etching from 1810. The illustration represents the ailments dropsy and consumption.

Advice manuals on preventing disease and maintaining a healthy constitution (ideas dating back to ancient times) became increasingly popular in the early modern period. Recommendations included a good diet, lots of physical exercise,

BEATING THE HEART: BLOCKBUSTERS & CLOT BUSTERS

One puzzling medical term, much used in the past but now obsolete, is 'dropsy'. The word literally means an excess of fluid, and may have been applied to a number of diseases in which an abnormal accumulation of fluid in the liver or heart could lead to death. One remarkable cure for 'dropsy of the heart' was discovered and promoted in the 18th century. William Withering (1741–99), a doctor practising in Birmingham, England, was given a recipe for treating dropsy by an old lady. The recipe contained a concoction of different plants, but Withering worked out that the vital ingredient was the purple foxglove (*Digitalis purpurea*) which, if used carefully and in small doses (for it is extremely toxic), can act as a powerful stimulant on the heart, as well as increasing urine flow and reducing oedema (pathological accumulation of fluid in the tissues).

When Withering died in 1799, his friends carved a bunch of foxgloves on his memorial. Digitoxin and digoxin – the active substances of the purple foxglove – are still used today to improve the speed and force of cardiac contractions.

An even older herbal treatment, derived from the bark and leaves of the willow tree, is also still used to treat heart disease, albeit in a synthetic form. The Roman encyclopedist Aulus Cornelius Celsus (25 BC–AD 50) described the benefits of *'boiled vinegar extracts of willow leaves for the relief of pain'*. In 1763 the Reverend Edward Stone (1700–68) of Chipping Norton, England, reported on the value of willow bark, which *'delights in moist or wet soil'*, to cure 'agues' (fevers) – then common in damp and marshy areas. In 1899 the pharmaceutical company Bayer patented 'Aspirin' (acetylsalicylic acid), a synthetic drug based on the active compounds found in willow bark. Bayer advertised Aspirin's safety by saying that the drug *'does not affect the heart'*. A century later, the benefits of low doses of aspirin (under medical supervision) to reduce blood clots and the risk of stroke, heart disease and death following a heart attack were recognized by medical science.

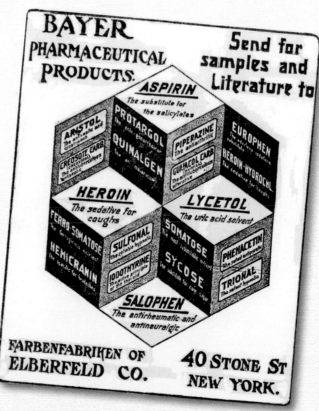

An early advertisement from the Bayer pharmaceutical company offers products including both aspirin and heroin.

moderate alcohol consumption and a balanced lifestyle. In 1763 James Boswell (1740–95), the biographer of Dr Johnson, was advised by his physician to take two or three brisk capers around the room upon waking. Boswell said this had the '*most agreeable effects*' and '*expelled the phlegm from my heart*'.

DETECTING ABNORMALITIES OF THE HEART

The practice of 'taking the pulse', as well as auscultation (the act of listening to the sounds generated within the body) and 'succussion' (shaking a patient to hear splashing noises within the chest) dated back to ancient times. 'Percussion' – tapping the chest wall with a finger and listening with the ear for reverberations – was described in the mid-18th century. The invention of the stethoscope in 1816 by René Laënnec (1781–1826) (see page 67) transformed the way physicians could 'hear' and detect heart abnormalities and valvular disorders.

A heart surgeon, photographed in 1956, makes adjustments to an improved version of his artificial heart–lung machine. This pioneering device enabled the functions of the heart and lungs to be maintained while the patient's own heart was stopped during surgical procedures.

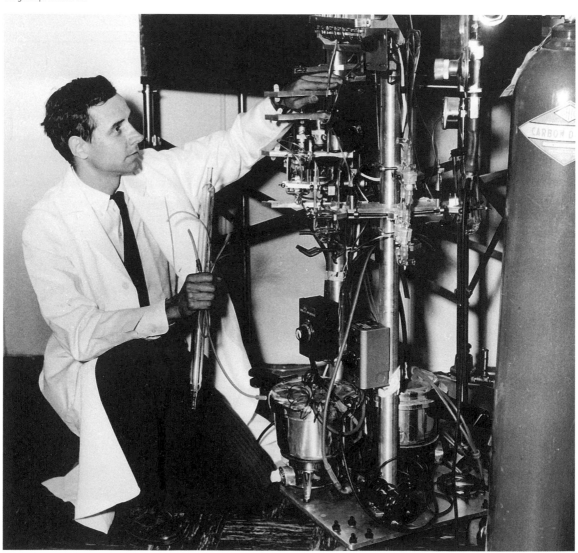

However, more sophisticated tools were needed, and in the second half of the 19th century attempts were made to obtain a graphical record of the heart's action, culminating in 1908 with the polygraph machine pioneered by James Mackenzie (1853–1925), a Scottish physician, for recording the pulse and its relationship to heart disease. In the early 20th century another new technique of measuring and recording the electrical signals generated by the heart's beat was developed – the electrocardiogram (which became known as ECG, or EKG in the USA). This transformed diagnosis and so began the scientific field of 'cardiology'.

A CHANGE OF HEART

The first formal use of the term 'heart attack', which accounts for a high proportion of all deaths from coronary heart disease, was not until the early 20th century. Heart attacks occur when one of the blood vessels to the heart becomes entirely blocked by a blood clot, whilst arteriosclerosis results from the narrowing of the arteries caused by deposits of fats and other substances. The risk of dying from a heart attack became increasingly apparent during the first half of the 20th century. In 1892 the Canadian physician William Osler (1849–1919) had described coronary heart disease as *relatively rare*. By the 1920s, however, one in eight deaths in the Western world was attributed to heart disorders.

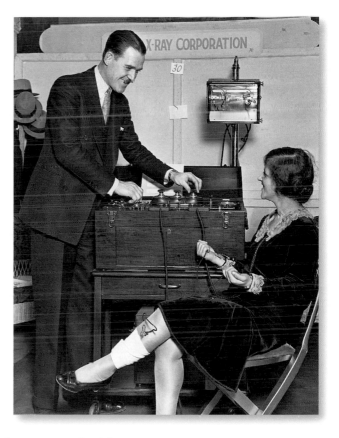

An electrocardiograph from the late 1920s. This device measures the electrical signals generated by the heart's beat, which are then reproduced visually in the form of an electrocardiogram. The electrocardiograph was initially an unwieldy contraption – needing five technicians to operate it – in which the patient had to place both hands and feet in buckets of water.

There had been huge improvements in surgery over the second half of the 19th century, following the introduction of anaesthetics, antiseptics and asepsis (see pages 76–79), but the heart had remained a no-go area. It was deemed just too risky to try to operate on the heart – although one or two brave surgeons did try to correct some cardiac defects.

In the 1940s, cardiac surgeons began to attempt bolder surgery of the heart and in 1944 the first surgical intervention for 'blue babies' (those born with congenital heart disease) took place. Fast procedures, surgeons showed, could be performed on a beating heart, but more complicated procedures required the heart to be stopped. The key innovation was the heart–lung machine, used in routine surgery from the late 1950s. This technology, along with body-cooling techniques (hypothermia), enabled surgeons to 'bypass' the heart, maintaining circulation and respiration artificially while surgery was conducted on the stopped organ.

The greatest publicity coup for cardiac surgery came in 1967 when Christiaan Barnard (1922–2001) in Cape Town, South Africa, performed the first human heart transplant. Barnard sewed the heart of a young woman, who had died

MAKING SENSE OF DISEASE IN THE PAST

Doctors in the past mostly had to rely on their five senses – touch, sight, smell, taste and hearing – to detect and diagnose outward signs of disease in the 'living' patient.

TOUCH: Feeling the pulse with the finger dates back to ancient times, and physicians would often remark on the regularity or abnormality of the pulse in a sick patient. Taking the pulse remains a hallmark of the medical profession. Touching the forehead (prior to the use of the clinical thermometer in 1714) was, and is still, used to detect fever. Finding out where it hurts and feeling for lumps and bumps were, and still are, classic ways of spotting abnormalities. But too much touching was often considered indelicate, and feeling beneath the clothes seemed undignified for a genteel physician.

SIGHT: Doctors have always needed a keen eye to spot and diagnose peculiarities – from rashes, blotches, pimples, pustules, running sores, ulcers, fleshy growths and changes in skin colour, urine and stools, to tell-tale signs of infection on the tongue, in the throat, eyes, ears, nose, or discharges from orifices of the body. *You look ill* remains a common phrase.

SMELL: One of the standard ways of checking for disease in the past was to sniff the patients' urine, stools, pus, perspiration or breath. Bad odours, fetid breath, pus-filled gangrenous sores, stinky stools, and other nauseous evacuations were key indicators that all was not well, and doctors' case notes usually contained detailed descriptions of their patients' smells. The smell of freshly baked bread from the skin or breath was supposedly indicative of typhoid; the smell of sweaty sheep was associated with smallpox; the odour of plucked feathers was linked with measles; while yellow fever patients supposedly smelled like a butcher's shop.

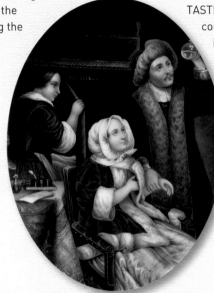

Examining a patient's urine has long been one of the physician's methods of detecting illness.

TASTE: Tasting urine was not as common as gazing at or sniffing it, but in 1776 Matthew Dobson (1735–84) demonstrated that the sweetness of the urine in patients with diabetes was due to sugar.

HEARING: Listening to the gurgles, coughing, creaking and croaking of the body were useful indicators for doctors. Auscultation – or the act of listening to sounds generated within the body – dates back to ancient times. Hippocratic writings describe 'succussion' – shaking a patient to hear splashing noises within the chest. Percussion – tapping the chest wall with a finger and listening with the ear for reverberations – was described in the mid-18th century. The invention of the stethoscope in 1816 transformed the way 'bedside' physicians detected abnormalities of the heart and chest and meant the physician could 'hear' what was going on inside while keeping a safe distance from the patient. Listening to the patient's own story – where it hurts – was, as it is today, a vital part of diagnosing disease.

in a car crash, into a recipient, Louis Washkansky. Washkansky died of pneumonia 18 days later, and the operation caused both sensation and controversy.

With the development of effective immunosuppressive drugs (following the use of cyclosporin) to prevent transplant rejection, heart transplants became routine. By the mid-1980s hundreds of heart transplants were being conducted, with many of the recipients surviving for over five years. As with other organ transplants, finding sufficient suitable donors continues to be a problem. Today around 3000 heart transplants are performed worldwide each year.

MENDING BROKEN HEARTS

Over the course of the past 50 or so years, a wide range of other techniques have been introduced, enabling surgeons to repair faulty hearts before a

'Louis Washkansky's heart came into full view – rolling in a rhythm of its own like a separate and angry sea, yellow from the storms of half a century, yet streaked with blue currents flowing from its depths – blue veins drifting across the heaving waste and ruin of a ravaged heart.'

CHRISTIAAN BARNARD DESCRIBES THE DISEASED HEART OF THE FIRST RECIPIENT OF A HUMAN HEART TRANSPLANT IN 1967

Members of Dr Christiaan Barnard's surgical team perform open-heart surgery in the theatre at Groote Schuur Hospital made famous by the 1967 Washkansky heart transplant operation.

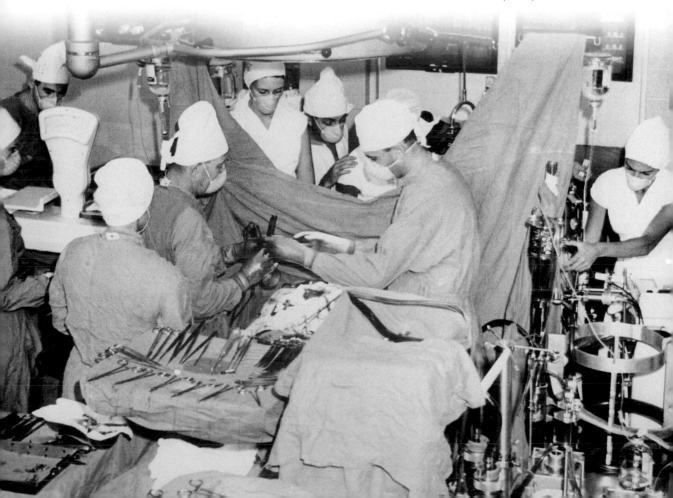

transplant becomes necessary. These techniques include the insertion of artificial pacemakers or defibrillators (electrical devices that maintain or restore regular heartbeat), balloon angioplasty (where a small balloon-like device is threaded through an artery to open the blockage), coronary bypasses, valve repair and replacement, and patch repair for congenital holes in the heart. New and non-invasive imaging methods – from ultrasound to CT and MRI scans – have also transformed the early diagnosis of heart disease.

In 1896 the British surgeon, Sir Stephen Paget (1855–1926), had written:
'Surgery of the heart has probably reached the limits set by Nature to all surgery; no new method, and no new discovery, can overcome the natural difficulties that attend a wound of the heart.'

Paget and others of his time would be amazed to see the sophisticated (and extremely expensive) state of the art equipment that now makes it possible to overcome *'the limits set by nature'*. A damaged or failing heart is no longer the death sentence it once used to be.

HEART-BREAKING FACTS

Some alarming statistics demonstrate the potency of cardiovascular disease (heart disease and stroke).

• Heart disease, together with stroke (caused by an interruption of blood supply to the brain either due to a blood clot in an artery or a burst blood vessel in the brain), is the leading single cause of death worldwide.

• There are 17.5 million deaths per year from cardiovascular disease – almost one-third of all deaths globally.

• Despite improvements in survival rates, in the USA, 1 in 4 men and 1 in 3 women still die within a year of a heart attack.

• 80 per cent of the global burden of heart disease is, today, in low- and middle-income countries. The double burden of infections and nutritional disorders plus chronic diseases, such as heart disease, cancer and diabetes, is of serious concern for the developing world.

• In the USA, about 652,000 people currently die each year from heart disease – 27 per cent of total deaths. In the UK, 120,000 people die from heart disease each year and in India in 2002 over 1.5 million deaths were attributed to heart disease, with a further 770,000 dying from stroke and 103,000 from rheumatic heart disease.

• In the UK, every two to three minutes someone has a heart attack.

• 12 million people are affected by rheumatic fever, which can lead to rheumatic heart disease.

• In 1900, only 1 per cent of the global population was over the age of 65 years; it is predicted that by the year 2050, some 20 per cent of the world's population will be aged 65 years and over – heart disease and cancer are predominantly, though not exclusively, diseases of the older age groups.

• Unless current trends are halted or reversed, it is estimated that over a billion people will die from heart disease and stroke in the first half of the 21st century.

TAKING ADVICE TO HEART

While surgical techniques have advanced dramatically in recent decades, there has also been a growing interest in understanding the underlying causes and possible ways of preventing heart disease. By the 1940s heart disease was the leading killer in the USA, raising many questions as to why it had reached such epidemic proportions. An important study – set up in the late 1940s in Framingham, Massachusetts – began to trace the lives of an initial cohort of 5209 healthy adult residents and examine them every two years. This and similar studies have highlighted significant risk factors for heart disease, including smoking, lack of physical exercise, diets rich in saturated fat and/or salt, heavy alcohol consumption, stress, obesity, type-2 diabetes, high blood pressure (hypertension) and high cholesterol levels.

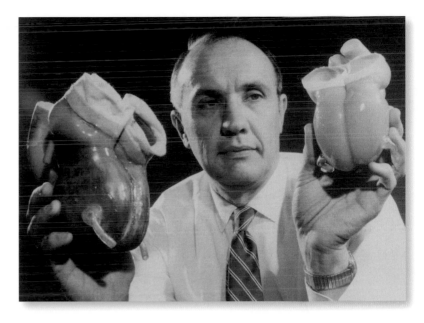

By 1968, an artificial mechanical heart (on the right) was small enough to be enclosed completely within the body – an earlier, larger, version is seen on the left. The human heart is composed of cardiac muscle – the strongest muscle in the body. It contracts rhythmically, under the control of the autonomic nervous system, pumping blood around the body. Unlike 'love hearts', a real heart is asymmetrical in shape.

The media and health-education campaigns now constantly remind people of the importance of adopting a healthy lifestyle to reduce the risk of heart disease or stroke, while a range of drugs is available for those identified to be at risk or to prevent fatalities from heart attacks (see Beating the Heart: Blockbusters & Clot Busters, page 241). Genetic susceptibility to heart disease also clearly plays a role, and scientists are hunting for the genes that might be linked to increased risk.

Rates of mortality from heart disease have fallen in a number of countries in recent years – for instance, by over 40 per cent in the past three decades in the USA, the UK, Australia, Canada and Japan – in part as a result of medical therapies and advances in life-saving interventions and in part as a result of reductions in major risk factors and taking advice on heart disease prevention. Nevertheless, cardiovascular disease remains the leading global cause of death and is now a serious problem in developing countries, where high-tech life-saving equipment is often beyond reach, and prevention and screening strategies are poorly established. Moreover, while heart disease is generally seen as a chronic non-communicable disease in the Western world, in developing countries infectious diseases such as rheumatic fever (a streptococcal infection) and Chagas' disease in South America (a parasitic disease; see pages 102–7) can lead to heart disease in both children and adults. '*Prevention is better than cure*' is an old saying, but in the case of heart disease it remains an important global message.

'All motions of sensation, including those produced by what is pleasant and painful, begin and end in the heart.'

ARISTOTLE, *PARTS OF ANIMALS* (FOURTH CENTURY BC)

GLOSSARY

Words in SMALL CAPITALS can be looked up elsewhere in the Glossary.

acute refers to symptoms or illnesses which are severe and intense for a short duration.

anaemia ('without blood') the medical condition anaemia can be caused by a diet low in iron, or may be triggered by parasites.

antibiotic a general term for a range of drugs, including penicillin, that are effective in treating BACTERIAL infections.

anti-contagionist a term used in the 19th century to describe a scientist or physician who did not believe that diseases were caused by CONTAGIOUS particles spread from person to person.

bacterial *See* bacterium.

bacterium (pl. bacteria) a group of single-celled microscopic organisms found everywhere in the environment and in the human body. Bacteria can live harmlessly in the human body but some may also cause serious infections, including plague, cholera and tuberculosis.

bejel a non-venereal form of syphilis, commonly a DISEASE of children, transmitted by close contact, occurring in the arid regions of North Africa, the Middle East and the eastern Mediterranean.

botulism first used in the 19th century to describe a DISEASE thought to be caused by eating contaminated sausage. It is now known to be caused by toxins produced from BACTERIA; although relatively rare, it can be fatal.

bronchitis an inflammation of the bronchi (the airways that connect the trachea, or windpipe, to the lungs) which results in a severe cough.

bubo a swelling in the groin which became a hallmark of bubonic plague.

chronic often used to refer to DISEASES that are protracted, persistent or recurring over time.

contagious a contagious DISEASE is one that might be transmitted by close touch or contact with an infected person.

diphtheria a severe and highly CONTAGIOUS BACTERIAL DISEASE, usually in children, that attacks the throat and nose.

disease (literally 'dis-ease' or absence of 'ease') the opposite of good health. In practice, the term is applied to any sickness, ailment or departure from sound health.

dropsy a condition that causes swelling in body tissues due to an accumulation of excess fluid.

dysentery a BACTERIAL or amoebic infection causing severe pain, usually accompanied by diarrhoea containing blood and mucus.

endemic a DISEASE that is not necessarily widely prevalent but typically found and always present among people of a particular place.

epidemic a DISEASE that affects a large number of people at a given time.

epidemiology the study of EPIDEMICS or DISEASES affecting groups of people.

febrile with fever.

germ theory a term often used to describe the theory developed in the mid- to late 19th century that DISEASES are caused by specific micro-organisms.

goitre a condition that gives rise to a swelling in the neck due to an enlarged thyroid gland, which may be caused by a number of factors, including iodine deficiency.

haemophilia an inherited bleeding disorder caused by a deficiency of a particular blood protein, known as Factor V111, which is essential to the process of blood clotting.

haemorrhage (adj. haemorrhagic; haemorrhaging) bleeding or blood loss. Haemorrhagic fevers typically cause bleeding internally (where blood leaks from blood vessels inside the body) and externally (from mouth and other orifices).

immunology the study of the immune system which plays a vital role in the outcome of DISEASE in an individual.

inoculation a term used initially for the practice of inserting matter from dried smallpox scabs into a person's body in the hope of providing long-term protection against the DISEASE; later superseded by VACCINATION.

in vitro the technique of performing an experiment in a controlled environment outside the living organism (e.g., in a test tube or other laboratory glassware).

Lassa fever an ACUTE viral HAEMORRHAGIC fever named after the town of Lassa in Nigeria, where a missionary nurse died from the DISEASE in 1969.

latent (n. latency) describes a period between initial infection and the time when the symptoms of a DISEASE become fully manifest.

Legionnaires' disease a pneumonia-like BACTERIAL DISEASE which was first recognized among delegates to an American Legion convention in Philadelphia in 1976.

Lyme disease a BACTERIAL DISEASE transmitted by infected ticks and named after the first recognized cluster of cases in Old Lyme, Connecticut, USA in 1975.

malignant (meaning 'born to be bad') most commonly used to refer to cancerous tumours that are likely to be serious or may spread and recur.

Marburg fever or Marburg HAEMORRHAGIC fever; a rare but potentially fatal viral infection named after the town of Marburg in Germany where the first cases occurred in 1967 in laboratories handling infected monkeys.

miasmatist a 19th-century term referring to a scientist who believed that DISEASES were caused by 'miasmas' or noxious vapours.

mumps a viral DISEASE, usually in children, causing swelling of certain glands, especially in the area between the ear and jaw.

palaeopathology the scientific study to detect signs of ancient DISEASES, most often from skeletal remains.

pandemic used to describe a DISEASE that is global, or that affects a significantly high proportion of people across the world.

Parkinson's disease a degenerative disorder of the central nervous system that often impairs the motor skills and speech. It is named after the British physician James Parkinson (1755–1824), who in 1822 described the condition as the 'shaking palsy'.

pasteurization a process of removing germs from liquids by heating, named after the French chemist Louis Pasteur (1822–95).

pestilence an EPIDEMIC of a serious DISEASE, typically infectious.

pinta a non-venereal form of syphilis which is transmitted by skin contact, often between children living in conditions of poor hygiene.

pneumonia a DISEASE of or pertaining to the lungs, often caused by BACTERIAL infections.

psychotic a psychotic episode usually refers to a profound mental aberration marked by loss of all sense of reality.

quarantine a term (meaning '40 days') first used by Italians to describe a period of isolation of individuals who had been exposed to an infectious DISEASE, with the aim of preventing its further spread.

relapsing fever a DISEASE transmitted by lice (louse-borne relapsing fever) or ticks (tick-borne relapsing fever).

rheumatic fever an inflammatory DISEASE which may develop after a streptococcal infection and can affect many parts of the body including the heart, nervous system, joints and skin. In the past it was a common cause of death in children and remains a leading cause of heart DISEASE in the developing world today.

rickets a DISEASE characterized by spinal deformity, twisting and bowing of legs, caused by a deficiency of vitamin D – which may be lacking in the diet – or inadequate exposure to sunlight.

rubella an infectious viral DISEASE, usually in children, known for its red rash. It is also called German measles, possibly because it was first described and identified by German physicians in the 18th and early 19th centuries.

sanatorium an institution or place of refuge for the care of people suffering from CHRONIC DISEASES such as tuberculosis.

scarlet fever a common BACTERIAL (streptococcal) DISEASE, especially in children, which is typified by a red rash and sore throat.

somnolent sleepy.

trachcostomy *See* trachcotomy.

tracheotomy a surgical procedure performed on the neck to open a direct airway through an incision in the trachea (windpipe).

tubercles various small anatomic lumps, including those which develop in the lungs as a result of infection by the *Mycobacterium tuberculosis* BACTERIUM.

vaccination *See* vaccine.

vaccine in the 19th century, the term vaccination was limited to the INOCULATION of a preparation derived from cowpox that protected people from smallpox. It was later extended more widely to describe similar measures taken to protect people against other DISEASES.

vector an intermediate 'vehicle', such as an animal, that is the carrier of an infectious DISEASE or an insect capable of transferring an infectious agent from one host to another.

virus a group of very small infective agents causing many DISEASES, including the common cold, influenza and AIDS.

WHO *See* World Health Organization.

whooping cough a highly CONTAGIOUS BACTERIAL DISEASE also known as pertussis, which is accompanied by a violent cough (that sounds like a 'whoop') and can be fatal.

World Health Organization established in 1948 with its headquarters in Geneva, Switzerland, the World Health Organization (the WHO) is a specialized agency of the United Nations (UN), acting as the directing and co-ordinating authority on international health.

yaws a BACTERIAL infection of the skin, bones and joints, related to the organism which causes syphilis.

INDEX

FURTHER READING

In condensing each of these rich and varied histories of 30 diseases into short chapters, I have had to generalize, simplify and touch only briefly on some of the continuing historical and academic debates. For those who want to explore the history of disease further there are many excellent sources in libraries and archives around the world, as well as on the World Wide Web. As a starting point, I would recommend any of the following reference works.

The Cambridge World History of Human Disease, edited by Kenneth Kiple (Cambridge University Press, 1993), is some 1000 pages in length and contains detailed descriptions of all the major human diseases. *The Encyclopedia of Plague and Pestilence from Ancient Times to the Present*, edited by George Childs Kohn (Checkmark Books, 2001), describes the major global epidemics. *The World Atlas of Epidemic Diseases* by Andrew Cliff, Peter Haggett and Matthew Smallman-Raynor (Arnold, 2004) is a mine of information and is illustrated with some excellent maps of the geographical distribution and spatial impact of epidemic diseases. The five-volume *Dictionary of Medical Biography*, edited by W.F. Bynum and Helen Bynum (Greenwood Press, 2007), is a valuable source of reference for discovering more about the world's greatest doctors and scientists. *Disease in the Modern World* by Mark Harrison (Polity, 2004) elegantly sets the history of disease within an international perspective. The two-volume *Encyclopedia of Plague, Pestilence and Pandemics* (Greenwood Press, 2008) contains in-depth entries from many of the world's most distinguished historians of medicine.

The Cambridge Illustrated History of Medicine, edited by Roy Porter (Cambridge University Press, 1996), *Western Medicine: an Illustrated History*, edited by Irvine Loudon (Oxford University Press, 1997) and *The Wellcome Trust Illustrated History of Tropical Diseases*, edited by Professor F. E.G. Cox (The Wellcome Trust, 1996), are all excellent books covering some of the broader aspects of the history of medicine. In addition, any of the numerous and stimulating books by the late Roy Porter, including *The Greatest Benefit to Mankind: a Medical History from Antiquity to the Present* (Harper Collins, 1997) and *Blood and Guts: a Short History of Medicine* (Penguin Books, 2002), are well worth reading. And for informative entertainment on this subject, the recent UK's BBC Radio 4 programme 'The Making of Modern Medicine' (available as BBC Audiobooks, 2007), written and narrated by Andrew Cunningham, is an enthralling six-hour listen.

For scientific and medical information on the current status of infectious diseases, the regularly updated *Control of Communicable Diseases Manual* (an official report of the American Public Health Association), edited by David Heymann, is a useful source, while the web site of the World Health Organization (www.who.int/) provides figures and facts on the incidence, prevalence and latest outbreaks of major diseases. I have used both these sources for estimates of the current global toll of each of the diseases.

There are many broad-ranging popular books on this subject, from Daniel Defoe's semi-fictional *A Journal of the Plague Year* (1722), Paul de Kruif's best-selling book *Microbe Hunters* (1926) and Hans Zinsser's classic study *Rats, Lice and History* (1935) to more recent compilations such as Kenneth Kiple's *Plague, Pox and Pestilence* (Weidenfeld & Nicholson, 1997), Laurie Garrett's *The Coming Plague – Newly Emerging Diseases in a World Out of Balance* (Penguin, 1994) and John Playfair's *Living with Germs – in Sickness and in Health* (Oxford University Press, 2004).

There are also many other fascinating books and articles which are too numerous to cite here but which are well worth discovering and reading.

Most of the research for this book has been carried out at the Wellcome Library for the History of Medicine in London, UK, which justly boasts that it is 'one of the most extraordinary libraries in the world' with a collection of over 2.5 million items on just about every possible aspect of medical history and spanning 3000 years. I wish I could have read them all!

AUTHOR ACKNOWLEDGEMENTS

I am indebted to my family, friends and many colleagues, students and scholars across the globe for sharing with me their ideas, knowledge and expertise over many years. I would particularly like to thank those who have so meticulously read, contributed to and commented on individual sections and chapters of this book at its various stages including Michael Alpers, Warwick Anderson, Virginia Berridge, Greg Bock, Linda Bryder, David Cantor, Andy Cliff, Frank Cooper, Frank Cox, Jacalyn Duffin, Peter Elwood, Myron Enchenberg, Tony Gould, Ian Glynn, Jenifer Glynn, Peter Haggett, Steven Hajdu, Anne Hardy, John Henderson, Rosemary Horrox, Margaret Humphreys, Kiheung Kim, Simone Kropf, David Lomas, Judith Lomas, Irvine Loudon, Maureen Malowany, John Manton, Malcolm Nicolson, Randall Packard, Steven Palmer, Janet Pickering, Carol Rawcliffe, Carole Reeves, Charlotte Roberts, John Skehel, Matthew Smallman-Raynor, Sue Smith, Patrick Wallis, Andrew Wear and Michael Worboys. Thank you for your generous input and your rapid responses which have been invaluable. If I have not been able to incorporate all your suggestions and changes – my apologies. And, of course, all remaining mistakes are mine alone.

My thanks, too, go to everyone at the Department of History and Philosophy of Science at the University of Cambridge, and the Wellcome Trust Centre for the History of Medicine at University College, London. These two academic departments, which are at the forefront of research into the history of medicine, have both generously appointed me as a Research Associate. St John's College, Cambridge, has also provided me with a stimulating intellectual environment while I have been working on this book. I am most grateful to the Author's Foundation of The Society of Authors which generously gave me a grant to enable me to conduct a number of aspects of the research for this book.

I would, moreover, very much like to thank the people who have worked so tirelessly and patiently with me to bring this book to fruition: Richard Milbank, the Publishing Director for non-fiction of Quercus Publishing, who has played a major role throughout; the team at BCS Publishing for the production of the book, including Ian Crofton who took on the onerous task of copy editing my script, Derek Hall and Virginia Carter for their final editing and captioning, Steve McCurdy and Martin Anderson for their help with the design and picture selection, Graham Bateman for his day-to-day management of the project, and Anna Smith of the Wellcome Trust Medical Photographic Library, who provided a rich source of ideas for the illustrations. Richard, Graham, Ian and the rest of the team, your input at the planning and production stages of this book has been terrific. Thank you all.

My sincerest thanks also go to two of my closest academic colleagues and friends – Anne Hardy and Maureen Malowany – who have encouraged me and contributed to this book in more ways than I could mention. Thank you both – you really have played a very special part in every aspect of this project.

Above all, I want to express my gratitude to my parents, the late Derek and Vera Schove, my sisters Ann and Hilary, my friend Roz and my mother-in-law Mabel, each of whom has given me so much help at various stages of my academic career. A special tribute goes to my husband Christopher (whose scientific knowledge, curiosity and insight are incredible and who, in spite of the many other demands on his time, read and gave constructive criticism on every single chapter) and to our sons Richard and William, who have been a fantastic support throughout this project and also kept me smiling. I dedicate this book to my family – I owe you all so much.

Mary Dobson

PICTURE
ACKNOWLEDGEMENTS

Wellcome Library, London
9; 10; 12; 15; 16; 17; 19; 20; 21; 22; 23; 25; 28; 29; 30;
33; 35; 36; 38; 39; 40; 43; 47; 48; 49; 50; 51; 52; 55;
57; 64; 65; 68; 73; 74; 77; 78; 79; 83; 84; 86; 88; 91;
96, 97 (top); 97 (centre); 98; 99; 102; 104; 108; 110;
111; 112; 113; 119; 120; 126 (top) Wellcome Images;
129; 133; 135; 136; 137; 138; 139; 146; 147; 149; 150
Audio Visual, LSHTM/Wellcome Images; 151; 153;
154; 157; 158; 159; 160; 161; 174; 175; 176; 179; 180;
193 Wellcome Library/John Wildgoose; 195; 198
Sasha Andrews/Wellcome Images; 209; 210; 211;
213; 214 (right) M.I. Walker/Wellcome Images; 217;
223; 225; 226; 232; 234; 236; 237; 239; 240; 244

Corbis
24 © Robert Holmes/Corbis; 26 © Bettmann/
Corbis; 41 © Hulton-Deutsch Collection/Corbis; 42
© Hulton-Deutsch Collection/Corbis; 45 © Stefano
Bianchetti/Corbis; 56 © Stapleton Collection/
Corbis; 58 © Hulton-Deutsch Collection/Corbis;
60 © Bettmann/Corbis; 61 © Hulton-Deutsch
Collection/Corbis; 63 © Corbis; 66 © Corbis; 67 ©
Bettmann/Corbis; 69 © Seattle Post-Intelligencer
Collection, Museum of History and Industry/
Corbis; 71 © Gideon Mendel/Corbis; 80 ©
Smithsonian Institution/Corbis; 82 © Jurgen Frank/
Corbis; 92 © Corbis; 93 © Nic Bothma/ epa/Corbis;
95 © Chris Hellier/Corbis; 101 © Robert Patrick/
Corbis Sygma; 103 © Hulton-Deutsch Collection/
Corbis; 105 © Balaguer Alejandro/Corbis Sygma;
107 © Balaguer Alejandro/Corbis Sygma; 114 ©
Gideon Mendel/ ActionAid/Corbis; 116 © Lloyd
Cluff/Corbis; 122 © Corbis; 125 © David Reed/
Corbis; 126 (bottom) © Bettmann/Corbis; 131
© Bettmann/Corbis; 141 © Nik Wheeler/Sygma/
Corbis; 142 © Corbis; 145 © Howard Davies/
Corbis; 155 © Karen Kasmauski/ Corbis; 163 ©
Bettmann/Corbis; 165 © Bettmann/ Corbis; 167 ©
Bettmann/Corbis; 168 © Bettmann/

Corbis; 169 © Bettmann/Corbis; 170 © Bettmann/
Corbis; 171 © Ramin Talaie/Corbis; 173 © Hulton-
Deutsch Collection/Corbis, 177 © Bettmann/
Corbis; 181 © Bettmann/Corbis; 182 © Nikola
Solic/Reuters/Corbis; 183 © Bogdan Cristel/
Reuters/Corbis; 185 © Gilbert Liz/Corbis Sygma;
186 © Charles O'Rear/Corbis; 188 © Corbis Sygma;
190 Patrick Robert/Sygma/Corbis; 191 Patrick
Robert/Sygma/Corbis; 196 © Karen Kasmauski/
Corbis; 200 © Gideon Mendel/Corbis; 202 ©
Reuters/Corbis; 203 © Reuters/Corbis; 204 © Byun
Young-Wook/epa/Corbis; 206 © Wang Bingyu/
EyePress/epa/Corbis; 214 (left) © Bettmann/
Corbis; 219 © Bettmann/Corbis; 220 © P.Ashton/
South West News Service/Corbis Sygma; 221 ©
McPherson Colin/Corbis Sygma; 227 © Bettmann/
Corbis; 228 © Bettmann/Corbis; 229 © Bettmann/
Corbis; 230 © Igor Kostin/Sigma/Corbis; 231
© Hulton-Deutsch Collection/Corbis; 235 ©
Sandro Vannini/Corbis; 241 © Bettmann/Corbis;
242 © Bettmann/Corbis; 243 © Underwood &
Underwood/Corbis; 245 © Bettmann/Corbis; 247
© Bettmann/Corbis

TopFoto.co.uk
37 © A World History Archive/TopFoto; 132
Corporation of London/HIP/TopFoto

Science Photo Library
121 David Scharf

Shutterstock
199

*Quercus Editions Ltd has made every effort to
trace copyright holders of the pictures used in
this book. Anyone having claims to ownership
not identified above is invited to contact
Quercus Editions Ltd.*

ISBN 978-1-4351-5166-6

Manufactured in China

6 8 10 9 7 5